An Orientation to
CHRONIC DISEASE
and DISABILITY

An Orientation to
CHRONIC DISEASE
and DISABILITY

EDITED BY JULIAN S. MYERS, PH.D.

Professor of Psychology
and Director of Rehabilitation Counselor Training
Graduate School, University of Cincinnati

The Macmillan Company, New York
Collier–Macmillan Limited, London

Third Printing, 1968

Library of Congress catalog card number: 65-23551

THE MACMILLAN COMPANY, NEW YORK

COLLIER-MACMILLAN CANADA, LTD., TORONTO, ONTARIO

Printed in the United States of America

PREFACE

The time has long since passed—if indeed it ever existed—when chronic disease and disability could be understood or treated solely as medical phenomena. Social, psychological, economic, and vocational factors are often of major importance in causing, intensifying, or prolonging illness. The converse is equally true: Prolonged illness and chronic disability affect the individual psychologically, socially, and economically; they influence his work adjustment, his educational accomplishment, and his family life. In other words, a chronic disorder is a highly complex condition, and the treatment and rehabilitation processes are equally complex.

The physician, no matter how competent and no matter what his specialization, cannot do the job alone. The increased variety and number of nonmedical professional personnel who in some way work with the chronically disabled bear testimony to this fact. A wide range of services for all types of disabled people is offered by the helping professions, as illustrated by groups such as rehabilitation counselors, caseworkers, psychologists, therapists, teachers of special classes, chaplains, administrators, nursing personnel, and medical service corps personnel in the armed forces. The list is not complete, but the needs of the disabled are far from being met.

This book was written to provide a background in medical information for the helping professions. Designed to provide a foundation on which they can base their skills, it does not purport to teach the specific skills —for example, counseling, casework, or teaching—per se. Nor does it intend to transform the reader into a diagnostician or medical practitioner. The major purpose is to enable the worker to function more effectively and intelligently in his professional role by helping him to understand chronic disease and disability. Our premise is that the worker cannot be of maximum help to the patient unless he is well aware of the nature and implications of the disorders with which he is dealing.

A second purpose is to provide a basis for improved communication among the health-related professions. This is a prerequisite for the team approach, which is lauded so frequently and practiced so rarely. The ability to pool information, share knowledge, coordinate objectives, and work cooperatively is necessary not only for the welfare of the patient and his family but also for the mutual respect of the professional disciplines concerned.

A third objective is to help the purchaser of medical services—for example, the rehabilitation counselor or the caseworker—develop a critical approach to the use of medical facilities. By understanding the standards of good medicine, by knowing what can or cannot be expected, and by knowing the questions to ask, the worker will become of increased value to his clients.

Along these lines we have tried to develop a book that can be used as a reference by the experienced worker and as a textbook by the student. The index has been designed to provide ready access to subject matter referred to in many chapters. In our writing we have tried to strike a balance between simplicity on the one hand and technical material on the other. Our focus is the intelligent professional worker with relatively little previous medical knowledge. We want this reader to follow the text without undue difficulty and yet be able to understand the average medical report as the result of his reading. Instead of preparing a glossary, we have explained many of the technical terms as we came to them.

We have tried to avoid making this a textbook on anatomy and physiology. However, it is not possible to understand disease processes and disabling conditions without some grounding in these subjects. The reader who finds that sections of some chapters tell him more about anatomy and physiology than he cares to know will find that he can still read profitably in the remaining sections which deal with specific disorders. Moreover, the reader may be pleasantly surprised at the amount of technical acumen that develops with practical experience.

Each chapter has been written by a specialist in that particular field. Medicine is not an exact science, and the reader may occasionally come across opposing points of view in his daily work. To the extent possible, however, we have tried to provide an authentic, authoritative presentation with a highly practical orientation. Illustrations have been selected to support the text and to aid in comprehension. The reader who prefers a different sequence of chapters than the one offered here will find that this poses no problem, for each chapter is a unit in itself. Bibliographies, where included, are only suggestive. The interested reader will do well to develop a personal annotated bibliography out of the tremendous literature that is available in the many subject areas covered.

Although this is not primarily a book on rehabilitation, the rehabilitation worker will find it helpful. In addition to the generic medical orientation which is so necessary, the reader will find a moderate emphasis on rehabilitation procedures and vocational implications. An authoritative supplement on mental retardation, made available by the American Association on Mental Deficiency, should be of considerable value to workers in this area.

Many friends and colleagues have helped in the preparation of this book. I would particularly like to thank Robert Hyde, M.D., Bernice Clark, M.D., Eugene Rappaport, M.D., and Gene Bocknek, Ph.D., for their assistance in preparing the manuscript. The authors would welcome suggestions and comments on how this book can be made more helpful to the reader.

J. S. M.

Pelham, New Hampshire

CONTENTS

IX

X

XI

XII

XIII

XIV

XV

XVI

I

INTRODUCTION AND OVERVIEW

Concern with the treatment and prevention of disease is reflected throughout the history of mankind. Primitive societies viewed deviations from health as evidence of supernatural influence and directed their efforts at the management of disease by propitiating, mollifying, or warding off the forces that were thought to be responsible for the disruption of man's usual or normal functional state. Such efforts were often identified with religious practices or rituals. Generations of experience and the recording of observations eventually resulted in the development of particular patterns of dealing with illness in many parts of the ancient world. The Bible contains references to practices designed to avoid disease. Various papyri from Egypt (3500 to 1700 B.C.) contain instructions regarding specific medical and surgical procedures. The code of Hammurabi (Babylonia, about 2250 B.C.) includes a section on medical practice, and in ancient Greece a number of temples were erected to Aesculapius, the god of health.

It is generally accepted that the basis for modern medicine began with Hippocrates (460–370 B.C.), a man of keen clinical acumen who evaluated his observations on health critically and identified disease with natural causes. The knowledge from Greece was carried to Rome and subsequently to the Mohammedan empire. During the Dark Ages, most physicians were monks, and knowledge was transmitted through monastery instruction. Scientific inquiry began in earnest with the Ren-

By HENRY J. BAKST, M.D. Professor and Chairman, Department of Preventive Medicine, Boston University School of Medicine; Director, Division of Health Conservation, Massachusetts Memorial Hospitals, Boston, Massachusetts.

aissance. At this time, further progress in medicine began to be characterized by the development of verifiable scientific knowledge.

MODERN MEDICINE

In looking back over the events that have taken place in medical history, it is apparent that progress has been a process of geometric progression in knowledge with the number of contributions to man's welfare increasing strikingly within relatively shorter periods as time went on. The twentieth century emphasized this pattern. New diagnostic techniques included endoscopy, refined developments in the use of x-ray, electroencephalography, electrocardiography, and cytological techniques for the early recognition of cancer. New drugs and new methods were introduced for the treatment and prevention of disease. Vitamins came into general use with advances in the knowledge of nutrition. The science of endocrinology expanded greatly; the phenomenon of allergy to specific substances was recognized; the sulfonamide and antibiotic drugs were introduced; and a number of world-wide diseases came under control, including malaria, diphtheria, typhoid fever, nutritional disorders, tuberculosis, and typhus fever. In surgery, aseptic techniques, anesthesia, new procedures, blood typing, and advances in the understanding of immunological reactions opened avenues for treatment and approaches that were hitherto undreamed of, such as modern heart surgery and organ transplants. New culture techniques and the development of the electron microscope permitted further understanding of virus diseases and the minute structure of cells. The discovery of radium and the development of radioactive isotopes are identified with a completely new approach to the diagnosis and treatment of disease.

Virtually the entire development of modern psychiatry occurred in the twentieth century. Sigmund Freud developed the technique of psychoanalysis, and the treatment of emotionally disturbed patients was carried on and improved upon by a succession of his followers. Shock therapy for mentally disturbed patients was introduced, and the concept of psychosomatic disease (physical manifestations of emotional disturbance) became firmly established. The contributions of the medical sciences, aided and abetted by social reforms and improvements in the standard of living, resulted in striking changes in the way of man's life and in a significant increase in his life expectancy.

In a most informative monograph Anderson and Rosen [1] have pointed out:

[1] Odin W. Anderson and George Rosen, *An Examination of the Concept of Preventive Medicine,* Chicago, Ill.: Health Information Foundation, Research Series #12, 1960, p. 3.

It is generally accepted now that disease always occurs in the same basic forms such as infection, disturbances of development and metabolism, trauma, and neoplasia. While these basic forms probably do not alter, their relative incidence and prevalence have varied and probably will continue to vary from time to time and place to place. The occurrence of disease in a given population at a particular time exhibits a characteristic pattern which can be identified in terms of its morbidity, mortality, and causation. In general, the pattern of disease is associated with a population's prevailing values and the level of social and technical development which has been attained.

The recognition of specific disease entities rather than a concept of medicine characterized by emphasis on symptoms and the knowledge of primary agents responsible for the causation of disease led to the control of many diseases due to micro-organisms. Also, it became possible to identify the problems of morbidity and mortality on a more precise basis. The simple cause and effect relationship, however, has given way to a more complex concept of multiple causation characterized by the interaction of agent, host, and environment. Thus, at any given place and in any given time, there are multiple factors which determine the general level of well-being of a population. These include biological strengths which may be fostered and weaknesses which may be supported, the health significance of cultural and psychologic characteristics, the level of scientific attainment which has been achieved, and the development of methods through which current knowledge may be applied.

MECHANISMS AND PROCESSES OF DISEASE

It is clear that a number of different interdependent mechanisms may be identified with the production of a variety of categories of disease. The invasion of the body by a *microorganism* through inhalation, ingestion, or inoculation may produce specific disease depending upon the nature of the organism, the characteristics of the host, and the environment in which this reaction occurs. Particular *genetic* characteristics may be associated with the transmission from generation to generation of susceptibility to certain disease, which may influence the growth and development of the individual or result in such problems as diabetes mellitus, gout, and certain forms of mental retardation. Other problems may be identified with the *physical environment* and result from exposure to excessive heat or cold, changes in oxygen tension, and mechanical trauma or injury. Certain manifestations of dysfunction may be associated with *emotional disturbances* (psychosomatic disease). On the other hand, the specific causes of a number of diseases—such as neoplasm, arteriosclerosis, and rheumatoid arthritis—still remain unknown.

BODY STRUCTURE AND FUNCTION

The various systems of the body, each complex in both structure and function, are interdependent and remarkably integrated, so that failure of one system to perform adequately for a given period of time will eventually result in interference with the ability of other systems to function effectively. While the various systems will be considered separately, this interdependent functional relationship must be borne in mind constantly.

CARDIOVASCULAR SYSTEM

Fundamentally, the heart is a pump that in the average individual contracts regularly about sixty to seventy times a minute 24 hours a day for the lifetime of the individual. Considering the present life expectancy at birth of about seventy years and occasional episodes of stress or exertion that would increase the rate, the average heart will beat at least three billion times during the average lifetime of an individual. This remarkable organ is located in the middle of the thoracic area with its apex extending well into the left side of the chest. It consists of four chambers, two atria (auricles) and two ventricles. The left atrium and ventricle are separated from the right-sided chambers by a septum or wall of tissue, and the atria are separated from the ventricles by valves (the mitral valve on the left and the tricuspid valve on the right). The ventricular chambers are enclosed by heavy muscular tissue which does most of the work of the heart.

The right atrium receives venous blood from the tissues and organs of the body. From there the blood flows by the tricuspid valve into the right ventricle. When the right ventricle contracts, the venous blood it contains is forced to the lungs via the pulmonary artery. At the base of the pulmonary artery is the pulmonary valve, which prevents blood from regurgitating from the pulmonary circulation into the right ventricle. Venous blood in the lungs gives up its accumulated carbon dioxide in exchange for oxygen. The left atrium then receives the oxygenated (arterial) blood, which flows past the mitral valve into the left ventricle. When the left ventricle contracts, the blood is forced into the aorta. Arterial blood is prevented by the aortic valve from regurgitating into the left ventricle. Immediately above the aortic valve are the openings of the coronary arteries, which supply the heart muscle with oxygenated blood and nutrient elements. Subsequent arterial branches from the aorta supply the rest of the body with fresh blood.

Heart function may be impaired as the result of a variety of processes. The organ or its main vessels may be malformed (congenital heart disease), or infection may injure the muscle (myocarditis), the protective sac surrounding the heart (pericarditis), or the valves (valvular heart disease). Disease of the coronary arteries (atherosclerosis) may result in a gradually decreasing flow of blood to the heart muscle (coronary artery heart disease) or obstruction of coronary artery (coronary thrombosis). The extra work demanded of the heart by long-standing elevation of the blood pressure may result in hypertensive heart disease.

Despite damage to the heart, with appropriate treatment most patients with heart disease are able to lead long and useful lives, and some may approximate normal life-spans. In some individuals, it may be necessary to restrict the extent of physical activity; in others, little or no restriction may be required. Many patients with heart disease are fully qualified for work, and some may engage in strenuous activity. In others, the presence of heart disease may require a change in the type of employment to one requiring less physical activity. Today the most common type of heart disease is due to atherosclerosis.

In the process of evaluating any type of heart disease, a careful history, physical examination, and a series of special laboratory procedures may be necessary (x-ray, electrocardiogram, circulation time, and others). A complete diagnosis of heart disease usually includes a statement of cause or etiology and a description of structural changes, physiological changes, therapeutic indications, and functional restrictions.

It should be borne in mind that this describes the condition as it is at the time the patient is evaluated. The condition may remain unchanged for an extended period of time or may change quite rapidly. Furthermore, for patients with certain types of cardiac damage a carefully supervised program of appropriate exercise may result in considerable improvement from the point of view of both prognosis and physical capacity for work. Of importance also is the need to evaluate carefully each individual to determine the extent and significance of fear or anxiety and its relationship to possible aggravation of symptoms. A majority of patients with heart disease can live entirely useful, productive, and active lives. The various types of cardiac disease, their manifestations, and problems of management will be discussed in more detail in the chapter on cardiovascular disease. The more common types include congenital heart disease, rheumatic heart disease, hypertensive heart disease, and arteriosclerotic heart disease.

Congenital heart disease is identified with structural abnormalities that develop during the process of fetal development and, if severe, may result in an admixture of venous and arterial blood or in interference with the flow of arterial blood as it leaves the heart. Various combinations of structural abnormalities may occur in a given individual. Many patients with congenital lesions suffer no significant functional impairment; and as a result of striking surgical advances, it has become possible to provide significant improvement in many children with marked congenital heart disease who otherwise would continue with limited functional capacities and poor prognoses.

Rheumatic heart disease is most commonly associated with infection from certain strains of streptococci. It is estimated that about 2 to 3 per cent of the population will exhibit such as response following streptococcal infection. Damage to the heart may involve the heart muscle (myocarditis), the heart valves (endocarditis), or the sac surrounding the entire heart (pericarditis), or any combination of these. The most characteristic lesion is mitral valvular disease resulting in mitral valvular insufficiency (mitral regurgitation) or thickening and hardening of the valve (mitral stenosis) interfering with the normal flow of blood from the left atrium to the left ventricle. In severe cases of mitral stenosis, the back pressure on the pulmonary circulation may result in an increase in vascular pressure within the pulmonary circulation.

Syphilitic heart disease most commonly involves the wall of the aorta nearest the heart (aortitis) and as a consequence of dilatation of the base of the aorta may produce aortic regurgitation. Weakening of the aortic wall may be associated with localized distention and sacculation in the involved area (aneurysm). The latter may rupture and result in a rapid fatal termination.

Various diseases, such as kidney disease or thyrotoxicosis, may be associated with elevation of the blood pressure. This is known as secondary hypertension. A more common form of elevated blood pressure is essential hypertension the cause of which is unknown. This may persist for many years and produce disease as the result of changes in blood vessels and consequently in the organs and tissues they supply. These changes characteristically impose an increased work load on the heart that eventually may result in hypertensive heart disease and reduce functional capacity of this organ. The course of the disease may be quite variable. It may run a rapidly progressive course or may progress slowly over many years. Since it is a generalized vascular process, the manifestations may be chiefly those associated with interference of blood supply to the brain, the heart, or the kidney. Many drugs are available for the management of hypertension; as a result, the course of this disease may be altered significantly. Secondary hypertension is controlled by treatment of the underlying disease.

The most common form of heart disease is that due to atherosclerosis with involvement of the coronary arteries. The extent of disease in these vessels determines the extent of reduction of blood supply to the heart muscle and, consequently, the ability of the heart to continue to function effectively. Normally the heart is able to increase its output of blood per unit of time as required by increased physical activity or emotional stress. Coronary artery disease decreases the capacity of the heart to respond adequately to these changing needs or diminishes the margin of cardiac reserve, resulting in a disproportion between supply and demand. This state of affairs may be associated with angina pectoris (coronary artery insufficiency) or myocardial infarction (coronary thrombosis or coronary occlusion). Most individuals survive such an acute episode; some are fatal. Repeated episodes may reduce the functional capacity of the heart and result in congestive heart failure.

The damaged heart my develop disorders of normal rhythm and produce further interference with functional efficiency.

PERIPHERAL VASCULAR DISEASE

There is an intimate relationship between cardiac function and the vascular system of arteries, capillaries, and veins through which the blood flows. The arteries carry blood from the heart to the organs and peripheral portions of the body and, by dividing into an extensive and fine capillary network, provide oxygen and necessary nutrients for the maintenance and function of the tissues of the body. The veins return the blood to the heart with carbon dioxide and metabolic wastes from the tissues and peripheral parts of the body. The venous blood is then transported to the lungs. The walls of the veins are thin as compared with the muscular coats of arteries and contain one-way valves that maintain blood flow toward the heart and prevent backward flow.

An inadequate flow of arterial blood to body tissue is known as ischemia. Often a relative lack of oxygen is associated with the production of pain in the area involved. In the lower extremities the production of such pain results from exercise or increased effort and may be relieved by rest (intermittent claudication). As a result of ischemia, skin may become cold, thickened, and discolored. If ischemia is prolonged, ulceration of skin and other changes may occur. Further progression of this process involves all the component parts of the area (bone, nerve, muscle, skin) and results in local necrosis or tissue destruction (gangrene).

The disposition of fats and calcium with scar formation in the walls of arteries and consequent narrowing of the lumen is characteristic of arteriosclerosis. Drugs that dilate the arteries (vasodilators) may improve the blood supply and reduce pain. Substances that will cause arteries to constrict (vasoconstrictors, such as tobacco) may result in diminution of the blood supply and increased pain. In some cases interruption of the sympathetic nerves may help to improve the blood supply. In others the use of human arterial or artificial grafts to replace diseased or blocked vessels or the actual removal of calcareous and fatty deposits may be necessary. Failure to improve the circulation in an extremity may require amputation.

Buerger's disease, thromboangiitis obliterans, is a generalized arterial disease with manifestations primarily affecting the lower extremities. The process involves a proliferation and accumulation of cells of the arterial wall, leading to a segmental narrowing and occlusion resulting in ischemia. The disease occurs commonly in males between the ages of 20 and 45. The course of the disease is variable, and its cause unknown. In contrast to Buerger's disease, arteriosclerosis occurs most frequently in an older age group.

Raynaud's disease most commonly affects women between the ages of 20 and 40 and is characterized by an overreactive response to cold, stress, and emotional factors, resulting in a functional peripheral vascular constriction. The diminution in the blood supply results in coldness, numbness, tingling, pain, and color changes of the skin in the involved area. The disease develops slowly; usually the impairment is not severe.

The formation of a thrombus or clot within a vein is known as thrombophlebitis. Usually this is accompanied by local pain, heat, and swelling. It may result from injury, irritation, infection, immobilization of the extremity, impaired blood flow, or an abnormal tendency of the blood to clot. Localized destruction of venous valves may result. The implications of the thrombophlebitis relate not only to the local change but to the fact that a portion of the clot, in deep veins particularly, may break off, flow freely in the blood, and eventually lodge in a pulmonary vessel (embolism). Sudden death due to pulmonary embolism is not unusual postoperatively or in immobilized patients if measures for the reduction in frequency of this complication are not instituted. However, pulmonary embolism may occur suddenly in the absence of clinically recognizable evidence of thrombosis elsewhere in the body. Thrombophlebitis itself, however, rarely results in significant disability.

The most common of peripheral vascular diseases is varicose veins. Weak-walled vessels, inadequate valves, infrequent muscular contraction, and pressure on the system of venous return as in pregnancy may result in venous incompetency. Discoloration of the skin and ulceration are not uncommon as a result of long-standing varicosities. Varicose veins, however, are usually not disabling. Elastic stockings may be helpful in providing relief, and in some instances surgical correction may be necessary.

RESPIRATORY SYSTEM

The respiratory system consists of the lungs and air pathways together with the thoracic cage, accessory muscles of respiration, diaphragm, and the various pathways by which nervous and chemical control of respiration is maintained. The process of breathing is involuntary but with a limited degree of voluntary control. An individual may train himself to hold his breath for limited periods of time but cannot maintain the state for a protracted period. The rate of respiration is affected by the physical and emotional state of the individual, the amount of air space available within the lungs, and the capacity to alter the size of the chest.

The lungs consist of three lobes on the right and two lobes on the left, which are separated by the area essentially in the midchest occupied by the heart and great vessels and the esophagus, trachea, and thoracic duct (the mediastinum). The lungs are covered by a thin layer of tissue (pleura) which is reflected back to cover the inside of the chest wall. The space between these two layers of pleura is at a pressure less than that of the surrounding atmosphere. This facilitates the entrance of air into the lung. Penetration of the pleural space, either from within the lungs or through the chest wall, results in a loss of the negative pressure in the pleural space and causes collapse of the lung on the affected side (pneumothorax).

The air passages (tracheobronchial tree) carry air to and from the tiny air sacs (alveolar spaces) in the lung with the final ramifications of this system, the bronchioles, opening into the alveolar spaces. The venous blood from the heart circulating around the alveolar spaces exchanges oxygen for carbon dioxide and thus provides the oxygenated arterial blood returning to the heart for circulation to the body.

The maximum amount of air that can be expelled after full inspiration is termed the vital capacity. The normal vital capacity ranges from 3,000 to 6,000 cubic centimeters and is quite variable with age, body build, and general state of health. The rate of expiratory flow of air may be measured as the maximum expiratory flow rate. A decrease of the timed measurement results from any constriction of the air passages (obstructive) or from limitation of chest motion (restrictive). The normal range of vital capacity for a given age and body build is known as the predicted vital capacity. Effective respiratory function depends on the displacement of air in and out of the lung and the transfer of gases, mainly oxygen and carbon dioxide, across the alveolar membranes. Interference with either ventilation or gaseous exchange affects respiratory function. The more common diseases that interfere with respiratory function and may result in disability are tuberculosis, asthma, emphysema, the pneumoconioses, and bronchiectasis.

An initial tuberculous infection or primary lesion is usually subclinical and often goes on to spontaneous healing. The small area that has been involved eventually may become calcified and may be seen by x-ray as a small calcified nodule. At times the primary lesion, however, may go on to further involvement of the lung, producing clinical disease as a result of the destruction of varying amounts of lung tissue and the development of cavitation or ulceration. This may be associated with coughing up of blood (hemoptysis). The involved areas heal by scarring but with some loss of usable lung tissue resulting. The degree of incapacity produced therefore depends on the amount of lung tissue destroyed. This may be negligible in some instances or extensive in others.

Bronchial asthma is characterized by intermittent paroxysmal attacks of shortness of breath that may last for brief or protracted periods (hours, days, or weeks); the cause is usually an allergic response associated with constriction of the bronchioles. In some instances asthma is apparently psychological in origin. Disability is dependent upon the severity, frequency, and duration of asthmatic episodes, the degree of functional impairment as measured by breathing tests between episodes, and the response to appropriate treatment. Long-term disability may result from the development of emphysema.

Severe disability from emphysema is usually due to the chronic obstructive type. The common complaints are shortness of breath, cough, and fatigue which result from diminished distribution of air and associated poor gaseous exchange. Chronic obstructive emphysema results from obstruction in the bronchial tree causing some of the inspired air to be trapped in the alveolar spaces, thus producing distention of the alveolar sacs. Elasticity of the lung is also diminished, so that greater effort is required in breathing. The chest becomes overinflated and less efficient, which may eventually lead to marked shortness of breath with insufficient oxygen drawn into the lung and inability to expel carbon dioxide adequately. Right-sided heart disease (cor pulmonale) may result from the consequent increased intrapulmonary pressure. The extent of disability produced may be measured by breathing tests and tests for the amount of oxygen absorbed in relation to the total air ventilated.

The term pneumoconiosis includes the chronic pulmonary diseases resulting from the prolonged inhalation of injurious dusts. The most important of these is silica, which penetrates the air passages, becoming lodged in pulmonary tissues and producing nodules that replace normal lung tissue. Disability is dependent on the amount of tissue involved and the consequent degree of interference with respiratory functions. Emphysema and tuberculosis are common associated problems.

Bronchiectasis is a chronic disease associated with structural changes in the bronchi due to inflammatory reactions and fibrotic changes. Localized dilatation of the affected bronchi results; characteristically the affected individual becomes increasingly susceptible to respiratory tract infections. In typical situations it is accompanied by a cough productive of copious amounts of purulent sputum. The disease may progress over many years and produce varying degrees of impairment of respiratory function dependent upon the extent of pulmonary tissue involvement.

MUSCULOSKELETAL SYSTEM

The ability of the body to make many complex and intricate movements results from the interdependent functional relationship of the bones of the skeleton and the body musculature. The physical independence produced by the highly developed function of bone and muscle may be lost when a bone is broken or when muscles are paralyzed or otherwise damaged. Bone, a viable tissue like other body tissues, makes up almost the entire skeleton. A small portion of the total skeleton, such as the joint surfaces, consists of cartilage, which is more elastic than bone. The skeletal structure of the body consists of the skull and spinal column and two girdles of bone, the shoulder and pelvic girdles, to which the upper and lower extremities are attached. The spinal column consists of individual bones (vertebrae) of which there are 7 in the cervical portion, 12 in the thoracic portion, and 5 in the lumbar area. Below the lumbar area are the sacrum and coccyx. Each vertebra consists of a body, a neural arch through which the spinal cord passes, and, projecting from the neural arch, the spinous process. Each vertebra articulates with the vertebra above and below and is separated from them by fibrocartilage (intervertebral disc). Twelve pairs of ribs are attached to the thoracic vertebrae in the back. The first seven of these are attached to the breastbone in the front of the chest (sternum). The next three are attached to the ribs above by cartilage, and the front ends of the last two are unattached.

The large bone of the upper arm is the humerus. The forearm consists of two bones, the radius and ulna. The shoulder girdle is formed by the collarbone in front (clavicle) and the scapula in back. The lower extremity consists of the main upper bone (femur) and two bones below the knee (tibia and fibula). The voluntary muscles are attached to the bony skeleton, and movement is possible as a result of their contraction or relaxation. Muscular function and coordination, when lost as a result of injury, disease, disuse, or malfunction, often can be restored by treatment of the cause and by appropriate exercise. Tendons are the tough, stringy tissue that connects muscle to bone.

The common disabilities of the musculoskeletal system include injuries resulting in breaking of bone (fractures) or dislocations, congenital defects such as clubfoot, diseases of the joints such as various forms of arthritis (rheumatoid arthritis, osteoarthritis), or disorders such as gout. Certain types of falls, jumps, lifting, bending, or twisting may compress the intervertebral disc, causing it to bulge backward and produce pressure on the spinal cord or spinal nerve roots. Infection of bone is known as osteomyelitis. Tuberculosis of bone, formerly fairly common, is seer nly infrequently today. Tumors of bone both benign and malignant are not unusual. It is important that the integrity of the musculoskeletal system is largely dependent on its use. Lack of normal stresses applied to the bones, disuse of muscle as in paralysis, is associated with the loss of calcium from bone (osteoporosis) and with rapid tissue wastage in unused muscles (atrophy). These are both common in advancing years with failure to maintain physical activity, but may also occur with metabolic disturbances.

GASTROINTESTINAL SYSTEM

The gastrointestinal tract includes all those areas concerned with the ingestion of food, its digestion and absorption, and the evacuation of the residue. Food chewed in the mouth (masticated) passes into the esophagus when swallowed. The esophagus passes through the diaphragm into the stomach. The process of digestion begins in the mouth through chewing and moistening; the action of the salivary enzyme (ptyalin) begins at this time. In the stomach, the hydrochloric acid and stomach enzymes (pepsin, renin, and lipase) continue the process of digestion. Food then passes on to the small bowel, which is divided into three parts—the duodenum, jejunum, and ileum. The portion of the small bowel nearest the stomach (duodenum) receives enzymes from the pancreas and bile from the liver. The intestinal juices secreted by glands in the wall of the small bowel also contain enzymes that further digest food or convert it into substances that can be absorbed into the blood. The first portion of the large bowel, or cecum, follows after the ileum. The cecum leads into the ascending colon, sigmoid, rectum, anal canal, and anal sphincter.

The principal diseases of the gastrointestinal tract are cardiospasm, diaphragmatic hernia, peptic ulcer, colitis, regional enteritis, hepatitis and cirrhosis of the liver, and neoplastic disease.

Cardiospasm, or spasm of the esophagus, may be painless or associated with severe pain which at times may be mistaken for angina pectoris. It is often accompanied by a sensation of obstruction to the passage of food. Persistence of this condition with an associated inflammatory reaction may result in the formation of scar tissue with permanent narrowing of the lower end of the esophagus. Cardiospasm may have an emotional basis.

Hiatus hernia or diaphragmatic hernia may occur when the opening in the diaphragm through which the esophagus passes to the stomach is too large. This permits a portion of the stomach to bulge through the diaphragmatic opening. If the opening is particularly large, some of the small intestine may herniate as well. The condition, to a minor degree relatively common in elderly people, is symptomless when the herniation is small. A similar situation may result when the esophagus is too short and causes constant tension, eventually producing herniation of the stomach through the diaphragmatic opening. Symptoms of distention, upper abdominal discomfort, and gaseous eructation tend to be worse in the recumbent than in the upright position. If the symptoms are severe and incapacitating, surgical correction may be necessary.

Peptic ulcer is a most common disease, occurring in about 10 to 12 per cent of the population. Ulceration, which may occur in either the stomach or duodenum, is seen more frequently in the duodenum. It is more common in men than in women. Ulcers are usually single in the duodenum but sometimes are multiple in the stomach. The characteristic symptom is a burning sensation occurring after meals and relieved by food. Symptoms of an active peptic ulcer are more common in the spring and fall of the year. Pain one-half to one hour after eating is more frequently associated with a gastric ulcer. Pain two hours or more after eating tends to be characteristic of a duodenal ulcer. Peptic ulcer usually responds to medical treatment. There are, however, four major complications. These are erosion of a blood vessel resulting in bleeding, erosion through the gastric or duodenal wall resulting in perforation and infection of the abdominal cavity (peritonitis), inflammation and swelling with scar formation resulting in obstruction, and finally intractability to the medical treatment. Various types of surgical approaches to these problems are common, including resection of a major portion of the stomach (subtotal gastrectomy).

Regional enteritis is a disease of the small bowel, particularly the ileum, which is characterized by inflammation, scarring, and narrowing of the affected portions of the bowel. It is associated with continuous or crampy abdominal pain, and there may be fever, diarrhea, bloody stools, and debility. The disease tends to progress slowly and irregularly; the complications of rupture, hemorrhage, perforation, or fistula formation may occur.

A common disorder of the large bowel is the syndrome of irritable colon. This is characterized by constipation and diarrhea, weakness, flushing, palpitation, and headache. It is thought to be psychogenic in nature and is rarely disabling. Ulcerative colitis, however, is charactized by the presence of multiple ulcerations in the wall of the large bowel. The disease may be mild or severe, and the common symptoms are diarrhea, weakness, fever, and bleeding with bowel movements. Malnutrition, weight loss, and anemia may develop; functional impairment of the individual may be quite marked. Serious complications of fistula formation, the development of abscesses, and perforation of the bowel may occur.

Hepatitis or inflammation of the liver may occur in several different forms. Acute infectious hepatitis is a viral infection resulting from ingestion of the virus; serum hepatitis is produced by the injection of a virus, usually by an inadequately sterilized needle that has come in contact with the blood serum of an individual who has had hepatitis, or occasionally as a result of blood transfusion. Hepatitis may also be associated with other infections and may be produced by certain chemicals. The symptoms are usually loss of appetite, nausea, vomiting, and marked fatigue. Jaundice usually develops, and the liver becomes enlarged. Sometimes, the spleen may be enlarged also. Recovery is the rule but sometimes with a protracted course. Some cases go on to a fatal termination.

Cirrhosis of the liver is a chronic, inflammatory disease associated with destruction of liver tissue and with scar formation. Portal cirrhosis is the most common type (Laennec's cirrhosis or alcoholic cirrhosis). It is most frequently seen as a dietary deficiency associated with chronic alcoholism. In the late stages of this disease, there may be abdominal swelling with fluid (ascites), jaundice, anemia, and striking loss of body tissue.

THE BLOOD

The blood consists of formed elements in a liquid medium or plasma. The formed elements are red cells (erythrocytes), white cells (leukocytes), and platelets (thrombocytes). The normal life-span of erythrocytes is about 120 days. New cells are released constantly from the bone marrow. Thus $\frac{1}{120}$ of the total number of red cells is replaced in every 24-hour period. Normally the number of red cells ranges from about 4.5 to 5.5 million per cubic milliliter of blood. The normal amount of hemoglobin carried by the red cells is 15 grams per 100 milliliters of blood. Usually anemia is considered to be present if the red count is below 4 million or the hemoglobin below 12 grams. The essential function of red cells is to carry oxygen from the lungs to the various tissues of the body and to take up carbon dioxide from the tissues. The carbon dioxide is then exchanged for oxygen when the red cells pass through the pulmonary circulation.

The white cells normally number between 5,000 and 10,000 per milliliter. There are several different varieties of these which have as their main function the protection of the body against certain infections or foreign substances. The platelets number 200,000 to 400,000 per milliliter and are important in the process of blood clotting through the release of thromboplastin.

The plasma is essentially water except for about 6 per cent by weight, which is largely protein and small amounts of other substances. These substances are important in cellular metabolism, in maintaining the proper concentration of water in the plasma, and in providing antibodies to protect the body against certain infections. The remaining substances are fats and carbohydrates and various chemical products of metabolism and electrolytes. The maintenance of the proper concentration of the various substances in the plasma is a complex interrelated process, involving the function of the kidneys, lungs, heart, and gastrointestinal system through intricate metabolic reactions. The various diseases of the blood include anemia resulting from hemorrhage or decreased production or increased destruction of red cells. An increased production of red cells results in polycythemia. White cells are increased in various infections and decreased in some toxic states. Thrombocytes are reduced in certain types of purpura. A striking neoplastic increase of various types of abnormal white cells is characteristic of different types of leukemia.

Pernicious anemia is a type of anemia due to inadequate red cell production. Vitamin B$_{12}$, one of the substances necessary for red cell formation, is not absorbed adequately from the intestinal tract in such individuals because of the absence of a necessary substance (the intrinsic factor). Iron deficiency anemias usually respond to an increased intake of iron. Aplastic anemia results from depression of bone marrow activity. This may be due to toxic substances, infection, or encroachment on marrow space by tumor.

Hemolytic anemia may be either acquired or familial. The former may be due to reactions such as are encountered at times with transfusions, erythroblastosis, or certain types of infections as well as with drugs and chemicals. There is a familial or genetic group of anemias which includes such diseases as spherocytic anemia, Cooley's anemia, and sickle cell anemia.

Polycythemia occurs in two forms, primary and secondary. The primary form (polycythemia vera) is characterized by the presence of an overactive bone marrow. The secondary form may develop as a result of prolonged exposure to low oxygen pressure or certain forms of chronic pulmonary disease that reduce the amount of oxygen available for the body. This is essentially a mechanism to compensate for oxygen lack.

URINARY SYSTEM

The main organs of the urinary system are the two kidneys of characteristic bean shape located just behind the lining of the abdominal cavity in each lumbar region. The functioning unit of the kidney is the nephron, which consists of a fine, minute arterial network, or small tuft or glomerulus, and system of tubules. Blood is brought to the glomerulus by an afferent arteriole and leaves by an efferent arteriole. The glomerular blood is filtered into a surrounding capsule, the glomerular capsule. Thus, the first step in urine formation is one of filtration. The glomerular filtrate, consisting of water, electrolytes, and waste products, then passes from the capsule to the convoluted tubule, Henle's loop, and finally to the collecting tubule. En route, through a selective process of reabsorption, some of the contents of the glomerular filtrate are returned to the blood stream. Also, other substances are secreted into the glomerular filtrate along this route. These various changes take place in such a manner as to maintain a constant composition of the blood. The final product of urine is the result of filtration, reabsorption, and secretion. The collecting tubules empty into the pelvis of each kidney, and then the urine flows down each ureter to the bladder. The bladder is emptied through the urethra.

There are literally millions of nephrons in the kidneys. When the body requires additional fluid, water is conserved by the process of reabsorption, and the urine becomes concentrated. When an excess of electrolytes and wastes must be disposed of, tubular reabsorption is diminished, making more water available to keep these substances in solution. Obviously the degree of urinary concentration or dilution is related to the daily fluid intake of the body. The ability of the kidneys to function effectively is reflected by their ability to produce a concentrated or diluted urine on demand. Thus, capacity diminishes as kidney function begins to fail. Kidney function may be impaired by vascular disease, damage to the glomeruli or to tubular function, or damage to kidney tissue as a result of infection, trauma, congenital malformation, or tumor.

Glomerulonephritis frequently follows an infection and, similar to rheumatic fever, has been identified with infection due to certain strains of streptococci. Most episodes of acute glomerular nephritis are mild, and although a number of glomeruli may be destroyed, the remaining functioning nephron units maintain kidney function usually without any clinically demonstrable evidence of insufficiency. Repeated episodes, or chronic glomerular disease, usually present an ominous picture with fatal termination which may result from progressive renal impairment. Sometimes chronic glomerular nephritis may start insidiously and is discovered accidentally. The disease is characterized by headaches, malaise, and edema, particularly about the eyes. Albuminuria and anemia are usually present, and the finding of red cells in the urine is typical. The blood pressure is generally elevated. The late symptoms may be associated with cardiac failure or cerebral vascular disease or renal failure reflected by increasing inability to dispose of metabolic waste products, resulting in uremia. The duration of the disease is quite variable; remissions and exacerbations are common; but in general each period of reactivation is associated with further renal damage.

Pyelonephritis is an infection of the renal pelvis almost invariably associated with concomitant renal infection. This may occur as a result of ascending infections from bladder to ureter to the kidney pelvis or as a result of local inflammation of the pelvis. To a greater or lesser degree functioning renal tissue is probably almost always involved. It is characterized by chills, fever, and the appearance of pus cells in the urine. Pain and particularly tenderness at the lumbar region are common. The course and the actual changes in the kidney may simulate chronic glomerulonephritis.

Atherosclerotic changes in the renal arterioles may result in degenerative changes in the glomeruli that are fundamentally ischemic in nature, producing impairment of renal function. Since this is apt to be part of a generalized vascular process, hypertension, cerebral vascular accidents, or heart disease may be part of the general picture.

"Nephrosis" identifies a syndrome consisting of edema, marked albuminuria, decreased serum protein, and an increase in plasma lipids. One form of this disease occurs in children and is associated with damage to the tubules and glomeruli; other types may occur during the course of chronic glomerulonephritis, with diabetes, and with certain toxic drugs and substances. Other kidney disorders include tuberculosis, stones (calculi), congenital malformations, vascular lesions, and tumors.

If for any reason the ureters become obstructed by a calculus, infection, scar formation, or pressure from outside the ureter, dilatation occurs above the level of obstruction. This may happen anywhere in the urine-collecting system from the bladder-ureteral junction to the kidney and produce dilatation in the collecting system of the kidney as well (hydronephrosis) with consequent impairment of renal function if the obstruction is not relieved. In the male, obstruction to bladder emptying may occur as a result of enlargement of the prostate gland at the bladder neck. This is a fairly common situation in older males and requires relief by surgical measures.

Disease of the urinary tract is significant because of impairment of kidney function due to interference with filtration, reabsorption, or secretion. In the late stages, it may result in uremia, which is essentially a reflection of inability to dispose of waste products of metabolism, a serious development. This condition is usually progressive but may at times occur in situations that are temporary and reversible.

ENDOCRINE GLANDS

The endocrine glands are ductless and produce hormones that are liberated into the blood stream. Through the action of these hormones, various metabolic functions are regulated. The endocrine glands include the pituitary, the thyroid, the parathyroids, the adrenals, the sex glands (ovaries and testes), the islet tissue of the pancreas, and several others, such as the thymus and pineal, which are of lesser clinical importance. Disease is produced as a result of either overproduction (hyperfunction) or underproduction (hypofunction) of hormones and often may be controlled by methods depressing glandular function, by actual removal of a portion of the involved gland in instances of hyperfunction, or by substitution therapy in hypofunction.

The pituitary gland consists of two parts, the posterior and anterior. Hormone action of the former is concerned principally with the regulation of water reabsorption by the kidneys and contraction of certain types of involuntary muscle tissue, such as the uterus in the female. Lack of production of this hormone results in the passage of copious amounts of urine (diabetes insipidus) and may be controlled by the administration of the antidiuretic hormone (vasopressin). The anterior pituitary gland regulates the function of other endocrine glands such as the thyroid, adrenal, and sex glands and also produces a hormone that regulates the growth of the body. Excess production of the latter hormone results in acromegaly (postpubertal) and in gigantism (prepubertal). Decreased production prepubertally results in dwarfism.

The thyroid gland regulates the rate of metabolic activity of the body through the production of thyroxin. A diminished production of this hormone leads to the development of hypothyroidism (myxedma). This is characterized by cold intolerance, lethargy, sluggish cerebration, slow heart rate, and increase in body weight as well as dryness of the skin and other disturbances of body function. Hyperthyroidism, associated with an increase in the metabolic activities of the body, is manifested by a rapid pulse, heat intolerance, nervousness, loss of weight, thyroid enlargement, and changes in the skin, nails, and eyes. In some cases the latter tend to become prominent, resulting in a characteristic stare (exophthalmos).

The parathyroids, of which there are four embedded in the thyroid gland, regulate calcium and phosphorous metabolism. Excess activity of these glands causes a rise in serum calcium, and diminished activity a lowering of serum calcium.

The adrenal glands are small, rest on top of each kidney and consist of two parts, a cortex and medulla. The medulla produces epinephrine (adrenalin) and norepinephrine, which are catecholamines. These cause an increase of the blood pressure, respiratory and heart rates, and the amount of sugar in the blood. Their production, controlled by the nervous system, is increased in fear, rage, and stress. The cortex produces hormones (steroids) that influence protein, sodium, and potassium metabolism and carbohydrate metabolism. Others influence the growth of hair and the development of the secondary sexual characteristics. Excess production of these hormones leads to Cushing's disease with obesity of the trunk of the body, a moon-face, plethora, and sometimes excessive growth of hair. This may be treated by surgical removal of the overactive gland. Addison's disease is associated with a decreased production of adrenal cortical hormones and is manifested by increased pigmentation of the skin and numerous membranes, low blood sugar, low blood sodium and high potassium, accompanied by weakness, fatigue, and weight loss, and frequently by gastrointestinal symptoms. The disease is treated by the use of adrenal steroids.

The islet tissue of the pancreas produces insulin. A diminished production or absence of this hormone results in diabetes mellitus, in which there is a disturbance of carbohydrate metabolism and also an interference with normal fat metabolism. This results in an increase in the amount of sugar as well as fat in the blood and the appearance of sugar in the urine, accompanied by symptoms of thirst, increased urinary output, hunger, and often weight loss. These metabolic defects, if uncontrolled, are associated with an increase in the amount of organic acids in the body and a disturbance in the acid-base balance. The disease may be controlled by the administration of insulin, or drugs that stimulate the production of insulin, and by dietary regulation.

Disability may result from the complications of this disease. The complications include arteriosclerosis, changes in the eye, neurological disturbances, and increased susceptibility to infection, particularly boils and carbuncles. Thus, amputation as a result of advanced vascular disease or gangrene, blindness as a result of diabetic retinitis, and the development of cataracts are major problems associated with the inadequate control of this disease. In addition, poorly controlled diabetes may lead to acidosis, coma, and death.

BRAIN AND NERVOUS SYSTEM

The nervous system consists of the brain and spinal cord, the peripheral nervous system, and the autonomic nervous system. Twelve pairs of nerves arise from the brain, and 21 pairs from the spinal cord. The nervous system controls all muscular movement of the body whether voluntary or involuntary; it is responsible for all conscious, subconscious, and unconscious thought and regulates many vital processes and the functions of the various body systems. The brain consists of four parts, the medulla oblongata, the cerebral hemispheres, the cerebellum, and the midbrain. The medulla, from which the last five cranial nerves emerge, is a continuation of the spinal cord. This area contains nerve centers concerned with swallowing, vomiting, breathing, speech, digestion, metabolism, and circulation. In it also are large bundles of fibers that originate in the two halves of the cerebrum which transmit impulses concerned with voluntary movement. These fibers cross to the opposite side, so that movement on the right side of the body, for example, originates from stimuli from the left half of the cerebrum.

Just above the medulla and continuous with it is the pons, which is made up of large bundles of fibers that spread toward the cerebellum and are responsible for skilled movement requiring the coordination of sight, hearing, muscular movement, and comparable related activities. A space within the pons is known as the fourth ventricle. The sixth cranial nerve arises from the floor of the ventricle. The cerebellum lies in back of the brain, with which it has many complex connections; it also has connections with the spinal cord. The cerebellum is essentially responsible for the coordination of complex movement into special acts. The midbrain is a small area between the pons and cerebrum. It is an important relay station for sensory impulses. It also governs some reflex muscle activities. The third, fourth, and fifth cranial nerves originate from this area. A large nerve to each eye (second cranial) meets just above the midbrain, and some of its fibers cross to the opposite sides. Vital functions, such as the regulation of the body temperature, metabolism, and heart rate, are controlled by cells of this region. The thalamus, located next to this group of cells, integrates sensations of different kinds. It is the seat of primitive consciousness, playing a role in the production of emotional responses. Primitive emotional responses that originate here are further elaborated and controlled by the cerebrum.

The two cerebral hemispheres represent the largest portion of the brain. Here is the seat of intelligence, and it is here that all sensory experiences are mixed and blended. The capacities for memory, emotion, and thought are dependent upon these areas. Visual impressions, hearing, speech, balance, smell, taste, judgment based on experience, and some of the most complex abilities of the mind are possible because of the remarkable capacities of the cerebral hemispheres. The impulses responsible for movement associated with these functions originate in the motor cortex of the cerebral hemispheres.

The first cranial nerve is associated with the sense of smell, and the second with sight. The third and fourth move the eyeball and control the pupil of the eye. The fifth cranial nerve carries sensation to the head and mouth and controls movement of the jaw. The sixth moves the eye to the side. The seventh carries impulses to the muscles of the face, and the eighth is concerned with hearing and balance. The ninth carries taste sensation to the back portion of the tongue and other sensations from the throat and mucous membranes. The tenth is involved with swallowing, talking, and slowing of the rate of the heart beat. It also carries fibers to the stomach, esophagus, intestine, liver, bronchi, lungs, and certain blood vessels. The eleventh carries fibers to some of the muscles of the neck which permit turning the head, and the twelfth goes to the muscles of the tongue.

Nerve tracts from the brain continue into the spinal cord. The spinal nerves emerge from each side of the cord between the vertebrae with each nerve attached to the cord by two roots, a motor and sensory root. The lower end of the cord terminates in a mass of nerve roots at the beginning of the lumbar area, known as the cauda equina.

The peripheral nervous system, in addition to the cranial and spinal nerves, includes the autonomic nervous system, which supplies nerves to most of the organs of the body that act automatically, such as the glands, heart, blood vessels, involuntary muscles, and internal organs. The autonomic nervous system, which receives fibers from the spinal cord, is connected by ganglia lying on each side of the spinal column. Fibers of this system are also connected with some of the cranial nerves.

Like other systems of the body, the nervous system may be affected by congenital and hereditary diseases, metabolic disturbances, and infection. Tumors may involve any part of the nervous system, and damage to this intricate system may occur as a result of trauma. Furthermore, any process that interferes with the blood supply to these tissues may result in various types of dysfunction, depending upon the location of the involvement. Hemorrhage or vascular thrombosis involving the left side of the brain may produce a right-sided paralysis of the body. Damage to the spinal cord in the lower cervical region may result in paralysis (motor and sensory) of all four extremities as well as impairment of gastrointestinal and urinary bladder functions. The problems of dealing with the disability and impairment of function resulting from nervous system damage are dependent mainly upon a process of re-education and retraining, with appropriate supporting devices when necessary. Impairment of the special senses, vision and hearing, may obviously result from disease or injury of the nervous system, but also can be produced by local disease or injury of the eyes and ears.

Psychiatric disorders include those which affect the mind and behavior of the individual. These may result from a variety of etiological factors concerned with failure of the mind to develop properly (mental retardation), from actual damage to the brain, and from numerous environmental experiences in the process of growth and development that condition the behavior of the individual. To a significant extent, the causes of mental illness and the factors responsible for mental disturbance reflect the difficulties of human existence. Healthy, well-adjusted, mature individuals deal with these difficulties without engaging in socially unacceptable behavior. Those who handle their problems in a less socially acceptable manner are apt to fall into the category of neuroses or sometimes psychoses. This represents an inadequate attempt to adjust to the various psychological and social forces with which they are confronted, or reflects their inability to deal with them effectively and appropriately. These various disorders may be classified as psychotic, psychophysiological (psychosomatic), psychoneurotic, and personality (character) disorders.

The psychotic reactions may be grouped as affective, involutional, manic-depressive, and schizophrenic. The psychosomatic disorders are generally those in which anxiety is expressed in terms of symptoms referable to organs or body systems served by the autonomic nervous system, such as cardiovascular, gastrointestinal, respiratory. The symptoms may actually be associated with physiological changes in the organs involved. The psychoneurotic disorders are less severe than the psychotic reactions and develop chiefly from efforts of the individual to deal with conflicts, tensions, or stresses by means of psychological defensive measures to control anxiety. These include the anxiety, dissociative, conversion, phobic, obsessive, compulsive, and depressive reactions. Finally, the personality disorders include disturbances of personality pattern, disturbances of personality trait, and sociopathic personality disturbance. These disturbances are characterized by patterns of abnormal behavior.

NEOPLASTIC DISEASE

New growths, tumors, or neoplastic disease may be divided into two broad categories, benign and malignant. They represent disorders of cellular growth and cellular reproduction. Benign tumors are usually encapsulated, do not invade adjacent tissue, but may, as they increase in size, produce symptoms as a result of the space they occupy or the pressure produced on neighboring tissues. The cells of malignant growths reproduce in a wild and uncontrolled fashion; they are usually not maturely developed and may either invade adjacent tissue or be carried to distant parts of the body to take root and grow where they lodge (metastases). Usually, the more immature the characteristic cell of a neoplasm is, the more rapid is the rate of growth of the tumor and the more rapidly does it tend to invade normal tissue.

The difficulties presented by malignancies are many. Fundamentally, they require nourishment for growth and consequently deprive normal tissues of sustenance. The increase in bulk alone may produce discomfort and pain, and the abnormal metabolism of cancer cells may produce a number of changes in the body such as weight loss, anemia, and weakness. Malignancies may spread by extension into contiguous tissue, or portions from the primary site may be carried off by the blood stream or lymph channels to produce secondary metastatic lesions elsewhere in the body.

Cancer has been produced in a number of different ways in experimental animals. Some strains of experimental animals have been developed that are highly resistant to the development of neoplastic disease, while others have been developed that are very susceptible. Excessive exposure to ultraviolet light is associated with an increased incidence of skin cancer in humans. Exposure to certain chemicals may be associated with the development of cancer of the urinary bladder, skeletal system, and lung particularly. Certain types of malignancy have been produced experimentally by the injection of materials isolated from sarcoma in fowls. It is probable, therefore, that malignant disease is not caused by a single agent and that different classes of cancer are produced by different causative agents. One of the difficulties involved in the identification of the causes of cancer in the human is the apparently long period of exposure to a causative agent before malignancy develops.

The various diagnostic facilities currently available, such as x-ray, biopsy, endoscopy, and cytological examination, however, permit diagnosis sufficiently early to provide for a relatively high degree of success in the control of this problem. In addition, the multiple methods of treatment—surgery, x-ray, chemical, and hormonal—offer considerable hope for a return to good health and activity for an extended period of time in cases where cure is not possible.

SUMMARY

The history of medicine provides an understanding of the steps through which man acquired increased knowledge of disease and of the constant struggle to improve health by the treatment, control, and prevention of illness. In recent years, increasing attention has been given to the process of improving man's functional capacity in the event of handicap or disability.

Certain agreed-upon standards have been established that make possible the classification of disease according to the structure or anatomical divisions of the body and the cause or mechanism by which disease is produced. The *Standard Nomenclature of Diseases and Operations* has been published regularly by The American Medical Association and provides an accurate and detailed classification. A growing body of scientific knowledge has required changes and revisions from time to time, but the general approach is essentially the same. The topographic classification is divided into ten main divisions and includes:

- Body as a whole
- Integumentary system
- Respiratory system
- Cardiovascular system
- Hemic and lymphatic systems
- Digestive system
- Urogenital system
- Endocrine system
- Nervous system
- Organs of special sense

The etiological classification includes diseases due to

- Prenatal influence
- Lower plant or animal parasites
- Higher plant or animal parasites
- Intoxication
- Trauma or physical agents
- Circulatory disturbances
- Disturbances of innervation or psychic control
- Static mechanical abnormality (obstruction, calculus, displacement, or gross change in form due to unknown cause)

- Disorder of metabolism, growth, or nutrition
- New growth
- Unknown or uncertain cause with structural reaction manifest (degenerative, infiltrative, inflammatory, proliferative, sclerotic, or reparative); hereditary and familial disease of this nature
- Unknown or uncertain cause with the functional reaction alone manifest; hereditary and familial disease of this nature manifest
- Undetermined cause

The expanding body of knowledge from the social sciences as well as the natural sciences has resulted in a deeper appreciation of the nature and meaning of disturbances to the individual to his family and to the community. Within this context rehabilitation is a complex process that for effective results must deal with forces that are physical, biological, psychological, and social.

An attempt has been made in this introductory chapter to establish a background of understanding that, hopefully, will provide an appreciation of the nature of some of the categories of disease that are associated with significant disability. No attempt has been made to be either complete or comprehensive. This will be the function of subsequent chapters.

BIBLIOGRAPHY

Anderson, Odin A., and George Rosen. *An Examination of the Concept of Preventive Medicine.* Chicago: Health Information Foundation, Research Series #12, 1960.

Cecil, Russell L., Robert F. Loeb, *et al. Textbook of Medicine,* 11th ed. Philadelphia: W. B. Saunders Co., 1963.

Goss, C. M. *Gray's Anatomy of the Human Body,* 27th ed. Philadelphia: Lea and Febiger, 1959.

Plunkett, R. J., and A. C. Hyden. *Standard Nomenclature of Disease and Operations,* 4th ed. Published for the American Medical Association. Philadelphia: Blakiston Co., 1952.

Rusk, H. A. *Rehabilitation Medicine.* St. Louis: C. V. Mosby Co., 1958.

Shryock, R. H. *The Development of Modern Medicine.* New York: Alfred A. Knopf, 1947.

II

DISEASES OF THE HEART
AND PERIPHERAL BLOOD VESSELS

Heart disease is by far the most important of all categories of disease ✓ in terms of mortality, at least in Western countries. In the United States in 1961 the National Office of Vital Statistics reported close to one million deaths due to cardiovascular disease, accounting for 54.6 per cent of deaths from all causes. The next most common cause, cancer, produced just over one-fourth as many deaths. Mortality data do not, however, provide the full story. Disability due to cardiovascular diseases, and in particular heart disease, probably involves many times the number of persons dying from these disorders.

THE HEART

[The heart is one of the most vital and at the same time most vulnerable organs in the body. It is the only organ that must do continuous mechanical work.] To accomplish this, the heart is provided with tissues and structures of a very specialized nature. The complexity of their arrangement and interrelationships, as well as the necessity for continuous performance of the heart, results in the peculiar vulnerability of this organ to a great variety of injuries and abnormalities.

ANATOMY OF THE HEART

EMBRYOLOGICAL DEVELOPMENT. In the early stages of development of the human embryo, the heart is a simple tube connected into the

By DAVID H. SPODICK, A.B., MD., F.A.C.P., F.A.C.C. Assistant Professor of Medicine, Tufts University School of Medicine; Senior Physician and Chief, Cardiographic Laboratory, Lemuel Shattuck Hospital; Clinical Associate in Medicine, Boston City Hospital, Boston, Massachusetts.

circulatory system. This tube enlarges and bends upon itself like the letter "S," after which its enlargement continues, and it becomes differentiated into a primitive chamber primarily for receiving blood, and another primarily for transmitting it, respectively the primitive *atrium* and *ventricle*. Later, each of these chambers becomes divided into two chambers by the *interatrial* and *interventricular septa,* and the atria become separated from the ventricles by the *atrioventricular septa,* so that the final four-chambered heart results. Concomitantly with

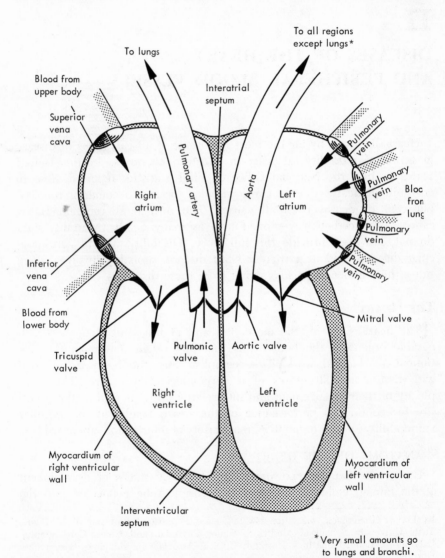

Figure 1. Schematic representation of the anatomy of the heart. Arrows indicate normal direction of blood flow. Endocardium and pericardium not included (see text).

the development of the heart chambers, the vessels entering the atria and those emerging from the ventricles form. Thus, the fetus normally has a fully formed and developed heart just before birth. However, while in the uterus, the fetus cannot have the adult-type circulation, which depends upon the lungs for breathing, since it cannot obtain air. In the uterus the placenta substitutes for respiration by interchanging fetal blood with maternal blood. Since both sides of the heart must preserve a balanced circulation, blood, which after birth goes into the lungs from the right side of the heart, is shunted across an opening in the *interatrial septum* (the partition between the two atria) into the left side of the heart. Failure of development or abnormal development of any of the structures, particularly of the partitions between the heart chambers, during fetal and embryonal life results in various forms of congenital heart disease.

THE CARDIAC CHAMBERS AND GREAT VESSELS. The fully formed heart (Figure 1) contains four chambers, the *right atrium* [1] and *right ventricle* (together called the "right heart") and the *left atrium* and *left ventricle* (together called the "left heart"). Blood returning from all regions of the body, excepting the lungs, enters the right atrium through the two *venae cavae*; the *superior vena cava* carries blood from the body above the level of the heart and the *inferior vena cava* returns blood to the heart from the body beneath its level. From the right atrium this "used" blood enters the right ventricle through the *tricuspid valve*, and from the right ventricle it is pumped into the *pulmonary artery* through the *pulmonic valve.* The pulmonary artery divides into right and left branches which carry the blood to the lungs. In the lungs this blood, which has given up a large amount of its oxygen supply to the body, is replenished with oxygen during its flow through tiny capillaries surrounding the lung *alveoli* (air sacs). From the lung it is carried via the *pulmonary veins* (two from each lung) to the left atrium. From the left atrium it passes into the left ventricle through the *mitral valve*; the left ventricle then pumps the blood through the *aortic valve* into the *aorta,* the largest artery in the body, which sends its branches to all regions.

SPECIALIZED CARDIAC TISSUES. The wall of the heart is composed mainly of muscle, the *myocardium*, which varies in strength, thickness, and distribution of its muscle fibers depending on the function of each of the chambers of the heart. The myocardium is especially thick, for example, over the left ventricle, which has the greatest pumping load, and is relatively thin on the atria, which do comparatively little active pumping. Around the outside of the myocardium is the *pericardium,* a double-layered sac, which provides protection and support for the

---

[1] Formerly the atria were incorrectly referred to as "auricles." The auricles are actually small ear-shaped projections of the atria.

heart and contains a fluid that helps to lubricate the heart movements, diminishing friction with the adjacent structures. The interior of the myocardium is lined with a very thin transparent membrane, the _endocardium._ The four *valves* are specialized structures of the endocardium situated between each atrium and ventricle and between each ventricle and its outflow artery, as described above. Normally, the heart valves, like valves in mechanical devices, permit only one-way flow and permit sufficient emptying of each chamber into its particular outflow artery. The myocardium contains within itself specialized conducting tissues: the *common atrioventricular bundle*, which divides into the *right* and *left bundle branches;* the latter ultimately keep branching into a very fine treelike arrangement, the *Purkinje network,* which is carried to all portions of the ventricular myocardium in the zone just below the endocardium. Similar specialized tissue is contained in two important circumscribed areas, the *sinoatrial* (SA) *node* and the *atrioventricular* (AV) *node*. The SA node is located in the right atrium near the point of entrance of the superior vena cava. The AV node is located at the junction of atria and ventricles just above and in connection with the common atrioventricular bundle. The *coronary blood vessels,* so named because they appeared to early anatomists to surround the heart like a crown, provide the circulation of blood to and from the heart. *Coronary arteries* are the first branches of the aorta after it leaves the left ventricle. The *coronary veins* collect the blood from the myocardium and return it to the right atrium.

PHYSIOLOGY OF THE HEART

The function of the heart is to provide continuous blood flow to the lungs and to all other portions of the body. It does this by acting as a pair of pumps—right and left—that normally work in almost perfect unison (Figure 1). The right ventricle pumps blood at relatively low pressure over the short distance to the lungs; the left ventricle must then raise this blood to a much higher pressure in order to perfuse the most distant portions of the body and at the same time provide much of the energy needed to bring the blood back again to the right side of the heart. To accomplish these tasks, the myocardium of both sides of the heart must be capable of contracting and relaxing rhythmically sufficiently often to keep all of the blood moving, and with such coordination that both sides of the heart move approximately the same amount of blood with each beat. The period during which the ventricles contract and blood is squeezed into the pulmonary artery and aorta is known as *systole;* the period during which the ventricles relax and receive blood from the atria is known as *diastole.*[2]

[2] Strictly speaking, these are *ventricular* systole and diastole. However, common usage omits the chamber name unless *atrial* systole or diastole are described.

The SA and AV nodes and the specialized conducting bundles act as a system that sets the rate of cardiac contraction (the heart rate) and normally controls the manner and sequence in which portions of the myocardium will contract. The SA node is the principal *pacemaker* of the heart. Normally it forms impulses, or electrochemical "signals," that stimulate the heart at a rate of between 60 and 90 beats per minute in most individuals. These impulses radiate through the atrial walls without requiring specialized conducting tissue. They reach the AV node where, after a slight delay, they enter the common atrio-ventricular bundle and are sent along the bundle branches to the myocardium of both ventricles.

Both sides of the heart move between 4.5 and 7.5 liters (about 5 to 8 quarts) of blood every minute in most normal individuals. This is known as the *cardiac output.* The portion of the cardiac output that is moved by each stroke or beat of the heart is known as the *stroke output* or *stroke volume*. Thus, a heart beating 60 times per minute with a cardiac output of 6 liters per minute would have a stroke volume of 1/60 of 6 liters, or 100 milliliters (about 3½ ounces), of blood.

Regulation of the heart is accomplished by a number of mechanisms, such as changes in the rate of impulse formation by the SA node or, in the presence of disease, default to other potential pacemakers, such as the AV node. Indeed, the heart has a hierarchy of pacemakers involving both nodes, portions of the nodes, specialized conducting tissues, and even the myocardium, which has an inherent rhythmicity, allowing it to contract independently if necessary. Normally the heart is regulated also by influences from the *autonomic nervous system*: the *sympathetic* nerves tend to increase the heart rate, while the *vagus* nerve (belonging to the parasympathetic nervous system) tends to slow it. Similarly *temperature changes*, as in fever, either increase or decrease the rate of impulse formation (and therefore the rate of cardiac contraction). Exercise, metabolic influences, and other moment-to-moment changes in the requirements of the body for circulation operate in a very complex feedback system, much like a mechanical servomechanism, to regulate both the rate of the heart and, frequently, the output per stroke. It is the task of the *coronary circulation* under all conditions to parallel the work of the heart by providing improved circulation during periods of increased demand.

RESPONSE OF THE HEART TO STRESS

It is apparent from the multitude of mechanisms for regulating the heart and the range of activity available to the heart that this unique pump has built-in capabilities for meeting various situations. When these involve very high or abnormally increased demands upon the heart for work, the extent to which the heart can meet these demands is known as the *cardiac reserve*. When abnormal demands arrive due to unusual metabolic loads, or mechanical strain upon the heart (such as having to contract against a high blood pressure), or actual damage to the myocardium (such as that due to decreased blood supply in disease of the coronary arteries), the heart may need to fall back on its normal reserve or ultimately resort to abnormal mechanisms in order to keep the circulation going. The simplest mechanism for meeting the demand for increased circulation is *tachycardia* (increased heart rate); by increasing the number of strokes per minute, the cardiac output will rise in proportion to the rate, as long as the stroke volume does not change. A more complex mechanism is *dilatation* of one or more heart chambers, which results from elongation of individual fibers of the myocardium; elongated fibers will, within limits, contract more strongly. Dilatation permits the heart to receive and expel a greater amount of blood. If the heart is subjected to unusual stress of almost any kind for a prolonged period, dilatation gives way ultimately to *hypertrophy*. This condition represents an increase in the thickness and weight of the myocardium and, to some extent, an increase in the number of muscle fibers, permitting, within limits, a stronger and more effective contraction. However, this mechanism tends to become inefficient because the coronary blood supply usually cannot keep pace with the enlarged, thickened myocardium. Thus, in the presence of chronic stress, hypertrophy ultimately gives way to a secondary dilatation. The latter indicates complete failure of all mechanisms designed to improve cardiac output and represents a late stage of heart disease.

Circulatory changes outside of the heart occur in order to support the heart when it is subjected to stress. These principally involve the smaller arteries, which tend to constrict in the presence of an abnormally low cardiac output and to dilate with a high cardiac output (a much less common situation).

PATHOLOGICAL PHYSIOLOGY: MECHANISMS OF HEART DISEASE

All categories of disease may involve the heart directly or indirectly and to a greater or lesser degree. Thus, in general, heart disease may be congenital, inflammatory, traumatic, neoplastic, or metabolic, the latter including conditions in which the oxygen supply is decreased.

MYOCARDIUM. The myocardium may be injured directly owing to physical trauma, but more commonly, injury is the result of decreased blood supply. Occasionally, inflammation due to infections or "allergic" mechanisms produces *myocarditis*. The myocardium responds, if the patient survives, by either localized or generalized scarring, involving the replacement of smaller or larger areas of myocardium by fibrous (scarred) tissues. This places the heart under a special handicap, because not only has it lost contractile muscular elements, but these have been replaced by rigid, nonfunctional scar. Commonly, such lesions involve the wall of a single chamber, usually the left ventricle, and ultimately result in hypertrophy and dilatation if that chamber cannot perform its function adequately. Involvement of individual chambers also occurs in congenital heart disease owing to abnormal communication between them—for example, persistence of a large communication between the atria (atrial septal defect), which is normal only in the fetus.

CORONARY LESIONS. *Atherosclerosis* and a few uncommon lesions like arteritis cause narrowing of the coronary arteries. If this process proceeds sufficiently far, the coronary arteries cannot transmit enough blood to nourish the myocardium, which is, therefore, placed at a disadvantage. This process occurs over a long period of time in the great majority of adults, although in most of them it does not cause critical narrowing. A more dramatic consequence of atherosclerosis is the change that it makes in the nature of the interior of the coronary arteries. Atherosclerotic lesions are laid down under the lining (*intima*) of the arteries as deposits of fatty material, rich in cholesterol, which irritate the vessel walls and ultimately become scarred as they increase in size; advanced lesions also contain considerable amounts of calcium (chalk). By roughening the lining of the arteries as well as by producing other physical and chemical changes, the process provides sites for formation of clots composed of elements of blood flowing over them. When clotting (thrombosis) occurs, the blood supply to regions of the myocardium is cut off more or less rapidly. This places the heart at a considerable disadvantage because it does not have the time to call upon its reserve mechanisms as efficiently as it might in more slowly developing lesions.

VALVES. Normally the valves permit one-way flow of a normal quantity of blood passing through the heart chambers and out the pulmonary artery and aorta. Inflammatory diseases and congenital abnormalities may alter the valves so they do not perform their functions properly. Basically, there are two types of valve lesion that may exist independently or concomitantly in the same valve or in several valves: *stenosis*, indicating a narrowing of the valve opening; *regurgitation*, denoting an abnormal opening during the time which the valve should be closed. Stenosis impedes the flow of blood and causes high pressures, mechanical strain, and ultimately dilatation and hypertrophy in the chamber of the heart "upstream" from the valve. For example, if the mitral valve is stenosed (mitral stenosis), the pressure in the left atrium will be high, and the left atrium may become enlarged and its wall thicken. In regurgitation, there is a backflow of strain on the chamber. If, for example, regurgitation occurs through the mitral valve (mitral regurgitation), strain is put on the left atrium somewhat like that of mitral stenosis, but there is also an undue burden on the left ventricle, which not only must expel blood into the aorta, but is also abnormally expelling blood back into the left atrium at the same time; in this circumstance the left ventricle also responds by dilatation and hypertrophy.

ENDOCARDIUM. The endocardium may become involved when diseases of the valve or myocardium are present. When these extend to the endocardium it may become infected or inflamed (*endocarditis*), or clots may form upon it—much as they form in sclerotic arteries—because it no longer presents an undamaged surface to the blood within the heart.

PERICARDIUM. Essentially the only cause of pericardial disease is inflammation (*pericarditis*), which may occur in conjunction with heart disease of the same causation or which may occur independently due to infections and, rarely, the presence of tumors. Acute pericardial inflammation usually causes distressing symptoms, but does not embarrass the function of the heart unless *cardiac tamponade* is present. This situation results when the injured pericardium pours forth a great amount of fluid into its sac, raising pressure around the heart which strangulates it, preventing the flow of blood into the ventricles. A similar situation occurs in *constrictive pericarditis* in which, in the absence of fluid, the inflamed pericardium slowly scars; the scar tissue contracts upon the heart and sooner or later strangulates it in much the same way as tamponading fluid.

SPECIALIZED CONDUCTING TISSUES. Involvement of the SA and AV nodes by disease produces *dysrhythmias* (arrhythmias) as a result of impairment of their pacemaker function. Under these circumstances abnormal pacemakers arise either in parts of the atrial myocardium or in the specialized conducting tissues of the ventricles. The most common important dysrhythmia is *atrial fibrillation*, in which there is grossly irregular beating of the heart owing to rapid formation of impulses in the atria in an uncoordinated manner. The AV node receives these impulses from the atrium at irregular intervals or at unequal strengths, and transmits them to the ventricles, which then beat irregularly. Interestingly, this dysrhythmia is compatible with life over very long periods. Less common, but very important, are dysrhythmias such as *atrial tachycardia* and *atrial flutter,* in which there is a rapid formation of regular impulses from the atrial myocardium, many or all of which are transmitted to the AV node. In the presence of disorders of the AV node (usually with the SA node intact) *atrioventricular block* may occur. Block refers to an abnormal delay in the conduction of impulses from the atria through the AV node to the ventricles. This may result in many of the atrial impulses being prevented from stimulating the ventricle so that there may be a ratio of two, three, or four atrial beats to each ventricular beat. More common than the foregoing, but usually much less important, are *ectopic beats* (extrasystoles). These do not necessarily depend on depression of pacemaker function, and may occur in normal persons. They become important when they are abnormally frequent, and suggest abnormal irritability of areas of the myocardium. Disorders of the specialized conducting bundles in the ventricles produce intraventricular blocks which cause a delay in the conduction of impulses to either the right or left ventricle or both (*left bundle branch block; right bundle branch block; "interventricular block"* respectively). Usually this does not cause sufficient incoordination to overtly impair cardiac function.

VASCULAR CHANGES. *Hypertension* (increased blood pressure) in the blood vessels into which the ventricles pump blood causes a strain of one or both sides of the heart because the heart must develop a higher pressure than that in the outflow vessels in order to expel blood into them. The blood pressure in the vessels of the pulmonary and systemic circulations depends partly on the thrust imparted to the blood by systole, but also upon the amount of blood (blood volume), changes in the blood vessel walls, regulation of vessel size by the autonomic nervous system, factors associated with the central nervous system, and various hormones. If hypertension in the outflow of one side of the heart is acute, the heart is placed at a serious disadvantage because it does not have adequate time to call upon its reserves. For example, if a blockage (usually due to a clot) suddenly appears in one of the pulmonary arteries, the pressure in that artery rises acutely, and the right side of the heart is acutely embarrassed. On the other hand, if the elevation in pressure is chronic, as is the case in the common form of arterial hypertension ("high blood pressure"), the left side of the heart ultimately adapts to this strain by hypertrophy.

ROLE OF EFFORT. Whereas the normal heart can support the activities of the muscles and the rest of the body during strenuous exercise, especially if the individual is "in shape," the diseased heart is at a considerable disadvantage in this respect. It is highly unlikely that even strenuous effort *per se* can cause heart disease; however, just as in normal individuals in various states of physical condition, different amounts of cardiac disease provide different thresholds at which effort may cause additional damage or may produce symptoms.

HEART FAILURE. A pathological condition common to all forms of heart disease is "heart failure." This may be defined as inability of the heart, for whatever reason, to maintain the circulation adequately in the face of a normal range of demand. In early failure, the heart may merely respond poorly to increased loads, such as unusually severe or sustained effort. Progressive failure goes through many gradations until even normal effort, such as walking or even eating, may precipitate signs and symptoms of cardiac distress. It is important to

point out that many persons with heart disease do not show much
evidence of heart failure, possibly because they do not indulge in
unusual exertion; others may have such rapid development of failure
owing to a massive insult to the heart that they never go through the
early stages, and relatively little effort causes disability.

Compensation indicates the operation of the cardiac reserve and
special mechanisms to offset some handicap that would otherwise produce overt failure. As mentioned previously, mechanisms such as _tach-
ycardia, dilatation,_ and _hypertrophy_ will operate, within limits, to offset
cardiac handicaps, given sufficient time to do so. Dilatation and hypertrophy each result in _cardiac enlargement,_ which may involve the
whole heart or, more commonly, one or two of its chambers. Once
enlargement is at hand, the presence of heart failure, even if compensated, has to be inferred. This is because an enlarged heart is
mechanically inefficient. It not only consumes more oxygen to do the
same or a smaller amount of work than does a normal-sized heart,
but now has deficient metabolic support because of the disproportionately small increase in the number of blood vessels to it. The latter,
plus the increased size of hypertrophic muscle fibers, exacerbates the
handicap because of decreased diffusion of oxygen and nutrients from
the blood into the myocardium.

Because most disease processes involve the whole heart, one side of
the heart only, or one side out of proportion to the other, heart failure
may be spoken of as left- or right-sided heart failure or "combined"
heart failure. When one side of the heart fails to pump adequately,
not only does it tend to contain an abnormal amount of blood, but
the pressure in the "feed line" entering it rises. Thus in "left heart
failure," there is increased pressure in the lungs and in the pulmonary
circulation; in "right heart failure" the pressure in each vena cava is
high, and through them the pressure in the veins all over the body is
raised. In both circumstances fruitless compensatory mechanisms produce an increase in the volume of blood in these circulatory distributions.
(Teleologically, this represents an effort to overcome the "blockade"
imposed by failure of that portion of the heart.) Both the increase in
pressure and the increase in blood volume contribute to the literal
"squeezing out" of fluid from the smaller blood vessels (capillaries)
into the body tissues. Collection of fluid in the tissues is greatly increased by the response of the kidneys to heart failure under the influence of certain hormones: there is an abnormal retention of salt
by the kidneys which would otherwise pass into the urine. This salt
retention aggravates the passage of fluid from the blood vessels into
the tissues, and is one of the most important factors perpetuating the
signs of heart failure. Accumulation of abnormal fluid in the tissues
is known as _edema;_ when associated with right heart failure it may

be seen first as swollen ankles, which may progress to swelling of great portions of the body. In left-sided heart failure, the changes are more dramatic: edema of the lungs (pulmonary edema), which may occur quite suddenly in some cases, causes impairment of breathing, and the patient literally will tend to drown in his own fluids unless treated.

The foregoing are frequently referred to as *congestive heart failure.* Another and less commonly encountered form of heart failure is *high output failure.* This can occur with or without intrinsic heart disease, and is due to an enormous demand that cannot be met for long even by a normal heart. This occurs in severe anemias, certain vitamin deficiencies (such as beriberi), hyperthyroidism, and abnormal communication between arteries and veins (in which the short-circuiting of large amounts of blood calls for an increase in the output of the heart to compensate for that portion of the cardiac output which has been recirculated without doing its task).

OBJECTIVE MANIFESTATIONS OF HEART DISEASE

DIAGNOSTIC PROCEDURES. After obtaining a history of complaints referable to the heart (see later, "Disability: Subjective Manifestations of Heart Disease"), the physician initiates an orderly progression of procedures designed to ascertain the presence of heart disease, to identify the type of lesion or lesions present (for example, disorders of valves, myocardium), and to determine the type of heart disease responsible for those lesions when this is possible. A large array of diagnostic methods are available, from familiar but important procedures such as the classic physical examination to the use of a variety of complex electronic instruments.

Physical Examination. This involves inspection and observation of the patient for signs of illness, some of which may have already been mentioned by the patient in his medical history. Attention is paid not only to the heart, but also to all areas of the body, because it is impossible to separate one organ system from another. Even the skin reflects changes due to heart disease, such as cyanosis, which gives it a blue color. Close attention, however, is paid to the chest wall where certain manifestations of cardiac distress may be observed. The pulse rate is taken, usually at the wrist (radial pulse), in order to ascertain how fast and how regularly the heart is beating; in some cases this must be compared with the rate of the heart itself as measured through the stethoscope (in atrial fibrillation, for example, many of the beats of the heart are weak and do not reach the radial pulse). The arterial blood pressure is taken, usually in the arm, in order to ascertain whether an excessive pressure is present in the arterial system supplied by the left heart; on the other hand, an abnormally low blood pressure—which is an uncommon event—under certain circumstances would also indicate cardiac distress. An attempt is made to evaluate heart size by percussion of the chest. In this procedure the air-filled lungs, which surround the heart, give a high-pitched note similar to that of a drum, while the heart itself produces a dull note because it is a blood-filled organ. At the same time, if the lungs are filled with fluid owing to failure of the left heart, they will give a dull to flat note because this fluid has displaced air. Following this, the stethoscope is used to evaluate the quality of the sounds produced by closing of the heart valves (heart sounds), to determine if there are any abnormal sounds and, above all, to find murmurs, which are noises principally caused by the flow of blood across abnormal orifices (for example, diseased valves, septal defects).

Roentgenographic Procedures. X-ray photographs are obtained of the heart to determine its actual size (percussion being subject to error) and its shape. *Fluoroscopy* is an x-ray technique in which the rays are passed through the heart on to a screen so that the physician may watch the actual character of the heart beat and may rotate the patient to various angles in order to better evaluate the individual cardiac chambers. These procedures are extremely valuable in locating certain valve lesions because of characteristic heart chamber enlargement and because certain valve disorders cause the laying down of calcium (chalk) in the valve which can be found roentgenographically. They also permit evaluation of the presence of fluid in and about the lungs and the presence of fluid or scarring in the pericardium.

Electrocardiogram. The electrocardiogram (ECG) is an extremely valuable procedure for determining the presence of acute and chronic injury of the heart, particularly in coronary artery disease and in conditions causing enlargement of individual heart chambers. It is indispensable for the identification of dysrhythmias, since it is a record of the electrical events associated with the heart beat. The ECG also identifies conduction abnormalities due to disease of the pacemakers (SA and AV nodes) and the specialized conducting bundles in the ventricles.

Other Graphic Procedures. Occasionally, other graphic procedures are required to further evaluate the patient. The use of these is growing in recent years, although in the majority of cases, they are not indispensable to adequate evaluation. These include the *phonocardiogram*, which is an electrical record of the heart sounds; the *electrokymogram*, which records the border movements of the heart; and the *ballistocardiogram*, which records the force of the various movements of the heart and the blood within it as transmitted to the rest of the body. The *apexcardiogram*, the *kinetocardiogram*, and the *vibrocardiogram* are all records of the changes and movements in the chest wall immediately in front of the heart (the precordium), as imparted to it by the heart movements underneath. The *vectorcardiogram* and the *vector ballistocardiogram* are used to depict the electrocardiographic and ballistocardiographic changes as they occur in three-dimensional space; these are of limited clinical value at present.

Cardiac Catheterization. Cardiac catheterization is a procedure by which small tubes and wires are inserted into the heart through various routes, generally via veins and arteries, so that a record of the pressure changes, the flow of blood, and sometimes the sounds made by the heart is obtained directly from within the heart. This also permits calculation of cardiac output per minute and per stroke as well as detection of abnormal communication between chambers of the heart and between the larger blood vessels. It is especially valuable in the diagnosis and localization of such lesions in congenital and rheumatic heart disease. It also permits the introduction into the heart of x-ray contrast material so that certain abnormalities of blood flow can be seen directly on fluoroscopy. A similar procedure, which does not require the catheter to enter the heart, is the injection of contrast material into the aorta just where it leaves the heart in order to outline the coronary arteries by x-ray (the value of this promising procedure is not yet completely established).

Other Procedures. Contrast materials may be injected into veins in order to obtain an *angiocardiogram*, which will outline the vessels entering and leaving the heart cavities as well as the shape of the cavities themselves on x-ray films. *Blood oxygen determinations* may be made in veins and arteries as well as directly from heart blood in order to determine whether there is too little or too much oxygen at certain points in the circulation. *Indicator-dilution studies* may be made without catheterizing the heart in order to ascertain the cardiac output and certain other data; this method involves injection of a known amount of a dye (or other indicator) into the blood stream and the sampling of the blood for the indicator when it reaches some point in the arterial system after it has left the heart.

OBJECTIVE SIGNS OF HEART DISEASE. In many cases heart disease may give no indication of its presence for a long period, other than the patient's complaints. However, the majority of patients display a spectrum of objective findings that can be determined by the physician during physical examination or by using one or more of the diagnostic procedures above. *Tachycardia* (heart rate in excess of 100 beats per minute) is a cardinal sign, particularly if it appears during the ordinary activities of the patient. At the same time, *bradycardia* (heart rate below 50 beats per minute) may be a sign of cardiac abnormality particularly in patients who develop *atrioventricular block. Dysrhythmias* and frequent *extrasystoles* are other definite indicators of cardiac abnormality. The presence of an abnormal blood pressure does not necessarily mean that the heart has been affected, although if a high blood pressure exists for a long enough period, signs of heart distress will eventually develop.

One of the most important manifestations is *dyspnea*—labored breathing either during exertion, during ordinary activities, or even at rest. *Cyanosis* indicates either a generalized or local decrease in the amount of oxygen in the blood. It may be due to the presence of fluid in the lungs because of failure of the left heart, or to slowing of the blood stream in areas relatively distant from the heart caused by poor cardiac mechanics. Under these circumstances, the tissues extract more oxygen from the blood during its slow passage through them; in such cases blueness is generally seen only in the fingers, toes, nose, lips, and ears. Cyanosis may also be due to abnormal communication between the sides of the heart, as in some forms of congenital heart disease, under which circumstance there is a flow of blood low in oxygen ("blue blood") from the right side of the heart into the left side of the heart, thus bypassing the lungs and entering the general circulation.

Edema, due to retention of salt by the kidney in heart failure as well as to increased pressure "upstream" from the side of the heart that is failing, may be seen in the legs and ankles in right heart failure; it may be found by x-ray and auscultation in the lungs in left heart failure. The tendency to pour out fluid into abnormal locations may be such that fluid also fills the abdomen (*ascites*) and the pleural cavities that surround the lungs (*pleural effusion*). Occasionally patients who have survived right heart failure for very long periods develop *anasarca* (dropsy), in which there is swelling of virtually the entire body due to edema, pleural effusion, and ascites.

DISABILITY: SUBJECTIVE MANIFESTATIONS OF HEART DISEASE

Patients are disabled by heart disease because it produces discomfort—that is, symptoms. Those who are fortunate enough to have heart disease without symptoms, and those who for one reason or another are not aware of the presence of heart disease, either will not be disabled or will not recognize the need for limitation of activity. Regardless of the type of heart lesion, symptoms and consequent disability are, in general, closely related—that is, the heart is relatively limited in its means of expressing distress to the patient. In virtually all forms of heart disease, symptoms and consequent disability arise from either (1) heart failure, (2) chest pain, (3) symptomatic dysrhythmias, and (4) psychogenic complaints.

Symptoms of Heart Failure, When the heart fails to pump adequately for the demands of the circulation, the patient may notice *weakness*, particularly upon effort, as well as *fatigue* and increasingly *easy fatigability*. With progression of disease this tends to appear even during normal activities. *Dyspnea* has already been referred to above; in general, this begins with exertion, dyspnea at rest indicates quite advanced heart failure. *Orthopnea* is very common in left heart failure because of the tendency to pour fluid into the lungs; this term indicates shortness of breath while lying flat, since gravity then tends to bring more blood and fluid to the lungs. Such patients must prop their heads up when lying supine so that gravity will aid the heart in draining fluid from the lungs. This is often measured in the number of pillows the patient must use at night (for example, "four pillow orthopnea" causes the patient to sit almost upright in order to sleep comfortably, and indicates serious distress). *Paroxysmal nocturnal dyspnea* refers to sudden awakening in the middle of the night because of rapid filling of the lungs; this may be provoked by lying supine, although in some cases apparently it is triggered by imperfectly understood mechanisms associated with the brain and certain reflexes. *Syncope* (fainting) occurs in some patients during exercise, as a result of either a great disproportion between the cardiac output and the demands of the muscles for blood, or inability to raise the rate of the heart (as in atrioventricular block), which effectively prevents the raising of cardiac output even without overt heart failure. *Abdominal pain* occurs in some patients with right heart failure because of congestion of the abdominal organs with blood that has "backed" upstream from the right atrium.

CHEST PAIN. Patients with a variety of heart diseases have various types of chest pain, most of which are rather vague and not clearly ascribable to the heart. The type of pain that is clearly of cardiac origin is known as *angina pectoris*. Typically, this is situated in the middle of the chest under the sternum. It has a squeezing or pressing quality and often is not very sharp (in fact, a squeezing or pressing sensation without real pain frequently occurs and is tantamount to the same thing). Anginal distress may radiate from the chest to the neck, the teeth, the shoulders, and the arms. Most characteristically, it radiates to the left shoulder and down the inside of the left arm, often ending in the left fourth and fifth fingers. It is important to emphasize that any portion of this kind of pain—for example, pain limited to the shoulder or arm or even the fingers—occurs in a number of patients in whom it is necessary to distinguish the presence of heart disease from disorders of the bones, muscles, and joints.

SYMPTOMATIC DYSRHYTHMIAS AND TACHYCARDIA. Most patients are not aware of most rhythm abnormalities especially when these have been present for long periods. However, the sudden onset of a rapid or irregular rhythm may be perceived by the patient as a sudden change or as a regular or irregular *palpitation* in the chest. Some patients are aware of extrasystoles, which commonly produce a feeling that the heart has stopped momentarily, followed by a strong thump. These can be very distressing even in the absence of serious heart disease. Symptomatic dysrhythmias and palpitations are usually produced on effort, but in critically ill patients they also occur at rest.

Disability Due to Complications. In the course of cardiac illness the presence of other diseases often causes more severe complaints and more objective findings than in patients who are free of heart disease. This is probably due to the extra strain thrown upon the heart and to the actual manifestations of these complicating disorders when added to those of the preexisting heart lesions. Lung disorders, for example, tend to throw an increased burden on the right side of the heart and to more easily provoke pulmonary edema in left heart failure. Patients with lesions of valves may develop clots upon the valves which then can leave the heart and travel through the arteries causing *embolism* (sudden blockade) of arteries in many other organs. The same patients can develop *bacterial endocarditis* due to the growth of colonies of bacteria upon the valves; these also cause embolism as well as fever and widespread dissemination of the bacteria, with subsequent infection throughout the body. Patients lying ill with heart disease for long periods of time will tend to develop thrombosis in the veins of the legs, which may result in embolism to the lungs (pulmonary embolism), a life-threatening situation that is a very common cause of death.

Psychogenic Symptoms. Patients who are aware of any form of illness are very likely to develop unexplained symptoms. In many instances, these are not associated directly with the disease or with changes in its course, regardless of how typical they seem. Some of them remain unexplained; others are associated with a definite anxiety state, anxiety neurosis, depression, or depression combined with anxiety. Frequently these disturbances are easily detected. On the other hand, in many patients it takes long observation to confirm them. In any event, the inference that a patient's symptoms are not "organic" must always be made on the basis of positive conclusions—that is, not merely by exclusion of disease or by a change in the course of an established disease.

Patients who know or believe that they have heart disease will often have brief, sharp pains in the chest which they will usually localize well to the left of center because of the common belief that the heart is located there. While heart disease can cause this type of pain, it is rather uncommon in organic conditions. Other individuals will develop chest pain radiating to the left shoulder and arm, exactly duplicating the radiation of typical angina pectoris. Another frequent psychogenic complaint is shortness of breath in the absence of signs of heart failure. This usually is an "air hunger" rather than real dyspnea. Yet another complaint is consciousness of the heart beat, commonly present at night—a time when the patient is free from external stimuli. This is to be distinguished from true palpitations which, however, also may be psychogenic.

GENERAL MANAGEMENT OF HEART DISEASE

The medical management (nonsurgical treatment) of all forms of heart disease is fundamentally similar. This is because the heart expresses distress or impairment of its functions in a limited number of ways, and because there are but a few classes of medications applicable to heart disease.

Many patients with mild forms of heart disease do not require active treatment. It is necessary only to limit the burden upon their heart, either to a reasonable extent (in those who do not have symptoms and signs) or to within the limits of tolerance (in those in whom excessive physical or mental activity will provoke signs of distress). Of course, in the acute phases of heart disease, more or less active treatment and restriction of activities is usually mandatory.

Rest is one of the principal recommendations for patients with heart disease. Frequently the patient will know his own limits and stay well within them. However, it is often necessary for the physician to lay out a program of permitted and restricted activities, which must be varied widely for the individual patient. Certainly once a definite heart lesion is present, virtually every patient will be forbidden to do any heavy work or engage in strenuous sports, but up to that point there is a wide variance in activities that can be tolerated. Psychic rest is always desirable, since not only can manifestations of heart disease— for example, angina, acute congestive failure, acute dysrhythmias—be provoked by psychic trauma, but it is now known that the process of *atherogenesis* (the laying down in arteries of atherosclerotic, cholesterol-filled deposits) may be accelerated by psychic stress. To this end, the patient has to be counseled by his physician with regard to family and occupational stresses. Frequently, sedatives such as phenobarbital are prescribed.

TREATMENT OF UNDERLYING OR PRECIPITATING CAUSES. It is always desirable to eliminate disease processes that either cause or provoke the signs of heart disease. In arteriosclerosis (particularly atherosclerosis) this is not yet possible, although many studies indicate that a prophylactic approach by altering the diet may be desirable. Medications for decreasing cholesterol and other fatty substances associated with the production of the lesions in the arteries are still in the experimental state. In congenital abnormalities of the heart chambers, the great vessels or valves, and in inflammatory lesions of the valves (such as rheumatic heart disease), surgical correction is often either palliative or curative. If the patient has high blood pressure, this may be reduced in the vast majority of cases. Concomitant pulmonary disease can often be treated if it is infectious; if pulmonary emphysema is present, special treatments and the elimination of smoking are needed. In the presence of an overactive thyroid gland (hyperthyroidism) "antithyroid" drugs may be used or, if unsuccessful, the thyroid gland must be removed. Severe anemias should be carefully diagnosed and treated in order to improve the blood supply to the heart. Similarly, nutritional deficiencies (uncommon in the Western world, except for alcoholics) should be treated with vitamins and proper diet.

TREATMENT OF HEART FAILURE. The medical treatment of heart failure is aimed at improving the function of the myocardium, particularly its ability to expel blood, by improving its contraction. The principal agents for accomplishing this are in the digitalis family of drugs. At the same time, it is necessary in many patients to combat the tendency to retain salt and water in the tissues. This is done by restricting the amount of salt in the diet and, occasionally, by also restricting water. The process is aided by the use of many different types of diuretics—drugs that promote the elimination of salt and water by the kidney. Just as salt tends to hold water in the tissues, salt put out by the kidney carries water with it and, in the presence of edema, tends to "dry out" the patient's tissues and lungs. In the presence of excess fluid in the pleural cavities surrounding the lungs and in the abdominal cavity (ascites), it is sometime necessary to insert a needle (paracentesis) to remove some or all of the fluid if it is causing distress to the patient.

Acute left heart failure is a life-threatening situation because the edema of the lungs may rapidly kill the patient in a manner analogous to drowning in salt water. This is treated by giving morphine or similar drugs rapidly. These frequently have a dramatically beneficial effect, the reasons for which are not completely known but may be associated with reflexes in the nervous system that may precipitate the acute attack. At the same time the patient is given oxygen. In appropriate cases, a phlebotomy is performed. This procedure removes blood via a needle placed in a vein; when the blood volume is expanded, the removal of an appropriate quantity tends to reduce the circulatory load on the heart. More often it is possible to obtain the same result by placing tourniquets on three of the patient's four extremities in order to trap blood in the arms and legs (this is known as "internal phlebotomy"). Patients with acute heart failure who have not taken digitalis, and those considered to have had too little, are simultaneously given rapidly acting drugs of the digitalis group.

TREATMENT OF PAIN. When chest pain due to heart disease is severe, frequently it will not respond other than to strong medication, such as *opiates* (for example, morphine and demerol). When it is anginal in character, medications of the nitrate group, particularly *nitroglycerin*, are used. Most of these are rapidly effective when given under the tongue, where they dissolve and enter the blood stream through the small vessels in the mouth. The action of the nitrates is not completely understood, and in many instances they act merely as a placebo. They appear to reduce the work of the heart, and may increase flow in the coronary arteries.

TREATMENT OF DYSRHYTHMIAS. Dysrhythmias are either acutely dangerous or chronically tend to impair the efficiency of cardiac action. In most instances, they either need to be converted to normal (sinus) rhythm or, as in the case of atrial fibrillation, frequently need only to be controlled. For this purpose *digitalis* is the principal drug used. Two other medications, *quinidine* and *procaine amide*, which are related to each other, are frequently useful. The latter must be employed with care, however, because toxic effects are relatively common. Recently, spectacularly good results have been obtained by *electronic defibrillation*: the heart is stopped by a powerful electric shock and restarted either spontaneously or by an electronic pacemaker.

TREATMENT OF SHOCK. Patients undergoing a sudden onset of certain cardiac disorders—such as arrhythmias, acute congestive failure, and acute myocardial infarction (see below)—may go into a condition of circulatory collapse known as *shock*. This requires extraordinary methods in order to support the output of the heart. For this purpose, certain drugs of the *pressor* group are used; these resemble *epinephrine* (adrenalin) in that they all tend to raise blood pressure. This results from an action both on the heart and on the blood vessels. The increased blood pressure results in better passage through the tissues, preventing irreparable damage. At the same time, most of these medications improve the contracting power of the heart. Epinephrine itself is not commonly used for this purpose, but agents such as norepinephrine, metaraminol, and related compounds are usually very effective.

CARDIAC SURGERY. The most impressive recent advances in the treatment of heart disease have been surgical. Many mechanical disorders of the heart and large blood vessels can now be partly or completely improved, either without cessation of cardiac activity or by stopping the heart (elective cardiac arrest or cardioplegia), while an artificial heart-lung apparatus (pump oxygenator) maintains the circulation.

The most successful cardiac operations are those that can completely correct abnormalities before their effects have irreversibly altered structure and function. Removal of the pericardium (pericardiectomy)—performed for constrictive pericarditis, recurrent acute pericarditis, or intractable cardiac tamponade—can be curative. Ligation (tying-off)of a congenital *patent ductus arteriosus* may restore the patient to perfect health if done early enough in life. Surgical implantation of internal or external *electronic pacemakers* can overcome the handicap imposed by dysrhythmias such as complete atrioventricular block, which cause the heart to beat too slowly to sustain adequate circulation.

Relief of rheumatic mitral stenosis by opening the narrowed valve (mitral commissurotomy or valvotomy) is the commonest procedure. Its success in a given case depends upon how badly the valve is scarred and calcified as well as the condition of the myocardium. In most patients a fair to excellent immediate result is anticipated, but some patients face restenosis, necessitating second and even third valvotomies within a few years. Aortic valvotomy, which has not been very effective in rheumatic cases, is quite successful in congenital aortic stenosis. Operations on the tricuspid and pulmonic valves are uncommon.

A promising beginning has been made in the field of *prosthetic valves*—mechanical replacements for stenotic or regurgitant heart valves. A number of procedures exist for "plugging" atrial and ventricular septal defects and for rechanneling blood flow in the presence of congenital abnormalities of the aorta, pulmonary artery, or pulmonary veins.

Operations for coronary artery disease are still in a developmental stage. Some, such as *internal mammary artery ligation*, have been done on thousands of persons, particularly in Europe, but have been worthless in controlled studies in which sham operations have shown no difference in subjective or objective results. The value of sprinkling powdered abrasives on the heart to stimulate new blood vessels via pericardial adhesions (*poudrage*) remains unproved. Removal of stenotic areas and clots from coronary arteries (*thromboendarterectomy*) has not yet been shown to be of value.

Rehabilitation of the Cardiac Patient. Few individuals are reduced to permanent inactivity by heart disease, even those with severe disorders. Thus, it is necessary to ascertain the extent of impairment in each individual. In general, once a patient is over an acute phase of his illness and is on a reasonable maintenance program of therapy (or under observation alone in those cases which do not require active treatment), his activity status with regard to his daily life and his occupation must be ascertained. In general, a graded program of activity is permitted over an individually determined period in order to observe the patient's tolerance. Sometimes, this is determined in work classification units, but more often it is the task of the individual physician or hospital clinic. When the patient can take up his occupation and normal life without distress, he is counseled to avoid excessive strain. When less than his previous activities are desirable, efforts are made with his employer, his family, and, if necessary, social service agencies, to provide modifications or even marked changes in his job and to provide help at home if this is necessary.

THE FUNCTIONAL AND THERAPEUTIC CLASSIFICATIONS OF PATIENTS WITH DISEASES OF THE HEART[3]

Functional Classification

NOTE: The classification of patients according to their cardiac functional capacity gives only a part of the information needed to plan the management of the patient's activities. A recommendation or prescription regarding physical activity should be based on information derived from many sources. The functional classification is an estimate of what the patient's heart will allow him to do and should not be influenced by the character of the structural lesions nor by an opinion as to treatment or prognosis.

Class I. Patients with cardiac disease but without resulting limitations of physical activity. Ordinary physical activity does not cause undue fatigue, palpitation, dyspnea, or anginal pain.

Class II. Patients with cardiac disease resulting in slight limitation of physical activity. They are comfortable at rest. Ordinary physical activity results in fatigue, palpitation, dyspnea, or anginal pain.

Class III. Patients with cardiac disease resulting in marked limitation of physical activity. They are comfortable at rest. Less than ordinary physical activity causes fatigue, palpitation, dyspnea, or anginal pain.

Class IV. Patients with cardiac disease resulting in inability to carry on any physical activity without discomfort. Symptoms of cardiac insufficiency or of the anginal syndrome may be present even at rest. If any physical activity is undertaken, discomfort is increased.

Therapeutic Classification

NOTE: The therapeutic classification is intended as a guide to the management of the activities of cardiac patients. It gives a prescription for the amount of physical activity which is advised for those in each functional class. From a practical point of view, it should be translated into terms of daily physical activity, such as walking a certain number of yards, climbing a specified number of stairs, lifting a certain number of pounds, and standing for an unlimited or limited part of the working day. For children it is necessary to individualize with permissible play programs, specifying the type and duration of outdoor and indoor activity which may be performed.

Class A. Patients with cardiac disease whose physical activity need not be restricted in any way.

Class B. Patients with cardiac disease whose ordinary physical activity need not be restricted, but who should be advised against severe or competitive efforts.

[3] Excerpted from *Diseases of the Heart and Blood Vessels—Nomenclature and Criteria for Diagnosis,* 6th ed., Boston: Little, Brown and Company, copyright 1964 by the New York Heart Association, Inc.

Class C.   Patients with cardiac disease whose ordinary physical activity should be moderately restricted, and whose more strenuous efforts should be discontinued.

Class D.   Patients with cardiac disease whose ordinary physical activity should be markedly restricted.

Class E.   Patients with cardiac disease who should be at complete rest, confined to bed or chair.

NOTE: The functional capacity of the patient does not always determine the amount of physical activity that should be permitted. For example, although a child at the onset of active rheumatic carditis may not experience discomfort on playing baseball, rest in bed is imperative. Such a patient would be designated as Class I (Functional), E (Therapeutic). There is frequently a difference between the amount of activity which a patient can undertake in terms of his functional capacity and that which he should attempt in order to prevent aggravation of his disease. The recommendation of physical activity is based not only upon the amount of effort possible without discomfort but also upon the nature and severity of the cardiac disease.

SPECIFIC FORMS OF HEART DISEASE

CONGENITAL HEART DISEASE. Congenital heart disease refers to disorders of the heart owing to anatomical (rarely, metabolic) abnormalities during the development of the embryo and fetus. In general, these involve abnormal communication between the right and left chambers of the heart; malformations of the heart and of the great vessels coming from and entering it; malformations of the heart valves; and abnormal communications between the great vessels. In most cases, the causes of these congenital conditions are not known. Infections of the mother (notably German measles) during the early months of pregnancy appear to have an important bearing on some types of congenital abnormalities. The commoner types of congenital heart disease are *atrial septal defect* and *ventricular septal defect,* which indicate an abnormal communication between the respective chambers. *Patent ductus arteriosus* refers to an abnormal persistence of the fetal communication between the aorta and pulmonary artery. *Dextrocardia* refers to a number of conditions involving the development of the heart more to the right rather than to the left, often accompanied by abnormalities of the heart chambers and vessels. *Transposition of the great vessels* refers to a variety of abnormalities in which the aorta and the pulmonary artery arise in whole or in part from the wrong ventricle. *Congenital valve abnormalities* include an abnormal number of valve cusps, stenosis, or insufficiency of certain valves. *Pulmonic stenosis* is the most common of these, and when combined with a large ventricular septal defect, this produces a complex known as the *tetralogy of Fallot.* In many instances, a number of congenital lesions are combined so that the presence of one requires ruling others out or in.

Congenital heart disease manifests itself by the presence of abnormal findings on physical examination which are usually present from birth, frequently in disorders of growth in children, and, when there is an abnormal communication with flow of unoxygenated blood from the right to the left side of the heart, as cyanosis. The latter may be present from birth ("blue baby") or may appear a number of years later. The most common congenital abnormalities found in persons who survive to adulthood are atrial septal defect and pulmonic stenosis.

The specific treatment of congenital heart disease is surgical correction, when this is possible.

ARTERIOSCLEROTIC HEART DISEASE (CORONARY HEART DISEASE). Coronary heart disease results from narrowing of the coronary arteries by atherosclerosis. This not only decreases the blood supply but predisposes to the presence of clots, which may or may not precipitate acute cardiac distress. Coronary heart disease may not be overt, in that its presence is not recognized in many individuals who eventually die of something else. Frequently, too, it combines with other forms of heart disease, notably hypertensive heart disease, so that the ultimate manifestations of both are inseparable. Coronary artery lesions are extremely common, and were found in a significant percentage of young, physically fit American soldiers killed on the battlefields of Korea. In recent years deaths attributed to arteriosclerotic heart disease among white males in the United States have been close to 300,000 per year.

Acute coronary heart disease is manifested by *acute myocardial infarction*. This is most often due to the presence of a fresh clot (*thrombus*) in one of the larger coronary arteries. In a significant number of cases there is no recent clot, but there is extreme narrowing, suggesting that the mechanism of infarction has been a discrepancy between the demands on the heart and the blood supply in particular regions. In either event, there is acute death of tissue (necrosis) in one or more zones of the heart, usually accompanied by anginal pain and frequently also by signs of shock, congestive failure, or dysrhythmia. It is a medical emergency of the first magnitude for which the patient usually must be hospitalized and given pain medication. Other signs of cardiac distress are treated as required. If the patient survives— the usual result in most episodes—the injury to the heart heals in a month to six weeks by the formation of scar tissue. *Chronic coronary heart disease,* on the other hand, may cause small scars in various areas of the heart, as well as large scars due to one or more myocardial infarctions. Eventually such hearts tend to dilate and hypertrophy and, with the passage of a variable amount of time, tend to become insufficient (if this has not already happened), requiring treatment for congestive failure.

The diagnosis of coronary heart disease is made on the basis of the patient's symptoms combined with electrocardiographic evidence of injury to the heart. There is no generally accepted specific treatment other than that for the manifestations of heart disease in general and prudent restriction of fat in the diet. The use of *anticoagulant* medications, such as Dicumarol, in order to prevent blood clotting is widespread. Their exact value is not yet established, even after more than a decade of extensive use. Estimation of their usefulness awaits the employment of large-scale controlled studies with rigorous statistical evaluation.

HYPERTENSIVE HEART DISEASE. Hypertensive heart disease develops because of the long-term effects of elevated pressure in the arteries into which the left heart must pump. It places strain on the left ventricle because it must raise the pressure of the blood to overcome that in the arteries, so that the left ventricle ultimately dilates and hypertrophies. These patients also have an apparently increased susceptibility to arteriosclerosis. Ordinarily, hypertensive heart disease is diagnosed by the presence of a blood pressure well above the statistically established normal ranges for age and sex. For most adults this means a sustained pressure above 150 systolic and 90 diastolic (expressed in millimeters of mercury). However, there is much variation, and psychogenic elevation of blood pressure is common, so that each case must be carefully evaluated. The presence of heart disease due to hypertension is determined from changes in the electrocardiogram, the chest x-ray, and examination of the heart. Treatment of hypertension has been spectacularly successful, and probably represents one of the most solid advances in the therapy of circulatory disorders. In the decade of the 1950's, reported deaths due to hypertensive heart disease diminished by 40 per cent. Treatment essentially involves the use of *antihypertensive* agents, such as rauwolfia preparations, medications which block the sympathetic nervous system, diuretics, and restriction of salt intake when this is necessary.

RHEUMATIC HEART DISEASE. Rheumatic heart disease is a result of acute rheumatic fever. The latter is due to an "allergic" type of reaction to components of certain streptococci that initially cause an upper respiratory infection, including a sore throat. A fair number of patients who have had rheumatic fever escape permanent cardiac impairment. However, if they have had a stormy course during the acute phase, it is likely that they will develop a valve abnormality. *Acute rheumatic fever* usually strikes between the ages of 8 and 15, causing a high temperature, much weakness, and considerable chest pain, as well as swollen, tender, red joints. During this phase the patient is usually placed on bed rest and treated with heavy doses of aspirin. The use of cortisonelike preparations (corticosteroids) in such patients often produces dramatic results, but their exact value is not yet clearly understood. The vast majority of children survive, but generally are kept at rest for a prolonged period, after which they are permitted to return to school with advice regarding physical activity restriction. After this they are observed at periodic check-ups to note any changes in their course.

Chronic rheumatic heart disease develops because the initial rheumatic inflammation has caused scarring and distortion of heart valves. Usually, the mitral valve or aortic valves or both are involved. The tricuspid and pulmonic valves are only occasionally involved. The usual conditions seen are *mitral stenosis* with or without *mitral regurgitation,* and *aortic stenosis* with or without *aortic regurgitation.* Diagnosis is made by a history of having had rheumatic fever (when this is available) and by physical examination, electrocardiogram, x-ray, and finally cardiac catheterization to pinpoint the location, nature, and severity of the valve disorder. Many of the valve lesions are amenable to surgical correction or palliation. Otherwise, patients must be treated for arrhythmias or heart failure or certain complications (see below) when these arise.

CHRONIC PULMONARY HEART DISEASE (Cor Pulmonale). A rising cause of cardiac disability is *pulmonary emphysema,* which appears to be associated with the great prevalence of cigarette smoking. This causes a diminution in lung function, principally because the lungs lose their "sponginess," and ultimately results in high blood pressure in the pulmonary artery (*pulmonary hypertension.*). This strains the right side of the heart in a manner analogous to that by which high blood pressure in the systemic arterial system strains the left side of the heart. It is diagnosed by the presence of advanced pulmonary disease, usually with right heart failure. Treatment is directed toward relieving any infections in the lung, spasm of the bronchi, and the manifestations of congestive heart failure.

ENDOCRINE HEART DISEASE. In the presence of thyroid disorders (either hyperactive or hypoactive thyroid), adrenal hyperactivity, and pituitary diseases, such as acromegaly, the heart may be either directly affected or unduly strained. Treatment is directed toward the relief of the abnormal glandular condition and of particular manifestations of heart disease.

UNCOMMON FORMS OF HEART DISEASE. Direct infections of the heart are quite common. In former years, *syphilis,* primarily affecting the aorta and aortic valves, was an important cause of heart disease. *Syphilitic (luetic) heart disease* is declining greatly with adequate treatment of syphilis and its incidental treatment (when it is unrecognized) during the administration of antibiotic agents for other infections. Diphtheria, too, once claimed a number of juvenile lives owing to inflammation of the myocardium (*diphtheritic myocarditis*) and heart block. However, it is quite rare today. Viral heart diseases, while still not very common, appear to be on the increase, especially in children, in whom the coxsackie viruses may cause myocarditis. Influenza viruses may affect the heart either directly or indirectly by causing lung lesions in the patient who already has an impaired heart. Parasitic heart disease is not common in the United States, although infestations with parasites such as trichinella (causing trichinosis) are quite common, owing to consumption of undercooked pork. Fortunately, trichinosis of the heart is rather rare. Malignant tumors rarely arise in the heart, although malignant tumors from other locations in the body occasionally metastasize to the heart. Because of the nature of these disorders, the course of disease is usually quite rapid and quickly resistant to treatment.

In recent years, it has been increasingly recognized that diseases of the connective tissues (collagen diseases) involve the heart rather frequently. Disorders such as rheumatoid arthritis, lupus erythematosus, scleroderma, and related disorders can cause severe cardiac impairment. Rheumatoid arthritis is the only very common member of this group, and its association with heart disease has only begun to be explored. In carefully analyzed studies a higher incidence of unexplained heart abnormalities is found in patients with rheumatoid arthritis than in comparable control groups.

PERICARDIAL DISEASE. Disease of the membrane covering the heart, the pericardium, is relatively common in many forms of heart disease, but it is usually silent and causes the patient no embarrassment. However, the pericardium may be quite inflamed with or without any associated heart lesion (acute pericarditis) causing pain very similar to or identical with angina pectoris, requiring careful observation and numerous electrocardiograms to make the differential diagnosis. When, following inflammation, the pericardium scars in a particular manner, the scar tissue may compress the heart, interfering with its function and closely mimicking the findings of congestive heart failure. This condition is known as constrictive pericarditis; frequently it can be cured by surgical removal of the scarred pericardium. Pericardial effusions may cause either acute or chronic cardiac tamponade (compression of the heart by excessive fluid in the pericardial sac).

COMPLICATIONS OF HEART DISEASE. Perhaps the most common complication of heart disease is drug toxicity, particularly that due to digitalis. This can often be very confusing because the symptoms of overdigitalization and those of insufficient digitalization may be very similar. It is usually necessary to withdraw digitalis and later readminister it if the need continues. Often digitalis toxicity is precipitated by the use of diuretics which wash out potassium in addition to salt (sodium chloride); a deficiency in potassium tends to cause even normal amounts of digitalis to become toxic.

Other complications include *bacterial endocarditis* (infection of damaged heart valve or endocardium) and *embolism* (the breaking up of parts of clots or foreign material in the circulatory system and their transportation to other areas where they acutely impede the flow of blood). Both these complications are most common in rheumatic heart disease. *Bacterial endocarditis* is recognized by the presence of microorganisms in the blood stream and is treated by the use of appropriate antibiotic agents such as penicillin. Embolism is recognized by the sudden appearance of signs and symptoms of occlusion of arteries somewhere in the body. This may involve the lung, the brain, the intestine, a leg, or one or both kidneys. Embolism is treated by the administration of anticoagulant agents, such as heparin or Dicumarol, and, where possible, surgical removal of the embolus or interruption of the sympathetic nerve supply in order to improve blood flow in the affected area.

Pregnancy produces a special kind of complication in that it normally burdens the heart owing to expansion of the mother's blood volume, changes in metabolism, and the needs of the fetus. The burden is greatest in the last three months of pregnancy. At this time the fetus has become quite large, and the need for a large cardiac output by the mother's heart is greatest. Many patients can be carried successfully through pregnancy in spite of various heart diseases (usually rheumatic because of the age group involved). In other cases, to save the life of the mother a therapeutic abortion may be necessary. The decisions involved require careful study of the patient and careful observation to detect signs of distress.

PERIPHERAL VASCULAR SYSTEM

This section deals with the blood and lymphatic vessels distant from the heart, exclusive of those in the brain, which form a special type of circulation. It deals particularly with the vessels of the lower extremities, since the vast majority of abnormalities affect these, with the notable exception of Raynaud's disease and diffuse connective tissue disorders.

GENERAL ANATOMY AND FUNCTION OF ARTERIES, VEINS, AND LYMPHATICS

Arteries are relatively thick-walled blood vessels that carry blood from the heart to the tissues, where they become successively smaller until they reach the size of *capillaries*, tiny microscopic vessels connecting with the *veins*. The veins begin as small tubes on the other end of the capillaries which continually join each other, forming larger and larger vessels carrying blood from the tissues to the heart. The veins are, in general, much thinner-walled than the arteries. The *lymphatic vessels* form a separate circulation which carries metabolic products and fluids from the tissues to large lymphatic ducts in the abdomen and chest; these ultimately empty into the large veins near the neck.

MECHANISMS OF PERIPHERAL VASCULAR DISEASE

Disease of any of the peripheral vessels is caused either by some form of injury, particularly inflammation, or by some form of impairment to the circulation within these vessels. In general, there are *five mechanisms* causing peripheral circulatory disorders: (1) *Stenosis*, or narrowing of a vessel, causes deficient circulation beyond the point of stenosis when the cross-sectional area of the vessel is narrowed beyond a critical point. (2) *Obstruction* causes interruption of circulation beyond the point of closure of the vessel; this is usually chronic, due to either the slow growth of clots within a vessel or pressure from outside. Acute obstruction occurs when a clot forms rapidly (usually due to some sudden injury or inflammation) or when an embolus obstructs a vessel that is too small for its passage. (3) *Inflammation* is a process of injury that may be caused by many factors, including physical trauma and infection; in many cases, however, inflammation appears to arise for unknown reasons. (4) *Aneurysm formation* results from chronic dilatation of a segment of a vessel because of weakening of its walls by a variety of disease processes. (5) *Arteriovenous fistula* is an abnormal direct communication between an artery and a vein.

In most diseases of the peripheral vascular system, factors such as aging, heredity, diabetes, and the presence of chronic diseases elsewhere play an important role in predisposing the patient to developing the abnormality. Physical trauma to the vessels is occasionally at fault. In the majority of cases, the actual disease process is imperfectly understood.

DISABILITY DUE TO PERIPHERAL VASCULAR DISORDERS

Disability in peripheral vascular disorders arises from the presence of symptoms or of direct or indirect complications of disease, such as surgical amputation of a limb. Pain results from interference with the circulation of muscles and nerves. When this is acute, the pain tends to be present at all times until relieved. In chronic disorders, pain typically occurs on effort when the greatest demands are made on the muscles. Pain may also be due to inflammation of the vessel itself, notably in the acute situation, when the relatively rapid interference with the circulation also may be due to swelling of the area involved by a circulatory disorder. The swelling results from an increase in fluid in the tissues (edema) which is the result of tissue injury, inflammation, or blockade of venous or lymphatic drainage of the part, or any of these in combination. Blockage of the venous or lymphatic drainage is analogous to the situation in heart failure in which impediment of the circulation at the heart causes fluid to build up in the tissues "upstream" of the particular heart chamber involved. Another mechanism of disability is destruction of tissue. This is the result of circulatory impairment of any type that not only causes death of tissue cells but predisposes the injured tissue to infection. Thus, there may be *ulceration* through the skin (a breakdown of the skin and inflammation of the underlying tissues) in areas of impaired circulation. When circulatory impairment is particularly advanced, there may be *gangrene,* which is essentially massive death of tissue.

DIAGNOSTIC PROCEDURES

The diagnosis of peripheral vascular disease is made on the basis of the patient's history, physical examination, and special procedures. A history of symptoms in a part, particularly sudden pain followed by swelling and inflammation, or a history of pain on use of the part which stops with rest is highly indicative of a circulatory disorder. Pain in the legs, thighs, or buttocks on walking which disappears rapidly on standing still is particularly common in chronic arterial disease of the lower extremities and is known as *intermittent claudication.*

Physical examination is directed at detecting abnormal skin color and temperature, particularly if these are unequal in one extremity as compared to the opposite extremity. The patient is also examined for abnormally increased, decreased, or absent pulsations of the arteries; here, too, any discrepancy between the two sides may be significant. The skin is inspected for ulcers or trophic changes. The latter usually involve changes in color or loss of hair, plus thinning and shininess of the skin, indicating diminished circulation to the part. Any edema must be evaluated as arising either from local circulatory changes, from heart or kidney disease, or from a combination of these. Occasionally, the physician will use his stethoscope to search for bruits, which are abnormal sounds due either to the passage of blood over unusual narrowings in the larger arteries, notably the abdominal aorta, or to the passage of blood through abnormal communications (*arteriovenous fistulas*).

The most important special procedures in confirming and locating peripheral vascular disorders are those using x-rays. Ordinary x-rays may show deposits of calcium in sclerotic portions of arteries; in advanced disease these may outline a whole artery. Special contrast substances may be used to outline the arteries, veins, and lymphatics by placing them into these vessels so that points of narrowing and obstruction are clearly shown. This not only may confirm a diagnosis but also may indicate an area for surgical treatment when this is possible.

Special graphic devices such as the *plethysmograph* give a record of the circulatory changes in a part. *Oscillometry* permits the actual measurement of pulsation of arteries in a given area. Occasionally, certain substances are injected to determine the circulation time between two parts of an artery or a vein; if there is sufficient impairment of circulation, it will take longer than normal for the given substance to reach a point "downstream" from the point of injection. Occasionally, too, special temperature measurements are made with *thermocouples* to detect significant differences in temperature in two different parts of the body. In the presence of inflammation, an abnormally increased temperature usually is present, while in the presence of arterial obstruction, decreased temperature due to decreased blood flow is the rule.

ARTERIAL DISORDERS

ORGANIC OBSTRUCTION AND NARROWING. The most common cause of significant obstruction and narrowing of the peripheral arteries is arteriosclerosis, the development of which is much like that of coronary arteriosclerosis. This disorder is most common in persons of advanced age, particularly men, and those who have diabetes. *Thromboangiitis obliterans* (*Buerger's disease*) is an unusual form of peripheral vascular disease involving rapidly advancing arteriosclerosis and inflammation of the superficial veins, which appears to occur in relatively young persons, nearly all of whom are smokers. In fairness, it should be stated that the existence of this condition as a separate entity is disputed, although most observers agree that it is entitled to special designation. In relatively few individuals, particularly women, diffuse connective tissue disorders (for example, lupus erythematosus and other disorders related indirectly to rheumatoid arthritis) cause chronic inflammatory diseases of the arteries and veins.

Acute occlusion of arteries is rarely due to traumatic injury with either interruption of the artery or clotting on its damaged surfaces. More commonly, acute occlusion is due to embolism that usually arises from clots on a damaged valve at the left side of the heart; occasionally large sclerotic lesions in the abdominal aorta dislodge either pieces of overlying clots or actual pieces of the sclerotic lesion, which are carried to smaller arteries of the lower extremities. Embolism is recognized clinically as a sudden change, usually painful, in the circulation of the involved area; in peripheral vascular disease it virtually always involves the lower extremities.

ANEURYSM FORMATION. Aneurysms (areas of extreme dilation and thinning) commonly form owing to arteriosclerosis of the abdominal aorta. They are much more rare in the smaller arteries peripheral to the aorta. Aneurysms of the abdominal aorta are important not only because they throw off emboli to the peripheral vessels due to clotting within them, but also because they may rupture, causing relatively rapid death due to hemorrhage into the abdomen. Signs of impending rupture usually call for immediate surgical treatment.

ARTERIOVENOUS FISTULA. Abnormal communications between arteries and veins rarely may be congenital. More commonly, they are caused by inflammatory disease or trauma, such as the passage of a bullet through an appropriate area. They are recognized by local signs of increased circulation in the venous system. If there is a large opening, the abnormal communication causes a strain upon the heart because of increased demands on both sides of the heart.

FUNCTIONAL DISORDERS. *Raynaud's disease* is a condition of unknown cause that occurs mainly in women between the ages of 13 and 40 and is usually limited to the hands and fingers. In this condition there is a sudden spasm of the small arteries supplying the fingers and hands which causes symmetrical symptoms and findings on both sides. Usually there is acute pain and sudden pallor which may be followed by a blue and then a reddish color. *Raynaud's phenomenon* causes essentially the same symptoms, though it need not be bilateral and symmetrical, and is usually a sign of other disease, such as scleroderma. In some cases these disorders are considered to have a psychogenic basis, although this is by no means definite.

TREATMENT OF CHRONIC ARTERIAL DISORDERS. The patient is generally counseled to avoid trauma, to care for superficial infections and burns immediately, and to avoid exposure to cold. Whenever possible, smoking is forbidden; this is mandatory in Buerger's disease and, indeed, for any young person with chronic arterial disease. Diabetes is treated intensively because this condition seems to predispose to the rapid advance of arteriosclerosis. When possible, surgery is employed to relieve or remove obstructions and to remove or support the walls of aneurysms. Frequently, it is necessary in such cases to introduce tubular grafts into arteries from which a relatively long segment has been removed in order to reestablish the circulation. These grafts may be made up of parts of blood vessels taken from other parts of the body, or plastic replacements may be made in the desired dimensions. One of the most effective treatments has been interruption of certain sympathetic nerves, a procedure known as lumbar *sympathectomy,* which allows the blood vessels in the area selected to dilate, thereby improving circulation to the part. Occasionally *endarterectomy* is done; this "reams out" areas of advanced disease with or without clotting, as well as the damaged lining of the vessel, in the hope that a new and intact lining will grow back. Where gangrene has occurred, surgical amputation is almost always needed, because gangrene implies irreversible death of tissue, which is then useless and prone to infection. Gangrene is particularly common in poorly managed, severe diabetes.

Various medications have been prescribed for the improvement of circulation in limbs; these may have been of value in individual cases, but their overall worth in chronic disease is still unclear.

TREATMENT OF ACUTE ARTERIAL DISORDERS. *Organic.* When an embolus blocks an artery acutely, the most direct attack is to remove it surgically (*embolectomy*). Whether or not this is done depends on the individual case. Certain other procedures may be used in order to dilate the vessels and improve circulation without removing the block. These involve *sympathectomy,* as in chronic disease, or *paravertebral block,* which produces a temporary sympathectomy. Similarly, sympathetic nerve-blocking medicines such as tetraethyl-ammonium bromide may be used, and agents such as Priscol, intended to dilate arteries, may be tried. For patients who have had an embolism, it is commonly necessary to provide anticoagulant treatment beginning with *heparin,* which rapidly acts to reduce the tendency of blood to clot (as well as having an as yet undefined action on the vessels themselves), and continuing more or less permanently with longer-acting agents such as *Dicumarol.*

Functional (Raynaud's). In Raynaud's phenomenon the treatment is for whatever underlying disease seems to be responsible. In both Raynaud's disease and Raynaud's phenomenon the patient is cautioned to avoid cold and to dress warmly. Interruption of the sympathetic nerve supply (sympathectomy) is done if necessary.

Amputation. Amputation is a drastic measure employed for specific reasons: (1) *Gangrene* (see above) is virtually an absolute indication for amputation. (2) *Uncontrollable infection* may necessitate amputation because of its production of more or less continual disability. (3) *Intractable pain* following extensive medical and surgical efforts occasionally warrants removal of the part. (4) When a limb becomes burdensome due to either *complete loss of function* or *contracture of muscles* (amounting to the same thing), it is often better for the patient to have a prosthesis, which will allow an approach to normal function of the part in many cases.

Arteriovenous Fistulas. Arteriovenous fistulas large enough to cause local circulatory disorders or to burden the heart must be closed or the circulation to them bypassed in some way. This is always a surgical procedure.

DISORDERS OF THE VEINS

VARICOSE VEINS. Varicose veins are due to dilatation and tortuosity causing impairment of function of small valves in the veins which normally limit backflow. This condition is of unknown cause, although there is a strong hereditary factor. It results in the appearance of large, more or less serpentine-appearing vessels under the skin (although the deeper vessels also may be involved). There is usually discomfort on standing for long periods, due to interruption of the venous circulation, and very commonly swelling of the feet, which is more noticeable in the evening than in the morning; this is because blood flow back toward the heart is improved during the night when the patient has his feet horizontally placed (neutralizing the effect of gravity). Varicose veins are subject to inflammation (phlebitis) and to clotting within them (phlebothrombosis), commonly combined as *thrombophlebitis.* They are particularly annoying to persons who have to stand on their feet for long periods, such as sales personnel, dentists, and waitresses.

Varicose veins may also be treated by the use of elastic stockings and bindings in order to support them, plus elevation of the extremities at times when the patient does not need to stand. If the symptoms become too far advanced, surgical procedures become warranted. This includes *ligation* (tying-off of the veins), commonly combined with removal of the diseased segments (stripping). Occasionally varicose veins have been injected with sclerosing solutions which are designed to scar them tight.

THROMBOPHLEBITIS. Thrombophlebitis is caused by the clotting of blood with consequent obstruction of a vein in which there has been inflammation, or in which inflammation appears to result during the formation of a clot. This is a particularly dangerous situation because such clots frequently break off in whole or in part and travel to the lung where they cause *pulmonary embolism* after passing through the right side of the heart. Pulmonary embolism, is a frequent cause of death in hospitalized patients. Indeed, patients confined to bed for long periods tend to develop phlebitis and clots in the veins of the lower extremities. Treatment involves prevention, when this is possible, including early ambulation of hospitalized patients, particularly following a surgical operation, as well as the use of elastic bandages and elastic stocking for patients confined to bed. The latter are also encouraged to move their toes and muscles as often as possible. In some cases, massage and physiotherapeutic procedures are added. Once the diagnosis of thrombophlebitis has been established, active treatment of some form is mandatory. Anticoagulant therapy on the same schedule as that of acute arterial embolism (see above) is immediately instituted. Where this is unsuccessful, or where thrombophlebitis recurs, ligation of the involved veins may be indicated. Where the thrombophlebitis is very painful and there is appreciable circulatory disturbance, a paravertebral block of the sympathetic nerves close to the spine is performed to avoid overlying skin ulcers and to relieve pain.

DISORDERS OF THE LYMPHATICS

ACUTE LYMPHANGITIS. Acute lymphangitis occurs in the presence of tissue inflammation generally, but this may be particularly severe with bacterial infection. It is treated in the same way as such infections—with appropriate chemotherapy, rest of the involved part, and either warm or cool applications as needed.

CHRONIC LYMPHATIC OBSTRUCTION. Chronic lymphatic obstruction is an uncommon condition that causes *lymphedema* owing to engorgement of the tissues with lymph that cannot exit by the usual channels. If this lasts long enough, fibrosis (scarring) of the tissues ensues, which may require surgical correction. Most lymphedema seen today is acquired following surgical operation involving the lymph nodes into which the lymphatic drainage of a part empties. For example, this may occur in women who have had a breast removed for cancer, necessitating the dissection of the lymph nodes in the axilla (armpit); following this, the arm on the involved side may swell chronically due to lymphedema. (A rare condition is *familial lymphedema* or Milroy's disease, which sometimes requires surgical management.) In addition to the surgical procedures for these conditions, the patient is encouraged to elevate the involved arm or leg in order to get better drainage of fluid, due to gravity, and to use elastic stocking or elastic bandages. Exercises may be prescribed in order to further improve drainage.

III

RESPIRATORY DISORDERS

Respiration, a requisite for life, includes the delivery of oxygen to the body tissues and the removal of the waste product, carbon dioxide, to the outside air. The respiratory system transports these gases between the blood stream and the outside air. The system consists essentially of tubular organs, which function as conduits to and from the blood stream, and of small air sacs at the end of these tubes, which are surrounded by capillaries. Gases diffuse between these air sacs and the capillaries.

ANATOMY OF THE RESPIRATORY SYSTEM

The conduit system consists of the nose, mouth, pharynx, larynx, trachea, and bronchial tree, each part of which has distinct additional functions to perform. The nose and its associated sinuses act as resonators for the voice, the area for appreciation of smell, and a filtering and humidifying system of the inspired air. The mouth and pharynx act as well in the process of alimentation. The larynx acts in the production of the voice. The tracheobronchial tree acts also as a humidifying system, the inner lining of which is composed of cells that produce secretions and of hairs (cilia) that carry semiliquid and particulate

By ROBERT H. JONES, M.D. Program Director, Coordinator of Rehabilitation, Assistant in Medicine, Massachusetts General Hospital; Instructor in Medicine, Harvard Medical School; Residency Training in Internal Medicine, Boston City Hospital and Massachusetts General Hospital; U. S. Public Health Research Fellow in Pulmonary Diseases, Thorndike Memorial Laboratory, Boston City Hospital, 1956–1958, Boston, Massachusetts.

59

matter upward from the depths of the tracheobronchial tree to the pharynx.

The trachea divides into two main stem bronchi, one to each lung. Shortly thereafter, each bronchus divides first into lobar and then into segmental bronchi. Each of the latter, accompanied by a pulmonary artery and vein, supplies a bronchopulmonary segment of lung tissue. The two lungs thus are divided into three lobes on the right and two on the left and are further subdivided into about ten segments on each side. The bronchi further subdivide into fine bronchioles, microscopic in size, which terminate in millions of air sacs called _alveoli._ The alveolar walls are composed of dense networks of anastomosing capillaries and associated reticular and elastic supporting fibers.

Each lung is enclosed in a thin membrane, the _pleura_, which continues from the central hilus of the lung around onto the inner aspect of the chest wall. The intervening space between lung and chest wall is called the _pleural cavity_ or space.

The lungs are bounded above by the structures of the shoulders and neck, laterally by the ribs and intercostal muscles, and inferiorly by the arched diaphragms, which are attached to the margins of the lower ribs laterally. The diaphragms act, by contraction, to increase the volume of the chest inferiorly, thereby producing inspiration. The intercostal muscles aid inspiration further by spreading and elevating the ribs to increase the volume of the chest laterally. Several accessory muscles in the shoulder and neck also aid by increasing chest volume superiorly. Expiration is passive at rest as these muscle groups relax and the stretched elastic tissues of the lungs return to their normal resting length. Active expiration is produced when abdominal muscles contract, producing superior displacement of the abdominal contents and therefore of the diaphragms; it is also produced by contraction of certain intercostal muscles that cause the ribs to again become approximated and lowered.

The lungs are supplied by two vascular systems. The bronchial arteries, arising from the aorta, carry oxygenated blood for nourishment of the lungs and are normally rather completely separated from the pulmonary arteries. The latter system brings poorly oxygenated venous blood from the right ventricle to the alveolar capillaries; pulmonary veins carry oxygenated alveolar capillary blood back to the left side of the heart.

The muscles of respiration are innervated by several groups of nerves that act in concert to produce coordinated movement of the respiratory apparatus. The diaphragms are innervated by the phrenic nerves, which originate from the third, fourth, and fifth cervical nerves in the neck; additional branches go to the lining of the heart (pericardium) and pleurae. Intercostal muscles receive their innervation from thoracic intercostal nerves; the neck and shoulder musculature receive their innervation from the eleventh cranial nerve and cervical nerves in the neck. Respiratory muscles in the nose, mouth, pharynx, larynx, and tongue are innervated by the fifth, seventh, ninth, tenth, eleventh, and twelfth cranial nerves. Sensations from the lungs and pleurae travel back to higher centers via the phrenic, vagus, intercostal, and sympathetic nerves.

Physiology of the Respiratory System

The ultimate control of breathing resides within the respiratory center of the brainstem. The center is stimulated by neurons from higher centers in the cerebral cortex which provide voluntary control of respiration and by neurons from the lungs and adjacent structures, as well as from such distant structures as joints and muscles. Respiratory center activity is also accurately and sensitively controlled by changes in the partial pressure of carbon dioxide and acidity of the blood bathing the respiratory center. In this manner, respiration is controlled so that the partial pressure of oxygen and carbon dioxide in the immediate environment of the body cell is always maintained within narrow limits in order to assure satisfactory cell function.

The respiratory system is figuratively composed of three parts: a muscle pump, which drives air in and out of the lungs; an air-fluid interface separated by a thin alveolar-capillary membrane, across which respiratory gases diffuse; and a second pumping system, which perfuses the lungs, bringing blood to and from the alveolar-capillary membrane. There are, therefore, factors of ventilation, diffusion, and perfusion, each of which can be measured and given normal values. Alterations of respiratory tissues by disease affect, variously, these three functions, often in characteristic fashion, with the result that measurement of these functions may frequently establish not only the type of disease but also its severity.

VENTILATION

The passage of air in and out of the lungs depends for its effectiveness upon the rate and depth of breathing as well as upon the speed of air flow. In addition, because the conduits of the respiratory system do not take part in gas exchange, it is that fraction of each breath which passes through this dead space to the alveolus that determines the effectiveness of that breath. Thus, the minute ventilation ($\dot{V}_E$) equals the product of the respiratory rate (f) and depth or tidal volume (V_t) of each breath: $\dot{V}_E = f \times V_t$. The effective alveolar ventilation ($\dot{V}_A$) equals the product of the respiratory rate (f) and the difference between the tidal volume and the volume of the dead space ($\dot{V}_A$) = f × ($V_t - V_d$).

The speed of air flow in and out of the lungs determines, to a certain extent, the respiration rate and tidal volume, and is itself determined by the patency of the conduit system. Where the conduit is normally patent throughout, resistance to air flow is small, as is the force required to push air through the tubes. Fast respiratory rate and large air flows are easily achieved. On the other hand, focal or diffuse conduit narrowing produces high resistance to air flow and requires a large force to push air through the tubes. This makes rapid breathing and rapid air flows difficult to perform, at the cost of high energy expenditure.

According to the above, a normal person might, at rest, breathe as follows:

$$\dot{V}_E = f \times V_t$$
$$5{,}000 \text{ cc} = 20 \times 250 \text{ cc}$$

Conversely, a person with airway obstruction might breathe:

$$\dot{V}_E = f \times V_t$$
$$5{,}000 \text{ cc} = 10 \times 500 \text{ cc}$$

with larger breaths at a slower rate. Each moves the same volume of air per minute and may consume the same amount of energy in so doing. However, to keep energy expenditure the same, the person with airway obstruction must produce a low rate of air flow and, accordingly, a slow respiratory rate, while increasing tidal volume in order to attain the same minute ventilation.

A person with either stiff scarred lungs, or one lung removed, produces a smaller than normal tidal volume. He takes rapid shallow breaths:

$$\dot{V}_E = f \times V_t$$
$$5{,}000 \text{ cc} = 25 \times 200 \text{ cc}$$

Finally, a person with both small or stiff lungs and increased airway obstruction might demonstrate the same rate and depth characteristics as normal but require higher energy expenditure in order to maintain the same pace.

Thus, different conditions produce particular and often unique breathing patterns that can be easily measured. At rest or with mild exercise, these patterns may not vary significantly one from another. However, when stressed to maximal performance, significant differences appear. It is under this latter situation that many tests of ventilatory function are made. The more common measurements are noted below.

The deepest breath a person can take is called the *vital capacity*. Normal values have been determined and vary according to the person's age, sex, height, and weight.

The maximal minute ventilation is termed the *maximal breathing capacity* (MBC). This test measures the strength, coordinated control and mobility of the respiratory muscle pump, the patency of the airways, and the distensibility of the lung tissues during a brief period of maximal effort. Normal values vary with age, sex, and body surface area.

Maximal expiratory flow rates are most commonly and easily measured in the "timed vital capacity" maneuver. The subject is asked to exhale, as rapidly as possible, a full breath into a special measuring device. Normal subjects exhale 75 per cent or more of the total in the first second of expiration, 85 per cent or more in the second second, and 95 per cent or more in the third second. Those with severe airway obstruction may produce as little as 20 to 30 per cent of the total in one second.

The results of these tests should be reviewed from two aspects. One should note the fraction of the maximal effort that is used in the performance of routine effort. And it should be noted how closely that maximal effort approaches predicted normal values. For instance, a healthy person walking at a slow rate of two miles per hour may breathe 15 liters per minute, have a MBC of 150 liters per minute, and a predicted MBC of 150 liters per minute. The walking ventilation requires only 10 per cent of his best ability, giving him a reserve of 90 per cent, and his MBC is 100 per cent of normal. On the other hand, a person with severe emphysema may utilize 15 liters per minute at the same slow pace, have a MBC of 25 liters per minute, with the same predicted MBC of 150 liters per minute. His walking ventilation requires 60 per cent of his best ability, leaving him with only a small reserve. Furthermore, his MBC is only 17 per cent of predicted normal. In this manner, two important views of functional ventilatory ability are obtained.

DIFFUSION

The process by which gases pass from the pulmonary alveolus through the alveolar-capillary membrane into the pulmonary capillary is called *diffusion.* This is a physical process that utilizes no expenditure of energy and depends upon the following factors: on the one hand, the difference in concentration of gas on either side of the membrane; the area of the membrane, and the solubility of that gas; on the other hand, the thickness of the membrane and the molecular weight of the gas. The greater the first three factors, the greater the diffusion capacity of the lungs; the greater the latter, the less it becomes. In most disease states the two variables most frequently altered by the pathological process are the membrane cross-sectional area, which is decreased, and the thickness of the membrane, which is increased. The diffusion capacity of the lungs can be measured, though only with expensive equipment. Normal values are now known.

VENTILATION-PERFUSION RELATIONS

The gaseous composition of both lungs and blood stream depends upon the volume of pulmonary capillary blood flow in relation to the volume of air flow to the lungs. Normally at rest, five liters of blood flow are matched by four liters of air flow per minute. Whenever this relationship is upset, the gas content of each is altered. When blood flow ceases to a portion of ventilated lung, normal parts of the lung are overventilated in order to assure normal gas exchange. When poorly ventilated portions are normally perfused, blood perfusing this area is not properly oxygenated or freed of its high carbon dioxide content. Other parts of the lung can "wash out" excess carbon dioxide but are unable to "push" sufficient oxygen into the blood stream to saturate the oxygen-poor aliquot as it mixes subsequently in the left ventricle. Thus, arterial blood going to the rest of the body is undersaturated. Evaluation of this defect can be made, though only with elaborate research techniques.

WORK OF BREATHING

The act of breathing requires energy to activate the thoracic muscle pump. For the normal person at rest, the equivalent of this energy requirement is small, amounting to about 3 cc of oxygen per minute. One reason for this is that work is required only during inspiration, while expiration remains a passive process. The chest and lungs are like a rubber balloon which requires that work be done to inflate it, but which deflates itself passively as the stretched elastic tends to return to its original smaller size.

With maximal efforts, both inspiration and expiration are active muscular processes. Accordingly, oxygen consumption rises sharply and may reach 2,000 cc of oxygen per minute.

In performing metabolic work at rest, about 2.4 cc of carbon dioxide are produced by the respiratory effort, while at maximal effort, a calculated 1,600 cc are produced each minute. Yet, this volume of carbon dioxide can be easily "cleared" by normal lungs.

In the severest forms of respiratory disease, the oxygen cost of breathing may assume a larger percentage of total oxygen utilization because more work is needed to move air through diseased lungs. In certain circumstances, the lungs cannot eliminate the large volumes of carbon dioxide produced by the metabolic effort. Carbon dioxide retention ensues and is often accompanied by arterial unsaturation.

The increased work of breathing in disease must cause a feeling of distress, and may be an important factor in the production of *dyspnea,* the uncomfortable sensation of difficult breathing.

CLASSIFICATION OF DISEASES ON THE BASIS OF PATHOLOGICAL PHYSIOLOGY

Many pulmonary diseases can be classified, on the basis of the pathophysiology produced, into one of four types of deficit: restrictive, obstructive, diffusion, or ventilation-perfusion imbalance. To be sure, there is often a mixture of the several defects. Also, major symptoms may arise from toxic aspects of the disease alone. Nevertheless, many diseases that produce long-term symptoms of respiratory distress in the vocational age groups are those which produce significant diffuse defects in either ventilation, diffusion, or perfusion.

RESTRICTIVE DEFECTS

Diseases causing restrictive ventilatory defects are characterized by a low vital capacity. These can be subgrouped into (1) those which decrease the strength of the muscle pump; (2) those which limit the maximal inspiratory volume of the thorax; (3) those which encompass and constrict the outside of the lungs with scar tissue; (4) those which stiffen the substance of the lungs with scar or edema fluid; (5) those which produce loss of lung substance.

The muscle pump is weakened in poliomyelitis whenever innervation of the diaphragm, abdominal, intercostal, or accessory muscles is involved. The same occurs following trauma to the cervical spinal cord to produce quadriplegia or quadriparesis. Such diseases as the Guillain-Barré syndrome, multiple sclerosis, amyotrophic lateral sclerosis, and progressive muscular atrophy also affect nerves innervating these muscles. Other diseases such as myasthenia gravis or muscular dystrophy may weaken the muscle pump by direct effect on the muscle. Diseases and conditions that produce a decrease in the volume of the thorax do so by limiting either rib motion or descent of the diaphragms. An instance of the former is ankylosing rheumatoid spondylitis; instances of the latter include pregnancy, ascites, pneumoperitoneum therapy in tuberculosis, and massive obesity.

A restrictive defect also occurs when scar tissue forms in the pleural space as a consequence of either infection (emphysema) or organized blood (hemothorax). Similarly, if the pleural space is filled with large amounts of fluid from a malignant tumor or right-sided heart failure, the volume of the lung or lungs will be decreased, often to the point of severe respiratory insufficiency.

Many diseases produce scarring within lung substance itself, thereby limiting lung expansion. Several of these may produce an associated diffusion defect which results in a more serious pathophysiological problem. These diseases will be discussed later. Others, such as an unresolved pneumonia, radiation fibrosis, silicosis, and sarcoidosis, may produce their effect primarily by reduction of lung volume. Here, the loss of vital capacity is usually not severe.

Tumors that infiltrate lung substance may destroy the tissue itself. Or they may cause bronchial obstruction, produce pleural effusion, or infiltrate and destroy a phrenic nerve with resulting significant decrease in vital capacity. Extirpation of this tumor mass may require sacrifice of an entire lung, which produces a 40 to 50 per cent reduction in vital capacity.

Some types of decompensated heart disease, such as mitral stenosis, may produce a restrictive defect by affecting all of the above-noted parameters: (1) a weak muscle pump because of arterial unsaturation or low cardiac output; (2) decrease in thoracic volume by ascites and an enlarged liver; (3) decreased lung volume by an enlarged heart and pleural effusion; and (4) stiffened lungs from lung edema.

In these conditions, there usually is little or no impairment of ability to perform light or moderate work until the vital capacity is reduced to about 50 per cent of normal. Further reduction to 30 per cent is accompanied by disability such that only sedentary work can be tolerated. At 15 per cent of normal, life may be threatened, even at complete rest.

During periods of stress from an infection or prolonged unaccustomed exercise, an otherwise moderate but compensated impairment may suddenly develop into gross respiratory insufficiency. Numerous examples are to be found each winter when respiratory infections abound. Frequently, old polio patients who maintain routine eight-hour workdays become so incapacitated that they require hospitalization and assisted breathing until the crisis abates. The insult may emerge in the form of fatigue from protracted ineffectual coughing or in connection with a decreased vital capacity produced by obstruction of a bronchus by secretions. Unless further lung damage occurs, these episodes of respiratory insufficiency are reversible. Unfortunately, function is often whittled down by each succeeding major infection until the person becomes totally disabled or succumbs during a crisis.

OBSTRUCTIVE DEFECTS

Those diseases that cause narrowing of the tracheobronchial tree produce obstructive ventilatory defects, manifested by decreased timed vital capacity and maximal breathing capacity. Obstructive emphysema and asthma are the most common diseases producing diffuse airway obstruction. This obstruction occurs principally in the smaller respiratory bronchioles; yet even the larger bronchi may partially collapse during forced expiration.

Isolated airways may be narrowed by lymph nodes or tumors compressing from outside the bronchus, by tumors growing within the bronchus, by aspiration of foreign bodies, or by thickened secretions retained within the bronchus.

A number of other diseases produce bronchiolar fibrosis and chronic inflammation, which ultimately lead to obstruction to air flow and other pathophysiological defects. Included here are chronic bronchitis, silicosis, tuberculosis, phosgene poisoning, and coal worker's pneumoconiosis.

The maximal breathing capacity may fall to 60 per cent of predicted normal with minor incapacity at moderate labor. Or it may fall to 15 or 20 per cent of predicted normal, at which level walking at the slow rate of two miles per hour demands the greatest effort, which can be maintained for only a few minutes at a time.

Intercurrent respiratory insults affect patients with these diseases in the same manner as those with restrictive diseases.

DIFFUSION DEFECTS

A number of rather uncommon diseases are manifested by dyspnea on exertion which is out of proportion to the observed slight decreases in vital, timed vital, and maximal breathing capacities. (In fact, these parameters of function are often within normal limits.) In most instances, there is x-ray evidence of diffuse pulmonary infiltrative disease. When associated with a proven diffusion defect, these conditions make up a group known as the *alveolar-capillary block* syndrome. Diseases that produce this picture include sarcoidosis and granulomatous diseases of unknown cause, beryllium disease, scleroderma, miliary tuberculosis, pulmonary lymphangitic carcinomatosis, Hamman-Rich syndrome, interstitial fibrosis of unknown cause, asbestosis, histiocytosis X (eosinophilic granuloma), pulmonary alveolar microlithiasis, sulfur dioxide poisoning, and radiation fibrosis.

The pathological processes produce stiff lungs and thickened alveolar-capillary membranes. With stiff lungs, shallow and rapid respirations are favored, and increased work in breathing may result during times of stress secondary to the increased effort required to stretch the fibrous tissues. The thickened alveolar-capillary membrane produces decreased diffusibility of oxygen into the blood stream. Initially, there is oxygen unsaturation only with effort; later, it may appear even at rest. Carbon dioxide, which is 21 times more diffusible than oxygen, always diffuses through the thickened membrane without difficulty. In fact, the blood carbon dioxide level is often low because of the persistent hyperventilation required to maintain adequate oxygen uptake.

Because this syndrome is uncommon and requires special equipment to demonstrate the defect, there have been few studies correlating the relationship between diffusion capacity and degree of impairment. However, where these studies exist, a fairly good correlation is found.

A strong presumptive diagnosis can be made by inference and exclusion whenever the following are obtained: dyspnea and arterial oxygen unsaturation on effort, essentially normal ventilatory studies, and diffuse x-ray changes.

VENTILATION-PERFUSION IMBALANCE

Ventilation-perfusion imbalance occurs whenever the proper ratio of air to blood flow to the lungs is altered by disease processes. In a disease such as emphysema, both types of aberration are found, some areas being poorly ventilated while others are poorly perfused. In large bullous areas (blebs), there is deficient blood flow because of destructive changes involving the pulmonary artery; conversely, a well-perfused area has limited ventilation because of airway narrowing.

In conditions such as pulmonary embolus, the various arteritides, and mitral stenosis, blood flow is decreased by obstruction of the vessel lumen or destruction of its walls. In lung cysts, the air spaces usually are poorly supplied with pulmonary capillaries and have variable communications with the bronchial tree. With good communication, dead space ventilation may be sufficiently large to require considerable hyperventilation of the remaining lung tissue in order to maintain normal oxygen and carbon dioxide tensions. With poor or intermittent communication, air may enter only during inspiration, thus creating a growing tension cyst that not only lacks effective pulmonary vasculature but also produces collapse of the adjacent healthy lung tissue. In this fashion, a situation may arise that is potentially fatal, although it may be corrected by surgery.

Using the routine pulmonary function tests described, this type of dysfunction usually cannot be properly evaluated, and more elaborate techniques are required for precise quantification of the defect.

PATHOLOGICAL PROCESSES

EXOGENOUS PIGMENTATION

Pigments enter the lungs from the surrounding atmosphere. They cause disease under the following conditions: when they are not filtered out in the nose or the mucosal lining of the bronchi; when they are small enough (0.5 to 12 microns) to pass into the terminal bronchioles and alveoli, but not so small that they act like a gas and can be readily exhaled; and when they have physical or chemical properties that cause an inflammatory response in the pulmonary tissues in which they reside. The important pathogenic dusts and the diseases they produce include silicon dioxide (silicosis), coal-dust (coal-miner's pneumoconiosis or anthracosis), bauxite fumes containing fine particles of alumina and silica (Shaver's disease), and diatomaceous earth (diatomite fibrosis). They also include pneumoconioses due to certain silicates such as asbestos (asbestosis), mica dust, and talc. Inhalation of beryllium compounds causes beryllium disease or berylliosis. Dust of bagasse, a vegetable residue of sugar cane, produces bagassosis, and cotton dust produces byssinosis.

Most of these dusts settle in alveoli where they are picked up by phagocytic cells to be carried back into the lymphatic system and then to regional lymph nodes where an inflammatory reaction and fibrosis occur. This sets the stage for obstruction of lymph flow, with subsequent pigment deposition and fibrosis in the lymphatics and alveolar walls themselves.

Not all exogenous pigments are pathogenic. Carbon, though it blackens lungs, causes minimal if any inflammatory reaction and no significant degree of fibrosis. Iron oxide, as produced in electric arc welding, does cause nodular lesions in the lungs, called siderosis. Though much like silicosis, this condition is benign, asymptomatic, and nonprogressive.

DEGENERATION AND INFILTRATION

In response to disease, changes occur in body cells and connective tissues that are indicative of at least temporary deterioration. An early change is cloudy swelling of the cells, thought to be produced by poisonous substances released by infectious processes.

With considerable severity, chronicity, or both, cloudy swelling progresses to other more important changes. Fatty degeneration is one such change involving alteration of both the amount of fatty materials and the type in and around cells. Hyaline is another degenerative material that appears in connective tissues, old scars, and where connective tissue is laid down as a part of chronic inflammation. A third type is mucinous degeneration, seen in epithelial cells that line the tracheobronchial tree, in which there is production of excessive amounts of mucus.

NECROSIS

Necrosis is cellular death, in terms of part or all of an organ, with continued life of surrounding tissues. In the lungs, it may be caused by trauma, heat, radiant energy, chemicals, bacteria, and loss of blood supply. A particularly striking example of necrosis due to vascular occlusion is the *pulmonary infarct.* This produces a wedge-shaped defect that is indicative of the shape and size of tissues supplied by that vessel. Its presence indicates the lack of collateral circulation to the region, else there would not have been cellular death.

The type of necrosis depends upon both the site and the nature of the insult. With necrosis in a pulmonary infarct, the affected area is white or anemic and looks grossly like coagulum, therefore the name *coagulation necrosis*. The area softens, swells, becomes granular, relatively dry, and friable; with time, it loses its fluid, shrinks, becomes more firm, and finally—unless a large area is involved—becomes completely replaced with scar tissue. Large areas in similar conditions become surrounded by a zone of fibrous tissue to become encapsulated.

The tubercle formed in tuberculosis undergoes a type of central necrosis that appears cheesy or caseous. The resultant *caseation necrosis* produces degeneration and death of cells, followed by replacement with fatty material. Necrosis is so complete that no remnant of the original tissue remains.

In abscesses or pneumonic exudates in the lung, a third type of necrosis is seen. The tissue becomes altered so as to produce fluid. This is called *liquefaction necrosis* and is the usual manner by which material is either absorbed or spilled into the tracheobronchial tree for expectoration.

CALCIFICATION

Areas of dense fibrosis, especially if hyalinized, and necrotic masses often become infiltrated with calcium salts. The resulting calcification is noted mostly in dense scars of old pleural infections and in tuberculous lesions in the lungs and mediastinal lymph nodes. It also occurs in certain fungal infections such as histoplasmosis and coccidioidomycosis.

INFLAMMATION

Inflammation represents the reaction between an injurious agent and the tissues in which it resides. The reaction can be either acute or chronic, exudative or alterative. The tissue response is composed of two parts, vascular and proliferative. In the vascular phase, there is an increase in blood flow to the area and an increased permeability of the capillary wall. This allows fluids and white cells to traverse the wall and surround or engulf injurious agents. In the proliferative phase, vascular endothelium and connective tissue cells proliferate into and around the reaction areas to form the eventual scar.

Exudative inflammations may be further subclassified into serous, fibrinous, hemorrhagic, and suppurative inflammations. Serous inflammatory responses contain serum, little fibrin, and few cells, and occur on pleural surfaces in response to chemical or sterile insults. Fibrinous inflammatory responses contain large amounts of fibrin, enmeshed within which are a moderate number of cells. These responses also occur on the pleural surface and are the type of exudate seen in the early stages of lobar pneumonia.

Hemorrhagic exudates occur when there is a bleeding diathesis (tendency) when the vessel wall is actually weakened or invaded by tumor, and in reaction to specific infectious organisms such as certain streptococci, the diptheria bacillus, and the tubercle bacillus in certain locations. A typical hemorrhagic pleural exudate is found where the pleura has been invaded by malignant tumor cells.

Suppurative inflammations produce pus, thick liquid composed mostly of both dead and living leukocytes. The consistency, color, and odor of the pus is related to the specific infectious organisms. The lung abscess is a typical form of a suppurative exudate and is a dangerous condition. If the abscess is not quickly resolved, it may extend, enlarge, and point into either a bronchus, a blood vessel, or the pleural space. People have been known to drown when a large abscess drained into a bronchus. Blood vessel invasion may seed the offending organism in remote parts of the body. Serious or fatal empyema may ensue if the abscess burrows through the pleural surface. If long-standing, the outer rim of the abscess becomes so thickly scarred as to be un-collapsible, even after the abscess has emptied. The thickness and consistency of this wall, as seen by x-rays, are often characteristic of specific bacterial or fungal infection.

Alternative inflammations are composed of the above-noted degenerative reactions in addition to exudation or cellular proliferation. Catarrhal inflammation is of this variety and occurs in the mucous membranes lining the tracheobronchial tree. The exudate is mucinous, with protein, white cells, and desquamated epithelial cells. The mucous membrane is thickened, reddened, and undergoes cloudy swelling, followed often by mucinous degeneration. The most frequent causative agents are the common cold, irritant dusts, gases, and chemicals.

Chronic inflammations differ from those of the acute variety in that they are often insidious, unlimited, and progressive. It is these characteristics which initiate progressive impairment and disability. The white cell infiltrate consists of lymphocytes and monocytes instead of polymorphonuclear leukocytes. There is usually an abundance of dense scar tissue and neovascularization, both of which create considerable hazards to the surgeon who is attempting reconstructive or palliative surgery. Chronic pleural infections are of this variety. Unlike acute infections, these often place a lasting and deforming stress upon the organ that is affected.

DISEASES

The following section does not include all diseases affecting respiration nor all the aspects of each disease discussed; only a thumbnail sketch is presented. For further more penetrating detail, reference to standard medical textbooks is indicated.

RESTRICTIVE DEFECTS

POLIOMYELITIS. This is an acute viral disease affecting the anterior horn cell in the spinal cord, with chronic sequelae. It is these residual effects that merit evaluation insofar as they affect respiration. In the spinal form, involvement of anterior horn cells from the upper third of the cervical spinal cord to the lower third of the thoracic cord can produce limitations of the respiratory muscle pump. Most serious is the complete loss of both phrenic nerves; these control the diaphragms, which contribute about 75 per cent of the power of the muscle pump. Less serious are isolated losses of the accessory muscles of respiration in the neck and shoulders, of the intercostals, or of the abdominal muscles. Yet when these are additive to paralysis of the diaphragms, the resulting impairment becomes progressively and strikingly worse.

There are two functional patterns of breathing that arise when certain combinations of muscle weakness appear. With weak diaphragms and intercostals, the vital capacity is greater sitting or standing than when lying down, because of the helpful action of the abdominal muscles in the upright position. In this position, the abdominal contents sag downward and out in inspiration but are pushed back in effectively by the abdominal muscles during expiration to force the diaphragms back up. While lying down, this favorable abdominal displacement does not occur; in fact, the diaphragms are already high in inspiration and cannot be further displaced. This strange situation allows some people to do sedentary work for a normal eight-hour workday when upright, while necessitating extra breathing apparatus at night.

On the other hand, patients with weak diaphragms and abdominals but fairly strong intercostals have a larger vital capacity when lying supine than when upright. They often need respiratory aids while sitting in a chair. In this situation, there is no assistance from the abdominal muscles during expiration. In the supine position, the abdominal contents press against the diaphragms to aid expiration, the intercostals having given additional assistance during inspiration.

In either condition, the vital capacity may vary with change of position by as much as 30 to 40 per cent.

When the brainstem is involved, the condition is called *bulbar poliomyelitis.* In this instance, loss of cranial nerve function or respiratory center control creates additional problems. The latter affection produces partial or total loss of all the central controlling mechanisms of respiration noted earlier in the chapter. Paralysis of cranial nerves affects speech, swallowing, or control of mouth and nasopharyngeal secretions. There is inability to prevent secretions and food from being aspirated into the trachea as well as ineffectual cough for raising these and intrinsic pulmonary secretions. Isolated bulbar involvement is infrequent; more commonly, it is mixed with spinal forms of the disease.

Clinical Course. Once paralysis has become established, it will either remain in this state or fade over the ensuing 18 months. The rate of recovery is fastest initially, with about 60 per cent of the total re-coverability occurring in the first three months, and 80 per cent in the first six months. After 18 months, any further return of function occurs as remaining muscle fibers become hypertrophied or as stronger ad-jacent muscles are substituted. Thus, a final functional picture evolves which, in the broad sense, is stable from that point on. And, insofar as this picture persists, one can then determine practicable goals for self-care, work, and recreation.

Unfortunately, with significant respiratory embarrassment, especially when a permanent tracheostomy is needed or bulbar paresis persists, the altered state has an increased affinity for recurrent pulmonary in-fections. In addition, poor habit patterns and poor environmental con-ditions (such as rapidly changing extremes in temperature and humidity, noxious gases, and dusts) may rapidly set the stage for the development of irreversible chronic pulmonary inflammatory processes. In this fashion, a stable picture soon may be replaced by one with progressive deteriora-tion and a shortened life-span.

Treatment. In the acute phase, special therapeutic efforts are shaped by each patient's needs and are aimed at maintaining optimal respira-tory exchange, elimination of secretions, and prevention of superinfec-tion. This may require only occasional encouragement to cough, or as much as tracheostomy, tank respirator care, and constant nursing coverage.

The tracheostomy tube, C-shaped and with various adaptations and fittings, is both a lifesaving instrument and a hazard. It is lifesaving in that it decreases the respiratory dead space by as much as 50 per cent, thus allowing the patient to breathe without respiratory aids. It also provides easy access to the tracheobronchial tree for suctioning of secretions. It is a hazard because it obviates the natural defenses of the upper respiratory system and allows dry, dusty, and bacteria-laden air directly into the lungs.

Successful handling of the respiratory cripple requires the use of various respiratory machines. Being of several types, they either push air into or out of the lungs, or suck it into the lungs. The "push" type is of two varieties: those which push it through the upper airways to aid the inspiratory effort; and those which push it out of the lungs by applying pressure on the abdomen through an expanding belt to produce an expiratory effort. The "suck" type is also of two varieties: one which sucks air out of the lungs through the upper airways in an expiratory effort; and one which produces inspiration by producing a relative vacuum either around the anterior chest and abdomen or around the entire body. The tank respirator is of the "suck" inspiratory, "push" expiratory type. The cuirass respirator, which fits around the anterior chest and abdomen, is similar but less effective. Similar to both of these is the "raincoat" respirator. With this device, the patient is wrapped in a covering that is held away from the chest and abdomen by a frame. The pneumobelt respirator is of the "push" expiratory type. Those respirators which are applied to the upper airways may produce both a "push" inspiratory and "suck" expiratory effect. Usually, only the inspiratory phase is used; expiration is allowed to occur passively.

Another useful device is the rocking bed, which rocks the patient through an arc of 20 to 60 degrees up and down. This motion puts the abdominal contents through directional movements that in turn move the diaphragm either up or down.

Special breathing exercises regularly performed help the establishment of a stable respiratory state. Such exercises include deep breathing and coughing each hour while awake, and performing postural drainage of the lungs every three to four hours during the day. Glossopharyngeal breathing (GPB), or "frog breathing," is a technique whereby the patient actively and repeatedly swallows air into his tracheobronchial tree. This procedure may convert a small vital capacity of 0.6 to 1.0 liters to as much as 3.0 to 4.0 liters. Used once an hour, it will provide a deep breath preparatory to an effective cough. Unfortunately, those who need this technique most—namely, those with bulbospinal polio—may not have the pharyngeal control to use it. Finally, a good therapist often can strengthen the existing musculature of the respiratory muscles. If this produces only a 5 to 10 per cent increase in vital capacity, it still is significant and makes a contribution to longevity. The net effect of all the efforts over several years time may be represented by a pliable chest that allows a large breathing excursion with little or no tracheobronchial secretions and few intercurrent infections. Without these exercises, the patient may develop a "frozen" chest wall with limited excursion, secretions, and repeated infections as frequent complications.

Avoidance of smoking and irritant dry air, sufficient rest, good nutritional intake, and prompt medical care of any respiratory infections will contribute greatly to the maintenance of a fairly stable state.

Surgical treatment referable to the respiratory system is limited, in the main, to fusion of part of the spine (cervical), or all of the spine in order to stabilize the skeleton, and to tracheostomy.

Prevention. Even though currently the use of oral vaccines appears to have effectively eliminated poliomyelitis in this country, it is too soon to accept this as a disease of the past. If nothing else, there remains the task of preventing further unnecessary deterioration in the present polio population.

OBSTRUCTIVE DEFECTS

ASTHMA. Asthma in Greek means "a panting." It refers to a chronic, episodic state characterized by cough, wheezing, mucoid secretions, and a sense of constriction of the chest. Changes occurring in the smaller and medium bronchioles consist of swelling of the bronchiolar wall, contraction of the smooth muscles in the wall to produce a constricted lumen, and the obstructing presence of thick tenacious sputum from the bronchial glands. The resulting reduction in airway size produces obstruction to air flow, chiefly in expiration—that phase of expiration in which the airways are at their smallest diameter.

The mechanism producing edema, smooth muscle contraction, and mucoid secretions is said to be the reaction of the bronchioles to a substance released by an allergic antigen-antibody reaction.

The allergic state is, at least in most cases, the underlying abnormal condition that triggers the "bronchospastic" response. It is believed that substances which formerly were well tolerated by the body begin to act like foreign substances. As antigens, they stimulate the production of antibodies. The resulting antigen-antibody reaction presumably produces a histaminelike material which in turn elicits the tissue reaction.

The "foreign" substances (allergens) most commonly producing the allergic reaction are organic dusts such as pollens, mold spores, animal danders, insecticides, feathers, and lint from fabrics. Other dusts, such as grains, flour, and vegetable seeds, usually become allergens after prolonged occupational contact. Some foodstuffs such as dairy products, fish, spices, nuts, and chocolates also become allergens.

These materials can, upon injection into the skin, produce allergic skin reactions, presumptive evidence that they are also allergenic on the bronchial mucosa. When suitably prepared, these substances can also be inhaled as test allergens. The resulting bronchospastic response is measured by changes in the timed vital capacity.

There are many asthmatics for whom there appears to be no such extrinsic allergen. Rather, these people appear sensitive to bacterial products, and have infections from these bacteria, either acute or chronic, which accompany or precede the asthmatic attack. The infection can be in either the upper or lower respiratory tree.

Because of this difference in etiology, asthma is divided by some into extrinsic versus intrinsic or infective groups. This grouping is of some therapeutic but little prognostic significance.

There is a third group of conditions under which susceptible asthmatics develop attacks for which no allergen is known. These include rapid changes in temperature or humidity, irritating gases, and violent exercise and emotional stress. These do not appear to be primary agents and fade in importance when the underlying sensitivity has been reduced.

Clinical Course. Asthma is a common condition with a strong family history that may strike either sex at any age. Usually, it appears first in childhood or middle age as a seasonal offender. Often it loses this seasonal specificity as time progresses, and it terminates as a chronic persistent problem. About 25 per cent of the childhood cases ameliorate and disappear during adolescence, but another 25 per cent or so become worse with prolonged and more persistent symptoms. Early in the course, there is a high incidence of the extrinsic type. These cases often become intrinsic or infective with time. A significant but unknown number of patients develop persistent changes that produce the picture of obstructive emphysema. The pattern then represents a combination of irreversible changes as well as reversible bronchospasm.

Attacks of asthma may be mild episodes of wheezing with little danger to life. These are easily reversed over an hour or so with or without medications. Severe attacks of status asthmaticus may last for days or weeks and even terminate in death. Here, the use of the entire therapeutic armamentarium may have little or only belated effect.

Therapy. There are four routes of pharmacological approach to the treatment of asthma: avoidance of contact with allergens; prevention of antigen-antibody interactions; interference, at the tissue level, with the utilization of the histaminelike product of the reaction; and chemical reversal of the histamine effect at the tissue level. The first mode of therapy, avoidance of contact, occasionally requires only avoidance or removal of the offending agent. More often, the allergen is inescapable during certain seasons of the year, as during the ragweed season. Frequently, the allergen is present constantly.

Under these latter circumstances, desensitization techniques are employed to prevent the usual antigen-antibody reaction, by development of a blocking antibody. Desensitization is often a long, slow process by which extremely small tolerated doses of the allergen are repeatedly injected. As tolerance is obtained, the dose is slowly increased until the patient can accept rather large doses of the allergen without reaction. Hopefully, this is accompanied by increased tolerance to the inhaled allergen.

In certain cases of specific-allergen asthma in the young, antihistamines are of value by interfering with the tissue utilization of histamine. However, these cases are infrequent, and often the sedative and secretion-thickening effects of the drug counterbalance its beneficial effects.

Usually, the most effective agents are those which reverse the histamine effect at the tissue level. These agents usually can be taken by the patient as needed, either orally or by inhalation. Occasionally, patients learn to give themselves subcutaneous injections of these medications. The single most effective drug is epinephrine. Similar drugs such as ephedrine and isoproterenol (Isuprel) are taken either orally or by inhalation.

When attacks are of sufficient severity, appropriate drugs must be given intramuscularly; if necessary, aminophylline is given intravenously either by direct injection or in an intravenous drip. When these measures fail to abort an attack, corticosteroids are used as a last resort. Occasionally, patients must be maintained on steroids as the only means of providing them with relatively bronchospasm-free states.

All these medications have potentially severe side effects. The steroids, which suppress endogenous adrenal hormone secretions, carry several possible risks with their use: peptic ulcers, edema, psychosis, osteoporosis and fractures, as well as worsening of the diabetic, hypertensive, and tuberculous states.

The successful control or amelioration of infective asthma may require, during acute infections, appropriate antibiotics. Occasionally, they can be used prophylactically with success during the wintertime when there is a high incidence of intercurrent respiratory tract infections. Desensitization techniques are also used by preparation of bacterial vaccines which are injected regularly in minute and slowly increasing doses.

For optimal management of his condition, the asthmatic must make certain concessions. He must live a life balanced with adequate amounts of rest and avoid high concentrations of allergens, physical fatigue, smoke, irritant gas, and dusts, even if this necessitates a change of occupation and residence. Often, the strict maintenance of the dust-free bedroom makes a major difference in the frequency or severity of symptoms. Such a room may require air conditioning in persistently hot, humid, or dusty periods of the year, and maintenance of dust-free curtains, blankets, pillows, sheets, furniture, and rugs.

Finally, control or amelioration of emotional factors may relieve or prevent occasional asthmatic attacks. There is little doubt that panic is the frequent companion of asthmatic attacks, much as panic often attends the underwater swimmer who feels he cannot surface on time. Development of the ability to relax in face of the inevitability of an attack will probably diminish the severe fatiguing respiratory efforts that superimpose excessive and unnecessary loads upon the requisite baseline demands. Certainly a well-known and proven pharmacological approach to the control of the attack will go far in allaying apprehension and panic. For those whose emotional problems interfere with additional areas of their daily lives, supportive therapy from their own physician or from a psychiatrist may help alleviate or temper the severity of the emotional responses and thus help control the asthma as well.

OBSTRUCTIVE PULMONARY EMPHYSEMA. Obstructive pulmonary emphysema is a diffuse condition characterized by abnormal inflation of the lungs and obstruction to air flow. It differs from asthma, which has a similar pattern of obstructed air flow, in that it is an irreversible condition resulting from tissue destruction. It is not a single disease resulting from one predisposing factor. Rather, it is a condition resulting from one of several possible conditions. Among several suspected predisposing diseases are asthma and chronic bronchitis. Also, patients with bronchogenically disseminated tuberculosis, sarcoidosis, and silicosis have functional and pathological entities indistinguishable from so-called idiopathic emphysema.

Microscopically, several types of changes are noted: (1) distention of alveoli and destruction of alveolar walls with resultant coalescence into larger blebs; (2) loss of elastic tissues in the lungs; (3) a paucity of pulmonary vascular channels with many of the remaining ones narrowed. It is believed by many, though strongly challenged by others, that the initial insult strikes the smallest bronchioles by means of infection of the bronchiolar wall and obstruction of its lumen. This produces distention of the alveolus, rupture of its walls, and loss of elastic tissues with subsequent rupture of vascular channels.

Physiologically, all the defects noted in the first part of this chapter are commonly present, excluding usually a severe restrictive defect. Most striking are the obstructive defects, poor and uneven mixing of inspired gases, ventilation-perfusion imbalance, and a diffusion defect of unknown amount. (The diffusion capacity measurement is difficult to interpret in this disease because of the lack of homogeneity of alveolar and pulmonary arterial blood gases.) Those investigators who measure the diffusion capacity do so because they feel it helps differentiate asthma from emphysema and because it has a prognostic value in emphysema.

Clinical Course. The disease is perhaps three to five times more common in males than females, strikes usually in the fifth decade, and is variably but inexorably progressive, with severe exacerbations accompanying either intercurrent bronchial or pulmonary infections or changes in meteorological conditions. The course of the disease commonly leads to death in the sixth or seventh decade with right heart failure (cor pulmonale) or severe ventilatory insufficiency.

Whereas dyspnea initially is noted only on moderate or severe exertion, it progresses to the point where climbing one flight of stairs or walking one block at a slow rate produces dyspnea. Later, there is dyspnea even at rest. The patient is often found pursing his lips and sitting or leaning forward in order to maintain the most efficient circumstance for easy breathing. Dyspnea, cough, fatigue and irritability are common symptoms associated, finally, with cyanosis and lethargy. Cough is often worse during the night or upon arising in the morning, is often paroxysmal, and becomes very distressing. Efforts to expel sputum may be so severe that they are occasionally followed by syncope (fainting), presumably because of momentary decrease or cessation of cerebral blood flow. Fatigue becomes a central symptom, along with irritability, as the patient finds it increasingly difficult, first to talk as he walks, then merely to walk at all. The patient's relatives often complain that his altered personality and coughing are major disrupting influences in family life.

Wintertime and periods of rapid temperature and humidity changes become trying times. The patient can predict the coming of rain much as can an arthritic. Presumably, an increase in relative humidity causes swelling of thickened, dry, retained secretions (as the secretions imbibe water and swell), which in turn causes increased airway obstruction or cough and dyspnea. As the secretions continue to imbibe, they finally loosen and are capable of being raised, with moderate relief of symptoms. Conversely, the low relative humidity of a heated room in the winter will allow secretions to become inspissated (thickened), tenacious, and difficult to raise, with a real danger that hard plugs will occlude a bronchus and precipitate either bronchopneumonia or pneumonia and perhaps an area of bronchiectasis.

A patient emerging from his heated home to venture into cold winter air will often feel as if his "tubes have shut down completely," being acutely dyspneic and uncomfortable. This leads some to shun the outdoors at this time of year.

Winter is also a time of increased incidence for upper and lower respiratory infections, both viral and bacterial. Epidemics of flu are potentially fatal for the severely incapacitated patient. Pneumonia, most commonly from *Hemophilus influenzae* or the pneumococcus, is just as dangerous.

These intercurrent episodes provide repeated insults to the tracheobronchial tree. Unfortunately, many of them produce irreversible changes. Patient, family, and physician all too often note that each episode is followed by a distinct step down in function.

Treatment. In order to interrupt this vicious cycle, patients have moved to places with warm dry climates such as Florida or Arizona. Such moves usually require large sums of money for people who are in their later vocational years and for whom vocational placement is difficult. Since medical relief does not always occur, such a move is occasionally catastrophic. Added to this, the annual influx of people to these areas with chronic disease and acute respiratory infections brings the patient again in contact with some of the problems he had left behind.

Though the condition is irreversible, much can be done for symptomatic relief and for slowing its progression. Treatment consists of the proper use of bronchodilators where bronchospasm is present; antibiotics when there is superimposed infection or when proper prophylatic measures will prevent wintertime infections; and moisture and expectorants when retained secretions are troublesome.

Postural drainage, properly performed, can make a significant difference in morbidity when secretions are otherwise not raised effectively. Drainage is enhanced when combined with bronchodilator and expectorant medications.

The patient with emphysema must make a number of concessions in order to help modify this disease. He must keep regular hours, avoid undue exposure to cold, and avoid fatigue and all respiratory irritant gases, smokes, and dusts which would stimulate further irritating secretions and inflammations.

When the patient develops severe decompensation with marked secretions, the judicious use of steroids may significantly reduce the inflammatory response and secretions, to the point where significant improvement is momentarily gained.

Some claim that the use of positive-pressure breathing machines, delivering air-oxygen mixtures, and bronchodilator drugs may be helpful symptomatically to the person who is hypoxemic. Several patients, previously bedridden, have been able to progress temporarily to mild ambulatory activities.

By the time that carbon dioxide retention and arterial oxygen unsaturation are chronically present at rest, cardiac failure soon intervenes, at which time appropriate additional medical treatment is indicated.

At this stage, tracheostomy is often performed, with frequent partial reversal of hypercapnia (high blood carbon dioxide) and hypoxemia. Nevertheless, the dangers attended by loss of protection from the upper airways, coupled with decreased ability to cough, may outweigh these advantages.

Finally, several drugs that artificially induce hyperventilation by central stimulation of the respiratory center have been used in order to reverse the end-stage arterial blood abnormalities. The results are equivocal and often equivalent to "whipping a tired horse."

There is a distinct difference, nonetheless, between respiratory failure that is endogenous and that which is exogenous—due to unwise use of respiratory depressant drugs or to overwhelming intercurrent infections. In the latter situation, judicious use of tracheostomy, respiratory stimulants, antibiotics, and bronchodilators may abate the crisis and allow the patient to return to a useful functional life.

DIFFUSION DEFECT

BERYLLIUM DISEASE. Beryllium disease, or *berylliosis*, has both acute and chronic manifestations, with associated dermatitis, conjunctivitis, nasopharyngitis, tracheobronchitis, and pneumonitis. In the pulmonary forms, the acute process is a dense pneumonitis with minimal fever, soon after contact with beryllium compounds. Cough, chest pain, and dyspnea on exertion increase over several days to a few weeks, after which many cases resolve or pass into the chronic phase. Other cases are fatal in the acute period.

The chronic form of the disease usually appears insidiously months to years after contact with beryllium dusts, often without any known preceding acute pneumonitis. Initial symptoms usually are nonspecific and include weakness, fatigue, and weight loss; later, cough, chest pain, and shortness of breath predominate. Finally, months or years later, the patient may become a respiratory cripple and succumb.

Initial contact with the dust may be direct, while grinding or cutting rods, coating fluorescent bulbs, or mining the compound. Often, the exposure is indirect; several patients worked as draftsmen or accountants in fluorescent lamp factories; a few people appear to have lived in proximity to a plant using beryllium compounds and have been in contact with exhaust gases from the factory. Known contact has been as short as one week and as long as several years.

The radiological picture of chronic beryllium disease is that of diffuse small nodular densities throughout the lungs, spreading out from the hilus of each lung. It is not a specific picture, and looks much like the x-ray of other granulomatous diseases.

Pathologically, small granulomas are seen. They consist of central fibrinoid material and peripheral mononuclear cells, surrounded by fibrous tissue. The lesions are located in alveolar walls, around bronchi and blood vessels, and in neighboring lymph nodes. They may be indistinguishable from the lesions of sarcoidosis.

Diagnosis is made on the basis of a good epidemiological history and the finding of beryllium in lung or skin tissue or in the urine.

The physiological abnormality, primarily an alveolar-capillary block, produces a diffusion defect. This defect and its consequences are fully discussed earlier in the chapter.

Treatment for the most part is symptomatic, though significant reversal of physiological abnormalities have been noted following the use of corticosteroids or ACTH in some cases. Antibiotics should be used whenever secondary infection is found. Finally, oxygen therapy will eliminate cyanosis and dyspnea at rest, and will temporarily prolong life. The key to proper handling of this disease lies in its prevention by education of industry, adequate venting of work areas where the compound is used, and prevention of beryllium-containing exhausts from contaminating the atmosphere.

VENTILATION-PERFUSION IMBALANCE

PULMONARY EMBOLISM. Pulmonary embolism is obstruction of the pulmonary artery, or its large branches, usually by a blood clot. The clot originates either in the right side of the heart, in the pelvic veins, or in the veins of the legs. Pulmonary emboli are found in about 10 per cent of all autopsies and occur clinically almost equally after surgery, during cardiac illnesses, and during noncardiac illnesses.

Pulmonary infarction is the process by which tissue death occurs in the lungs following embolic occlusion of the pulmonary artery. It is characterized pathologically by hyperemia, followed by cloudy swelling, fatty degeneration, and necrosis, with subsequent slight scar tissue formation. Infarction follows embolism in a majority of noncardiac cases and in almost all cardiac cases.

Other forms of pulmonary emboli are fat emboli, following fracture of a long bone; air emboli from introduction of air into a vein or from the "bends"; septic emboli, from infected foci involving veins; and tumor emboli, with clumps of tumor cells arising from tumor invasion of veins.

Massive embolism without infarction may be fatal almost instantly. It is not known why this should occur, for surgical ligation of an artery similar to one that has been occluded is unattended by such fatal sequelae. It is almost as though the entire pulmonary vasculature were sent into spasm when one small portion was blocked.

Smaller emboli with infarction often produce chest pain, which is sometimes continuous and oppresive, sometimes sharp and found on inspiration alone. This is associated with fever, prostration, cough, and hemoptysis (blood expectorated from the tracheobronchial tree). The symptoms may abate over several days, leaving few or no sequelae; or, in the presence of severe underlying pulmonary or cardiac disease, the patient may afterward notice further loss of reserve.

The pathophysiology of the acute episode is discussed elsewhere in this chapter. The length of time following initial insult during which the ventilation-perfusion imbalance persists is not known, but it must last for many hours. During this time, analysis of the difference in carbon dioxide tension between pulmonary and arterial blood gases provides a rough estimate of the amount of imbalance and thus provides presumptive evidence of the presence of an embolus. Such evidence has been used to set the stage for an immediate embolectomy, a risky procedure not frequently performed.

It can be speculated that soon after the acute episode, that portion of the lung which was ventilated but not perfused presumably either becomes involved in the necrotic process and is no longer ventilated, or again becomes perfused as the "vascular spasm" that accompanied the embolus disappears.

There are infrequent cases of multiple pulmonary emboli in which there is progressive loss of the pulmonary vascular bed, with associated dyspnea, cyanosis, and cor pulmonale. There is insufficient area for diffusion of oxygen as well as for perfusion, with a resultant strain on the right side of the heart because of the paucity of channels through which blood can travel.

Treatment of the acute condition, except in that rare situation where the embolus can surgically be removed, consists of prevention of further emboli. The prophylactic attack is three-pronged: prevention of blood stasis in the lower extremities or pelvic region with appropriate exercises several times daily, and use of elastic stockings or bandages which further prevent blood pooling; anticoagulant therapy, using either or both heparin and Coumarin or related drugs to prevent further intravascular clotting; and vein ligation when the original focus of a prior embolus is known and anticoagulant therapy has not succeeded.

MIXED DEFECTS

SILICOSIS. Silicosis is an occupational disease caused by inhalation of air containing silicon dioxide, which produces fibrotic nodules, usually 2 to 5 mm in size, throughout both lung fields. The disability continues to progress for several years after contact with the dust has ceased and consists of a moderate restrictive defect, a significant and at times incapacitating obstructive defect, or infrequently a relatively pure diffusion defect which may be equally incapacitating. Contact with the dust necessary to produce recognizable lesions varies from 1 to 2 years, under conditions of extremely high concentration, to 10 to 15 years at lower concentrations. Mining industries handling silica-bearing rocks, granite quarries, ceramic industries, glass manufacturing plants, and industries making or using abrasives and sand blasting are a few of the more than a hundred industries listed in 1942 by the U. S. Department of Labor as involving possibly hazardous exposure to silica dust.

The diagnosis of silicosis depends upon the finding of a positive exposure history, x-ray findings consistent with the diagnosis, and objective demonstration of ventilatory impairment. A lung biopsy that demonstrates a high free silica content is good corroborative evidence of the diagnosis. Yet the mere presence of silica does not establish the diagnosis, for it is often found in normal lung tissue.

The differential diagnosis must include diffuse nodular tuberculosis, sarcoidosis, static carcinomatosis, and siderosis. These diseases produce radiological findings similar to those in silicosis, but symptoms, signs, and occupational histories will help differentiate them.

A major complication of silicosis is superinfection with tuberculosis. In the past, the incidence of combined diseases was very high, and there has been experimental evidence suggesting actual increased virulence of the tubercle bacillus on the silicotic lung. The diagnosis must be suspected when a person with slight or moderate impairment develops cough, fever, sweats, and weight loss with a moderately rapid alteration in the course of the disease. Furthermore, asymmetry of lesions, gross conglomerate lesions and cavities suggest this complication. The diagnosis must be established by the finding of tubercle bacilli in the sputum.

Treatment of silicosis includes removal from the offending dusty environment, use of bronchodilator drugs and other modes of therapy useful in ameliorating the effects of emphysema, and the cautious use of corticosteroids. However, when using steroids, the danger of provoking a flare-up of concomitant tuberculosis demands that the patient either be placed simultaneously on antituberculous drugs or be watched closely and continuously for evidence of tuberculous activity.

It has been proposed that the inhalation of grease-free aluminum powder in proper particle size has both protective and therapeutic value in silicosis. Yet, the results have not been accepted as being uniformly beneficial.

Most emphasis should be placed upon prevention of this disease. Adequate mask protection, venting techniques, and antidust measures can hold the contact to a safe minimum level. Nevertheless, constant inspection and supervision of known exposure sites must be maintained, and close periodic examinations of workers in the field is necessary.

Bronchiectasis. Bronchiectasis, a disease which may eventually produce a restrictive defect with or without an admixed obstructive defect, is primarily a disease of the bronchi. By definition, there is widening of the bronchial lumen, as demonstrated by the use of special x-rays, bronchograms, where radiopaque dye is instilled into the tracheobronchial tree. In a few advanced cases, the widening, which maybe saccular, tubular, cylindrical, or cystic, can be seen on routine chest films. Upon examination, the bronchial wall shows chronic catarrhal inflammation, decrease or absence of bronchial ciliated epithelium, and loss or weakening of the deeper supporting bronchial muscular and elastic tissues. Occasionally, changes are so severe that cartilage is lost, and all that remains is a fibrous tube covered with epithelium.

There are two additional associated pathological findings. These include peribronchial and parenchymal fibrosis and anastomoses of the bronchial artery with the pulmonary artery system. The bronchial arteries arise from the aorta, provide nutrition to the tubular structures of the lungs, and in health do not show functional anastomoses with the pulmonary system. In this disease, however, rich anastomoses are found at the pulmonary precapillary level.

The cause of bronchiectasis is not entirely resolved, but appears to spring from several sources. These is evidence that many cases are congenital and are associated with other congenital abnormalities. Other cases have been seen to occur after obstruction from foreign bodies, tumors, and lymph nodes at the base of the lung and from pneumonia.

In these cases, infection behind the obstruction seems to be the agent producing bronchial wall destruction.

Bronchiectasis appears to be a waning disease in America, perhaps because pulmonary infections are treated more thoroughly and effectively, both medically and surgically. The disease is found in both sexes and in all age groups.

Clinical Course. The progression of this disease varies considerably with the amount of underlying disease and the success of medical or surgical treatment. It was formerly thought to be a disease associated with a 10- to 15-year survival from onset of first symptom. This, however, was in the preantibiotic era. Currently, there are patients known to have lived a similar length of time without demonstrable progression. Therefore, it must be assumed that a normal life-span is possible.

Symptomatology. There are three prominent symptoms: bronchorrhea (cough, productive of large amounts of purulent sputum), hemoptysis, and episodes of recurrent localized pneumonitis. Bronchorrhea is a manifestation of infection, mucous degeneration, catarrhal inflammation, and loss of ciliated epithelium which would otherwise be carrying secretions back up the bronchial tree in a constant conveyer belt fashion. Hemoptysis, which may be severe and troublesome, is attributed to the abnormal bronchial-pulmonary artery anastomoses, and occurs in perhaps 50 per cent of the cases. Recurrent episodes of localized pneumonitis represent both the cause of more bronchiectasis and the result of present disease.

Treatment. The initial approach to the problem should be medical. This consists of postural drainage, expectorants if secretions are thick and raised with difficulty, sufficient fluid intake to keep secretions loose, good general nutrition, and proper antibiotic medicines at appropriate times. Postural drainage must be performed so that the affected segments or lobes are effectively drained by gravity three to four times daily. Proper positioning, for 15- to 20-minute periods, requires that the physician has identified the offending area and has instructed the patient in the proper body placement so that the offending bronchus is drained by gravity. Antibiotics are most useful for handling acute flare-ups, in preparation for surgery, and in limiting or decreasing the seriousness of the chronic phase.

Surgery offers the only definitive cure for this disease and yet is applicable only in localized disease, where either segmental or lobar resection may be performed. Yet, even resection may be attended with new difficulties: either prior undiagnosed bronchiectatic areas may flare up, or the restrictive defect resulting from ablative surgery may be as disabling as the prior symptoms. The former complication will not arise unknowingly if proper bronchography has previously outlined all bronchopulmonary segments. The dyspnea from ablative surgery will be minimal when proper selection and minimal extirpation have been exercised.

TUBERCULOSIS. Tuberculosis is an infectious disease, occasionally acute but usually chronic, which may strike almost any tissue of the body and which currently manifests itself predominantly by pulmonary infection. It is a relapsing disease and still should be considered essentially as incurable.

Bacteriology. The tubercle bacillus is a bacterium of the genus *Mycobacterium,* which contains other parasitic and saprophytic bacteria. Two related bacilli are the avian and bovine strains. The avian is pathogenic in birds but rarely in humans; the bovine is pathogenic in both cattle and humans. The bovine bacillus formerly was a serious source of extrapulmonary human tuberculosis but caused pulmonary disease only in about 6 per cent of the cases. Today, bovine tuberculosis is largely eradicated in the United States.

One characteristic of the genus is its affinity for certain dyes, notably carbol fuchsin, which becomes fixed in the lipid coat of the bacteria and cannot readily be removed, even by acids. This has lead to the term "acid-fast" bacillus. Another characteristic is the viability of the bacillus in the absence of heat or sunlight, where it may remain for months or years. In direct sunlight, it is killed in a few hours, and by boiling it is killed in minutes.

Pathology. In the human lung, the tubercle bacillus causes a progression of pathological changes. The earliest lesion may be an exudate within the alveolus, made up of mononuclear cells, with little damage to lung tissue. At this stage, the lesion is essentially reversible. It, however, may progress to a granulomatous lesion composed of epithelioid cells ringed with fibrous tissue. The granuloma is destructive of normal pulmonary tissue. It may either resolve and be replaced by scar tissue or undergo central caseous necrosis.

If the caseous material remains intact, it will become a site for future calcium deposition, which may entirely replace the caseous lesion, with the tubercle bacillus often entrapped within. If the caseous material becomes liquefied, it will be extruded through the bronchus, leaving a fibrous-walled cavity lined with caseous and granulating debris, a rich breeding area for the tubercle bacillus.

The cavity may remain in open communication with the bronchus for years. Occasionally, its opening is occluded and the cavity refills with liquefied and caseous debris to become a solid-appearing tumor by x-ray. It is unusual, without treatment, for the cavity to close, resolve, and be replaced entirely by scar tissue.

Spread of the tubercle bacillus from the above lesions is either by direct extension via the bronchus to adjacent or distant parts of the lungs, or via the lymphatics to the regional, mediastinal, and even cervical lymph nodes. Finally, the lesion may invade local blood vessels to seed many distant areas of the body. If the invasion is massive, the result will be *disseminated miliary tuberculosis,* an extremely dangerous and fatal condition if untreated.

Natural History. The natural history of tuberculosis is not uniform and predictable but rather a complex picture with many variables. The disease varies clinically in severity and type from one age group to another. The highest incidence of generalized disease occurs in early childhood, while chronic pulmonary tuberculosis characteristically is first seen in the second and third decades. After the fourth decade, primary infections often are indolent and slowly progressive. At the same time, mortality rates vary directly with increasing age; in the United States in 1950, it was 9 per 100,000 in the first year of life, dropping to 2 by age 10 and rising to 40 per 100,000 at age 60.[1] There are also differences in mortality rates by race, suggesting constitutional or racial differences in natural resistance. In the United States, mortality rates for nonwhites is three times higher than that for whites; American Indians and Chinese in the United States have a tuberculosis death rate twice that of Negroes, who in turn have a higher death rate than whites. Pregnancy and malnutrition often aggravate tuberculosis, and intercurrent disease, such as uncontrolled diabetes mellitus, predisposes to severe tuberculosis. Finally, ignorance, poor housing, and overcrowding all influence the incidence and severity of the disease.

Since the turn of the century, there have been temporal changes in the seriousness of tuberculosis, with lowering of both the new case and mortality rates. In 1900 in the United States, the death rate was 200 per 100,000; in 1953 it had dropped to about 15 per 100,000; and by 1956, it had dropped further to less than 10.

The new case rate has dropped irregularly and less strikingly from 100 per 100,000 in 1930 to 70 per 100,000 in 1952. In certain areas, such as Minneapolis, the drop has been more striking: 47 per cent of grade school children had positive tuberculin tests in 1926, 19 per cent in 1936, 8 per cent in 1944, and 4 per cent in 1954.[2]

Whereas 40 years ago, the majority of people had positive tuberculin tests by early adulthood, the prevalence of positive reactions now is much lower in all except those who are in the older age brackets. (These older people undoubtedly are carrying with them the prevalence of their youth.) For example, one study in Minnesota in 1960 showed

[1] J. Katz and S. Kunofsky, "Trends of Tuberculosis Morbidity and Mortality," *Am. Rev. Resp. Dis.,* **84**:217, 1961.
[2] J. A. Myers, "The Natural History of Tuberculosis in the Human Body (IV. Behavior of Tuberculosis Among Elderly People)," *Am. Rev. Resp. Dis.,* **85**:232, 1962.

that a positive tuberculin test was found in 0.3 per cent of those 0–5 years of age, in 2.2 per cent of those 15–19 years old, in 27.5 per cent of those 50–59 years old, and in 44.8 per cent of those 60 years or older.[3]

Reasons for the decrease in new cases and mortality undoubtedly stem from many changes which have occurred over the past 60 years. Notable among them have been more effective case-finding techniques, eradication of bovine tuberculosis, better social conditions, and improved forms of therapy.

Even though the picture of tuberculosis is much brighter than it was even ten years ago, there are two disturbing facets to the problem. The first relates to case findings. Though the increased use of tuberculin skin testing and survey x-rays brings much latent or overt disease to light, it is disappointing that most of the cases thus found represent moderate to far-advanced disease, with only about 20 per cent being at the minimal stage.[4]

The second facet relates to relapses. Even with modern drug coverage and surgery, the relapse rate within the past decade has been reported to be 8 per cent in two studies and as high as 25 per cent in a third study.[5] At this point, the true long-term relapse rate under good drug and surgical care is not yet known.

Allergy and Immunity. Knowledge of different responses to infection at various age levels gave rise to speculation that there was a change in host defenses with increasing age. It also became apparent that an earlier but not quiescent infection seemed to provide increased resistance to further infection. It was believed that there were few host defenses present in the childhood primary case. Because of this, it was reasoned, there were minimal symptoms, mild local lung reaction, and diffuse dissemination in many cases. Conversely, when reinfection did occur, host defenses were high: there was intense local pulmonary reaction and a paucity of diffuse hematogenous spread.

The reasons for these variations with age and prior infections have not been made clear. However, these findings stimulated thoughts concerning allergy and immunity in tuberculosis. In relation to allergy, original observations by Koch in guinea pigs demonstrated that after an initial infection, injection of tubercle bacilli into the skin caused an intense local reaction, which was markedly different from the initial reaction. Subsequently, when tuberculin, the protein extract from tubercle bacilli, was injected into the skin of humans who had no prior infection, no skin reaction occurred. However, with prior infection, an intense local allergic reaction occurred at the site of injection.

[3] *Ibid.*, p. 243.
[4] *Ibid.*, p. 239
[5] *Ibid.*, p. 242.

There developed from these findings the tuberculin skin tests, using either OT (old tuberculin) or PPD (purified protein derivative), the latter being more stable and reliable. The positive response does not indicate active tuberculosis; it may indicate that tubercle bacilli are harbored somewhere in the body; it definitely indicates that there has been an infection at some time in the past. A negative response indicates that, except in certain circumstances, the patient has not had a tuberculous infection. False negatives occur with poor technique, in the first few weeks of tuberculosis before hypersensitivity has developed, in certain cases of overwhelming disease, during an eruption of measles and perhaps some other exanthematous diseases, and in less than 1 per cent of the patients who have had tuberculosis.

In relation to immunity, the same observations by Koch gave rise to the speculation that vaccine containing live, killed, or attenuated strains of tubercle bacilli might confer immunity. One vaccine, BCG, a living culture of attenuated bovine bacilli developed by Calmette and Guérin, has been found to confer some degree of immunity to humans. Though quite safe, it has been decided for several reasons [6] that in this country it should not be used except in areas where contagion is high and control measures are poor.

Symptomatology. Early cases produce few symptoms, the largest single reason why new cases are advanced before coming to medical attention. The symptoms are usually those only of fatigue and malaise, especially at the end of the day, associated with mild weight loss and mild evening temperatures. Only with bronchial involvement or progression to liquefication of caseous material does cough and sputum production become significant. This is associated with worsening of prior symptoms, higher evening temperatures, and sweating. Hemoptysis, usually small in amount, occurs as blood vessels in tuberculous cavities are weakened or ulcerated. Copious bleeding is not rare, though fatal hemorrhage is. Pain, a symptom of pleural involvement, may arise at any time during the course of the disease and persist for variable periods of time depending upon the underlying pathology.

Prognosis. The eventual outcome of the disease is closely related to the severity of symptoms, the type and extent of lesions, and the size of cavities. It is also related to the ability of the patient to follow a well-conceived program of treatment. Unfortunately, a sizable reservoir of disease resides in a group of the population who cannot maintain a proper program of rest, sanitarium care, and constant intake of proper medications. Equally unfortunate is that many patients and

---

[6] "Report of Ad Hoc Advisory Committee on BCG to the Surgeon General of the United States Public Health Service," *Am. Rev. Tuberc. and Pulm. Dis.*, 76:726, 1957.

physicians place excessive faith in modern drugs and surgical procedures, with the feeling that permanent cure has been obtained and the need for close follow-up no longer pertains.

Treatment. In the past 60 years, treatment of tuberculosis has changed radically, with maintenance of many older forms of therapy, at least in principle, and with the addition of newer approaches as pertinent. The basic modality is rest of both the total patient and the involved lung. The latter is effected by collapse therapy. Originally, this was obtained either by introduction of air into the pleural space (pneumothorax) or abdomen (pneumoperitoneum) or by crushing the phrenic nerve on the involved side to produce a paralyzed elevated diaphragm. Later, resection of ribs (thoracoplasty) was performed, with collapse produced by the loss of the overlying bony structures. Currently, the same effect is also produced by extrapleural and extraperiosteal plombage, a procedure whereby the ribs are maintained intact, the rib lining (periosteum) stripped away and displaced inward against the lung, with the subsequent space maintained by placement of material into the space. Lucite spheres are often used for this purpose.

In the mid-1940's, streptomycin was first used as a chemotherapeutic agent to retard and arrest the growth (bacteriostasis) of the tubercle bacillus. Since that time, PAS (para-aminosalicylic acid) and isoniazid have been developed as additional mainstays of drug therapy. Various combinations of these three agents are now used with good effect. Still, a true bactericidal drug is not available.

Following the development of drugs, it became possible to remove quiescent, stable, and well-defined areas of infected lung, thus further reducing the threat of future relapse. Surgical resection of lungs, lobes, or segments then became part of the standard armamentarium. The extent of surgery is defined both by the type and extent of disease and by the limitations imposed by the ability to safely remove the least amount of lung tissue possible in order to retain maximal functional lung tissue.

Complications. Aside from the possible side effects of drug therapy, which include deafness (streptomycin) and peripheral neuropathy (isoniazid without pyridoxine coverage), complications arise as the result of scar tissue formation. These include distortion of structures, limitation of motion of the chest wall or lung, and loss of parenchymal substance. Here, the loss of vasculature may exceed that of ventilating lung, yielding ventilation-perfusion imbalance. Narrowing of bronchi, as a result of endobronchial tuberculosis or adjacent parenchymal pathology, may be of sufficient magnitude to decrease air exchange and abet retention of secretions in the affected lobe or segment. Fibrothorax or parenchymal scarring may produce a significant restrictive ventilatory defect. Finally, Gaensler [7] found that "among 1,533 patients with pulmonary tuberculosis studied over a ten-year period, 61 per cent had chronic obstructive emphysema; and a survey of 200 patients hospitalized in a sanitarium revealed an incidence of emphysema of 44 per cent. For this reason, it is important to obtain pulmonary function studies when patients with prior moderate or severe disease contemplate returning to more than sedentary work.

Perhaps equally severe a complication is development of the stigma of being contaminated. This is felt by both the patient and the public. Relatives and acquaintances fear that they will contract the disease. Yet, the fear of contagion far exceeds the actual infectivity of the disease when proper control measures are instituted. The good physician and related personnel can do much to educate the patient and family about these matters so that the adverse emotional reaction is minimized.

CHRONIC BRONCHITIS. Until recently, chronic bronchitis had been viewed in the United States as an unimportant condition characterized as chronic cough or "bronchial trouble," which had no serious sequelae. However, the British have long recognized it as a definite and respectable disease with even lethal consequences. In this country, interest has grown as a relationship has been showed between smog, other types of polluted air, and cigarette smoke and chronic productive cough. Also, as diseases such as lobar pneumonia and tuberculosis have declined in importance, investigators have become aware of a link between chronic bronchitis and emphysema. This has been accompanied by much reliable evidence linking smoking and its associated chronic bronchitis with bronchogenic carcinoma. It is because of these latter two possibilities and complications that this entity is discussed.

Chronic bronchitis has also suffered from a paucity of definitive investigations because of the lack of a precise and acceptable definition. One usable definition states:

> It is a disease characterized by prolonged productive cough either of insidious onset or beginning with a major acute respiratory infection. Cough and sputum are almost invariably worse in the winter, worse in the morning and worse with changes of temperature, foggy weather, and with exposure to smoke and dusts. The disease is slowly progressive, worse after each major infection and may lead to obstructive emphysema. [8]

In its earlier stages, it is reversible if the offending irritant is removed. ✓

The above definition does not imply that ventilatory insufficiency

---

[7] E. A. Gaensler, "Evaluation of Pulmonary Functions: Results in Chronic Obstructive Lung Disease," *Ann. Rev. Med.,* **13**:323, 1962.

[8] E. A. Gaensler and I. Lindgren, "Chronic Bronchitis as an Etiologic Factor in Obstructive Emphysema," *Am. Rev. Resp. Dis.,* **80**:187, 1959.

is necessarily present. In fact, it may be argued that ventilatory impairment signals the earliest clinical phase of obstructive emphysema. However, in regard to smoking and chronic bronchitis, Gaensler found, in review of the literature, that "every epidemiologic study . . . showed both a higher prevalence of respiratory symptoms and a lower mean ventilatory capacity in smokers than in non-smokers." [9]

As public health officials and the lay population became more aware of the consequences of pollution of the inspired air, reactive changes have been forthcoming, with the result that many affected urban areas now have developed intensive air pollution control programs. Also, there have been extensive alterations in cigarettes and smoking habits.

REHABILITATION

Rehabilitation of chronic respiratory disease is related to the medical, physiological, sociological, and psychological characteristics of each disease and of each patient and, additionally, is represented by the application of that which has gone before. There are no unique characteristics or applications in this set of disorders.

Notwithstanding, there is a feeling that these diseases lend themselves to special handling because objective tests can frequently and easily quantify the degree of impairment. The mistake frequently made is to equate physiological impairment with the feelings of disability of which the patient or client complains. The impairment actually may bear little or no relation to its interpretation by the patient. Therefore, the problem resolves into the need to assess the degree of impairment caused by the disease and by the individual's reaction to the disease. Once this differentiation has been made, effective therapeutic plans can be laid.

BIBLIOGRAPHY

Cecil, Russell L., Robert F. Loeb, et al. Textbook of Medicine, 11th ed. Philadelphia: W. B. Saunders Co., 1963.

Comroe, J. H., R. E. Forester, A. B. Bubois, W. A. Briscoe, and E. Carlsen. The Lung, Clinical Physiology and Pulmonary Function Tests. Chicago: The Year Book Publishers, 1955.

Hinshaw, H. C., and L. H. Garland. Diseases of the Chest. Philadelphia: W. B. Saunders Co., 1956.

Karfner, H. T. Human Pathology. Philadelphia: J. B. Lippincott Co., 1949.

Knowles, J. H. Respiratory Physiology and Its Clinical Applications. Cambridge: Harvard University Press, 1959.

[9] Gaensler, "Evaluation of Pulmonary Functions," p. 323.

IV

BONE, JOINT, AND MUSCLE DISORDERS

The musculoskeletal system is simply a mechanical device for dealing with the three dimensions of space and the force of gravity. It is what enables man and all creatures to get about in space. In addition, especially in the case of man, space may be fashioned to the individual's liking. The musculoskeletal system operates on a few simple physical principles. The framework is composed of _bone_, a connective tissue modified by the deposition of calcium salts which specifically makes its parts rigid. The various parts of this framework must move in relationship to each other and therefore are joined together by other forms of connective tissue, cartilage and ligament, the chief property of which is flexibility. These flexible junctions are designated _joints_. The muscles produce the motion. _Muscle_ consists of a certain type of protein, the most important property of which is that, when stimulated in certain ways, it contracts or diminishes its longitudinal dimension. Depending on how the muscles are attached to the bones, this action produces certain movements.

The controlling mechanism of this elaborate mechanical device is the nervous system, which may be considered an enormously complex computer. It takes information that has been provided by the various senses—visual, auditory, olfactory, gustatory, tactile, proprioceptive, balance—combines this with information that has been stored in memory, analyzes the data available, and initiates appropriate action. A simple example is suggested by the way in which the neuromusculoskeletal

By JOEL C. GOLDTHWAIT, M.D. Visiting Physician, Robert Breck Brigham Hospital; Assistant in Medicine, Harvard Medical School, Boston, Massachusetts.

system deals with gravity. In the inner ear is the organ of balance, which not only sends information to the brain about the position of the head in relation to gravity, but also produces data concerning the motions of the head in space. Sensory nerves from all the joints and muscles transmit to the spinal cord and brain information on stretch, tension, and position—in other words, the relationship of the different parts of the body to each other. This is known as *proprioception*. The sense of touch enters the equation (for example, pressure on the soles of the feet), and vision combined with memory provide additional data. On the basis of this information, a decision is reached, and the commands of the brain and spinal cord are carried to the muscles through the motor nerves. Decision for action may be reached at a simple level involving only a single segment of the spinal cord or may necessitate participation by all levels of the central nervous system, up to and including the cerebral cortex, the seat of the intellect. An example of action on a simple level is the knee or ankle jerk. The muscle is suddenly stretched by a blow on its tendon and in turn contracts, a basic antigravity mechanism. Action of a more complicated sort would be illustrated by a circus acrobat walking the length of the tight wire.

The discussion of bone must start with a description of cartilage, since the majority of the bones of the adult skeleton have their origin in the fetus as cartilages of similar shapes. *Cartilage* is a tough elastic substance which is strong enough to form the entire skeleton in many of the fishes. It consists of a matrix, in which are scattered cartilage cells, enclosed by a layer of perichondrium which merges with the surrounding connective tissue. Cartilage develops from primitive mesenchymal or connective tissue in areas called centers of chondrification. Why these develop in the positions appropriate for the subsequent arrangement of the skeleton is entirely unknown. Bone develops relatively late in embryonic life, after the muscles, nerves, vessels, and many of the organs have been formed. Membrane bones, those of the face and skull, are formed directly from connective tissue. Cartilage bones, which include most of the others in the body, are formed first in the cartilage. In both these situations, chemical change of a type not entirely clear takes place in the original tissue, and so-called bone matrix is formed. Soon after its formation, the matrix attracts certain calcium salts, following which ossification takes place. This process is carried out by the periosteal tissue; a dense layer of cortical bone forms the shaft or *diaphysis*. Within the substance of the bone the process is carried out in such a fashion that a network of spicules, the so-called cancellous or spongy bone, is formed. Cells called osteoblasts and osteoclasts line up on the surfaces of these spicules, the former making bone, the latter destroying it, so that the architecture is continually being changed in response to growth and to mechanical stresses and strains that affect the bones.

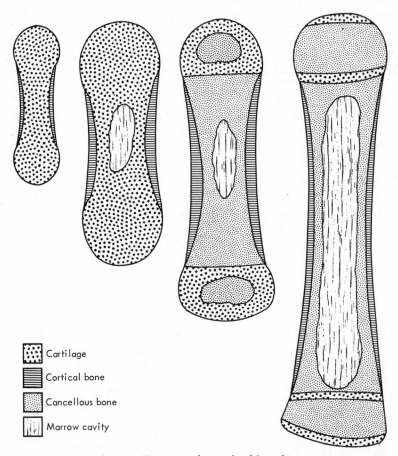

Figure 2. Diagram of growth of long bones.

Growth in length occurs chiefly through the activity of the uncalcified cartilage. At each end of the cortical bone that forms the shaft there is a rounded mass of cartilage. Cells in these masses divide, form longitudinal rows, and as ossification takes place at the inner end of these rows, new cells are formed at the outer. Thus the shaft increases in length. After a time osteogenic tissue appears within the cartilage masses, and small areas of bone are formed known as *epiphyses.* Between the epiphysis and diaphysis a layer of cartilage remains which allows for further growth of the older child and adolescent. In the adult this too becomes ossified. It should be emphasized that adult bone is not simply an inert structural material, but living tissue whose mineral composition fluctuates under the influence of the other body functions. Trabeculae of bone constitute a calcium store readily available for the maintenance of the calcium requirements of other tissues when the exogenous supplies are deficient.

Bones may be joined in two ways. If the connection is made by fibrous tissue, as between the bones of the skull, or by modified cartilaginous tissue, as between the vertebral bodies, only limited motion is present. This joint is known as a *synarthrosis*. In the majority of the joints, however, the connective tissue between the bones remains loose in texture, and early in fetal life a cleft forms within it containing tissue fluid. This is the joint *cavity.* It is bounded by the opposing articular cartilages at the ends of the two bones and by the joint *capsule,* a continuous curtain connecting their sides. As the joint develops, the perichondrium disappears where the articular cartilages on the bone ends come in contact with each other. The joint capsule develops into an outer fibrous layer, thickened areas of which are called *ligaments,* and an inner layer, *synovial tissue,* which in effect lines the joint. A specialized protein called *mucin* develops in the joint fluid to provide adequate lubrication for the opposed cartilage surfaces.

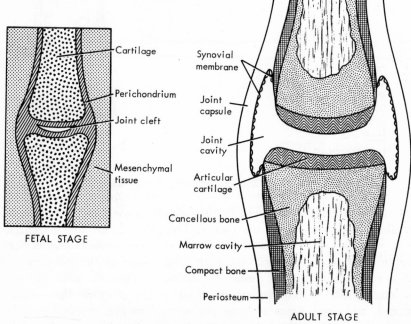

Figure 3. Diagram of the development of a diarthrodial joint.

Muscle develops early in fetal life from the same mesenchymal tissue that later gives rise to cartilage and bone. Mesenchymal cells become immature muscle cells through a process that is not understood;

these muscle cells in the embryo grow out to develop into the future muscles of the body and limbs. As the cells become older they become filled with fibrils which run the entire length of the cell; the nuclei move to the outer surface. The most conspicuous characteristic of skeletal muscle is that the fibrils are composed of alternating light and dark portions, so arranged that the dark parts of one fibril are located beside the dark parts of the next. Thus, light and dark transverse bands pass from one side of the fiber to the other giving a striated appearance and accounting for this term being applied to skeletal muscle. The striations coincide with the physical dimensions of the proteins of which the tissue is made. These proteins, actin and myosin, combine when the muscle is stimulated, forming a complex that is unstable in its extended or resting state and dissipates energy by either shortening or increased tension. Energy-utilizing chemical reactions then occur which return these proteins to their original condition. Thus is chemical energy transformed into mechanical work.

DISEASES OF BONE

CONGENITAL

Osteogenesis imperfecta is an inherited generalized disorder in which osteoid in bone and collagen in connective tissue are not properly formed. It is characterized clinically by abnormalities in a variety of organs in the body. These may occur in various combinations and in various degrees of severity. The most prominent feature of the disease is multiple fractures occurring with minimal trauma. These are particularly prominent in childhood; they occur less frequently after puberty. Bowing of the legs, dwarfism with shortening of the legs, a large head with flattening of the base of the skull (platybasia), and thinning of the bones (shown by x-ray) are features of severe cases. Loose-jointedness is prominent with easy dislocation of joints. The sclera of the eye may show blue discoloration. Progressive deafness is entirely similar to that which occurs in otosclerosis.

Achondroplasia, one of the causes of dwarfism, is characterized by the appearance, shortly after birth, of short fingers, arms, and legs, and a large head with prominent forehead, pug nose, and prominent jaw. These individuals have normal intelligence and often pleasant dispositions. The defect responsible for this disease is not known. The problem consists of retarded growth of bone at the epiphysial plates at the ends of the bones of the limbs, and premature ossification and fusion of the bones at the base of the skull. There are many other congenital defects of skeletal ossification. (For a complete discussion of this topic, the reader is referred to textbooks of orthopedic surgery or pathology.)

FRACTURES

Trauma is an integral part of man's existence in the three dimensions of space, and as related to the skeletal system, trauma of significance manifests itself as fracture of bone. Aside from the catastrophic trauma that occurs in automobile, train, and airplane wrecks, explosions, falls from high places, and so on, accidents generally follow certain patterns, and certain injuries are commonly seen. The collarbone (clavicle), being fixed at either end, buckles in the middle when force is applied in an inward direction, as in falls upon the point of the shoulder or upon the outstretched rigidly held arm. Fractures of the upper end of the humerus are produced in the same fashion. The shaft of the humerus is broken by violence of a direct sort, but torsional strains, even muscular effort as in throwing a ball, may produce spiral or very long fractures. Falls upon the outstretched arm produce a variety of fractures about the elbow joint. The condyles of the humerus may be broken in several ways; the olecranon may be separated from the ulna by forced contraction of the triceps; the head of the radius may be crushed or split. Fractures of the bones of the forearm are generally the result of direct trauma and are a common fracture of childhood. The most common fracture, caused by a fall on the outstretched arm, is the so-called Colles' fracture of the wrist, in which the lower end of the radius is displaced backward. This type of injury may also fracture the carpal scaphoid, one of the bones of the wrist. The meta-carpals are broken by striking a blow with the hand closed in a fist. Broken fingers are caused by direct violence as from a car door or from a blow that violently flexes or extends one of the phalanges. At the point of flexion or extension, either an extensor or flexor tendon pulls a fragment of bone from the articular surface. This is the so-called "baseball finger."

In the lower extremity, fracture of the pelvis is produced by direct violence of a severe sort, such as a crush between cars or the passage of a heavy vehicle over the body. A variety of breaks in the region of the femoral neck are produced by falls in which an elderly individual does not react quickly enough to check the fall by putting out an arm. Fractures of the shaft of the femur and fractures about the knee joint are due to direct violence. The "bumper fracture" is a product of modern times in which a blow on the lateral aspect of the knee, commonly by an automobile bumper, causes the lateral femoral condyle to compress the lateral tibial table. Fractures of the tibia, and less commonly both tibia and fibula, are caused directly or by falls in which there is twisting of the lower leg resulting in a spiral break. Fractures of the tibia and fibula at the ankle, Pott's fracture, are produced most commonly by turning the ankle out (eversion and abduction). Turning the ankle in (adduction), a much more prevalent injury, produces as a rule only sprain of ligaments. Fractures of the heel (*os calcis*) result from a fall in which the patient lands on his heel. Breaks of the metatarsals and toes are caused by direct trauma. Fractures of the ribs, jaws, bones of the face, and skull are similarly caused. Fractures of the spine most commonly consist of crushed vertebral bodies produced when the patient falls in a sitting position with the spine flexed.

Aside from displacement of bony fragments produced by the injury, the surgeon must deal with the forces applied to these fragments by various groups of muscles. This is an important factor to be considered when fractures are reduced to anatomical position and immobilized awaiting the healing process. The manipulation involved in reducing or setting a fracture is dependent on the amount of displacement present. This may vary from none at all to marked degrees of shattering (comminution).

Healing takes place through organization and scarring of the hematoma about the broken ends of bone. In this fibrous tissue, new bone (callus) is formed both inside and outside the previous limits of the skeleton. Once firm union is obtained and the part is again put to use, the bone is gradually remolded into its original form. If, for some reason, immobilization during the healing process is not complete, or if bits of soft tissue are interposed between the bone ends, callus formation will be hindered, a condition called nonunion. When one immobilizes a fracture limb in plaster, one necessarily immobilizes the joints adjacent to the fracture site, and this, due to some little understood property of joint tissue, results in temporary immobility when the plaster is removed. Physical therapy, with emphasis on active exercise, will restore motion in a matter of several days to several weeks.

INFECTION

Acute osteomyelitis is a destructive invasion of bone, periosteum, and marrow by pyogenic (pus-producing) organisms. Ninety per cent of all cases are due to the staphylococcus, and the remainder are caused by a variety of organisms: streptococcus, gonococcus, pneumococcus, typhoid and colon bacillus. Osteomyelitis may occur following a compound fracture, but in general it is secondary to a focus of infection elsewhere in the body. With the widespread use of antibiotics that has prevailed in recent years, osteomyelitis is less frequently seen than in the past. Presumably the spread of organisms has been prevented by the drugs. The disease occurs most commonly in the first decade of life. Clinically the patient complains of severe pain associated with marked spasm of muscles, limiting motion of the affected part. The systemic symptoms—fever, rapid pulse, and general prostration—may be alarming. Pus formation under the sensitive periosteum is the chief source of pain, the bone itself being insensitive. Once proper drainage is established, the pain is relieved to a great degree. Surgical intervention is now routinely preceded by antibiotic, fluid, and transfusion therapy; in many cases this treatment instituted early will make surgery unnecessary. In the differential diagnosis one must consider cellulitis, trauma, acute rheumatoid arthritis, and rheumatic fever. Osteomyelitis may become chronic under several circumstances. Probably the most common is the continued presence of dead bone (sequestrum) in the depths of the abscess cavity. Extension of the infection into a joint or persistence of sinus tracts connecting the infected area with the outside may also lead to chronicity. On rare occasions, skin from the surface may grow into the sinus tract and partially line the abscess cavity itself. Other factors promoting chronicity are inadequate antibiotic therapy and the presence of other disease, reducing the patient's resistance. In general, the chronic case yields only to a combined medical and surgical program: careful choice of antibiotic based on the sensitivity of the infecting organism, and wide opening of the involved area to provide adequate drainage of purulent material and removal of all nonviable tissue. When the time-consuming process of healing is completed, mobilization and rehabilitation of the patient may be carried out.

Tuberculosis of bone is a form of chronic osteomyelitis which practically always develops secondary to pulmonary or alimentary tract infections. Since tuberculin testing of dairy herds and pasteurization of milk have become standard public health practice, alimentary tract infection with the bovine strain of the tubercle bacillus has all but disappeared, and secondary infection of the skeletal system, once common in childhood, is now a rarity. Bone lesions caused by the human strain are entirely similar and generally occur in cases of advanced pulmonary tuberculosis. Tubercle bacilli are carried to the skeleton by the blood stream. Except for vertebral lesions, in the majority of cases of bone tuberculosis a joint is also involved. The question of the exact location of the initial focus has never been clearly settled. Synovial or joint tuberculosis very promptly extends into the adjacent bone, and bone tuberculosis almost invariably involves the adjacent joint.

In the spines of children, the tuberculosis lesion appears in the center of a vertebral body. In the adult, foci originate in the ligaments over the anterior aspect of the spine and spread backward into the adjacent vertebral bodies. In either case, one gets collapse of vertebral bodies and dorsal angulation of the spine. The disease is suspected when an indolent infection is present, producing a certain pattern of bone destruction on x-ray. The diagnosis is made by obtaining tissue from the involved area, by either needle or open biopsy, and recovering tubercle bacilli or observing characteristic tuberculous granulation tissue under the microscope.

The antituberculous drugs have markedly improved the outlook. At the present time, tuberculous osteomyelitis and arthritis caught early may be completely eradicated by a program of bed rest, a good diet, and immobilization of the part in combination with one, two, or all three of the most commonly used drugs—streptomycin, isoniazid (INH), and para-aminosalicylic acid. Surgery still holds a place in the treatment of the more chronic lesion where scar tissue and caseation have appeared, but the use of the drugs makes it possible to apply the principles of surgical debridement of necrotic tissue and drainage of the abscess without fear of spreading the disease. Surgical fusion of large joints to make the healing process more certain is still performed if significant destruction is present. As may be seen, treatment of this disease is also a time-consuming process; the mobilization and rehabilitation of the patient are often long delayed.

Lesions of the third stage of *syphilis* (gummas) may occur in bone. With penicillin treatment so effective, one is not apt to encounter even tertiary syphilis, let alone a gumma in bone, but one should be aware of the fact that this does occur.

There are various infectious fungal diseases that may involve bone— *actinomycosis, blastomycosis,* and *coccidioidomycosis*—but the primary infection in each instance is elsewhere, and the bone disease is secondary.

NUTRITIONAL DEFICIENCIES

There are two diseases of bone classified as vitamin deficiencies: *rickets* (osteomalacia in the adult), due to lack of vitamin D, and *scurvy,* due to lack of vitamin C. In children these diseases are seen rarely at present, and then as the result of only the most abject deprivation. The difficulty in rickets is that calcium and phosphorus salts are not properly laid down in the areas where bone is growing; enlargement of the costochondral junctions and of the ends of the long bones of the extremities, bowing of the legs, and pelvic deformities result. Chronic kidney disease, through a disturbance in calcium and phosphorus metabolism, can cause a change in the bones similar to that of rickets, which is called *renal rickets.* It represents another cause of dwarfism and is fortunately rare. In the adult, osteomalacia, when severe, can cause deformities of the bones similar to those of rickets in children. It is seen in certain countries in Asia where the diet is deficient in calcium and vitamin D, where many pregnancies and prolonged lactation early in life are the custom, and where women spend a secluded existence indoors out of the sun. In the United States it occurs only as a result of intestinal disease where absorption of fat and secondarily of vitamin D is prevented.

Scurvy in infants manifests itself as subperiosteal hemorrhages which are very tender. Scurvy in adults in past generations was commonly associated with the extreme dietary deprivation of long sea voyages. At the present time it is seen only in alcoholics whose food intake is extraordinarily limited; it is manifested by changes in the skin and in subcutaneous hemorrhages. It rarely reaches the stage of osteoporosis, loss of teeth, and failure of wound or fracture healing.

RETICULOENDOTHELIOSES AND LIPID STORAGE DISEASES

In this group of diseases where the causation is unknown, the lesions consist of destructive granulomas in bone which clinically must be differentiated from neoplasm. Eosinophilic granuloma, Hand-Schüller-Christian disease, and Letterer-Siwe disease are primarily granulomas. Gaucher's disease, Niemann-Pick disease, and solitary xanthoma show primarily deposits of unusual types of fat. Only eosinophilic granuloma, solitary xanthoma, and Gaucher's disease have their onset and prove to be problems in adult life. The first two are strictly localized to the skeleton; the third shows characteristic lesions in liver, spleen, and deep lymph nodes in addition. Since the skeletal involvement must be differentiated from neoplasm, surgical intervention for biopsy is the usual practice; occasionally the lesion may be excised completely. Aside from this, there is no effective treatment.

ENDOCRINE DISEASES

There are a variety of diseases of endocrine glands that produce alterations in the skeleton. Excess secretion of growth hormones by the pituitary gland occurring prior to puberty produces *gigantism*, the skeletal system increasing in all dimensions. Such excess secretion occurring after puberty produces a condition known as *acromegaly*, in which the bones increase in bulk but not in length. The patient in the advanced stages presents a picture bordering on the grotesque, with coarse facial features, lantern jaw, massive hands and feet, barrel chest, and dorsal kyphosis. Excess secretion of adrenocorticotropic hormone (ACTH) by the pituitary (Cushing's disease) produces excess secretion of cortisone by the adrenals. Marked osteoporosis (decalcification of the bones) follows, often with compression fractures of the vertebrae secondary to minimal trauma. Lack of pituitary secretion in childhood produces not only dwarfism but lack of secondary sex characteristics. This is the childlike or "little orphan Annie" type of dwarf. Another type of dwarfism, *progeria*, in which the patient, even as a child, takes on an aged appearance, is thought to be related to pituitary deficiency.

Hyperthyroidism produces excess excretion of calcium and osteoporosis, but usually the disease is recognized and treated before this stage is reached.

Hypothyroidism in childhood (cretinism) is another cause of dwarfism. This is easily treated with thyroid but is often associated with other defects, particularly mental retardation.

The parathyroid glands control the balance of calcium and phosphorus in the body. Excess secretion of the hormone produces high blood levels of calcium, increased calcium excretion in the urine, and decalcification of bone in a pattern known as generalized *osteitis fibrosa*. If the patient has a good intake of calcium, the bone changes may not appear; the disease will then manifest itself through calcium stones in the kidneys. Treatment is surgical; removal of an adenoma or hyperplastic parathyroid glands results in cure. Diminished secretion of parathyroid hormone is characterized by the rather dramatic symptom of tetany convulsions but produces no bone disease.

Excess secretion of cortisone by an adrenal cortical tumor or hyperplasia will produce Cushing's syndrome with the same effect upon the skeleton as the pituitary condition (Cushing's disease) described above. Treatment is surgical. The same changes are produced by long-continued administration of cortisone-type drugs for chronic arthritis or asthma.

There are no characteristic bone lesions associated with the masculinizing or virilizing effects of another type of adrenocortical disease called the *adrenogenital syndrome* or with the lack of adrenal secretion, *Addison's disease*.

The only significant bone lesion associated with the gonads is the osteoporosis that occurs fairly commonly following the menopause in women and also occasionally in older men. This condition presents itself with the symptom of back pain and may go on to compression fractures of the vertebrae. Treatment consists of replacement of the appropriate hormone, estrogen or androgen.

PAGET'S DISEASE

Paget's disease is a localized disturbance of bone growth in which the microscopic architecture of the involved area is disrupted by rapid bone destruction and repair proceeding concomitantly. The process may be minimal and asymptomatic, involving only part of one bone. Under these circumstances it is an incidental finding when x-rays are taken for some other reason. It may also be extensive, involving most of the bones of the body. If extensive, the gross architecture of the bone is affected, and one sees characteristically increased size of the skull and bowing of the legs. Pathological fractures may occur. It is a disease of the middle years; severe involvement is fortunately rare, since no effective treatment is known.

PULMONARY HYPERTROPHIC OSTEOARTHROPATHY

This syndrome consists of the deposition of new bone in the periosteum around the shafts of the bones of the extremities. There is also nonspecific nondestructive inflammation of the joints and clubbing of the fingers, a situation where the nails became widened, brittle, and dome-shaped, curving over the ends of the fingers. This disease is caused by conditions of the lung, either chronic suppurative disease or tumor. The mechanism is unknown, but interestingly, if the lung disease can be eradicated either surgically or otherwise, the osteo-arthropathy will disappear.

NEOPLASM

Bone tumors are classified on the basis of their microscopic structure, the principal component tissue dictating the name. This is not an entirely satisfactory method of classification, but will have to do until more is known about the cause of these growths. In general, the benign tumors appear as asymptomatic masses, whereas the first symptom with malignant tumors is pain, which in the early stages may be intermittent. Physical examination is of little help in diagnosis, but many tumors show a characteristic appearance on x-ray, and the actual presence or absence of a bone tumor can be easily determined by this means. However, for an accurate diagnosis, surgical biopsy with microscopic examination of the tissue is necessary. In general, the rehabilitation worker will encounter the bone tumor patient where an amputation of the affected limb has been performed and a prosthesis is being used. It should be recalled, however, that the most common cause of malignant tumor in bone is spread or metastasis from origins in an internal organ. Breast, thyroid, lung, prostate, and kidney are common sites. Treatment depends on the nature of the growth; local excision, amputation, or radiation therapy are all used in appropriate situations.

ASEPTIC OSSEOUS NECROSIS

Nearly every secondary epiphysis and many of the primary epiphyses in the body have been observed to be the site of *aseptic osseous necrosis*, a condition also called *osteochondritis*, in which, for some unknown reason, the bone dies and is gradually replaced by new bone. Rapid growth is believed to make the epiphysis more vulnerable. Primary epiphyses become involved during infancy and childhood, secondary epiphyses during puberty, the period of their most rapid growth. The common areas involved are the capital epiphysis of the femur, the tibial tubercle, the primary and secondary epiphyses of the patella, the tarsal navicular, the second metatarsal head, the apophysis tuber of the *os calcis,* the head of the humerus, and the primary and secondary epiphyses of the vertebral bodies. The chief symptom produced by these conditions is pain; the diagnosis may be suspected if this is localized characteristically. Essentially, however, this is an x-ray diagnosis, and the course of the disease from onset to complete healing can be followed very nicely on films. The most important feature of treatment is that the affected area must not be subjected to any mechanical stress, since in the regenerative phase the bone is soft, and distortion of the contour is possible. This is particularly important where articular surfaces are involved, since even though healing appears to be taking place anatomically, minor derangements may cause degenerative arthritis to appear years later.

Osteochondritis dissecans is a similar process pathologically which occurs most commonly in young adults. A segment of bone adjacent to joint cartilage becomes necrotic. If undisturbed it may remain in its bed and subsequently regenerate. It may, however, drop into the joint and become a loose body. Treatment in this condition, as in epiphysial involvement, consists of protection of the joint so that healing may take place. However, if the fragment becomes loose and interferes with the mechanics of the joint, it should be removed surgically. Aseptic necrosis of bone may also occur related to certain fractures and dislocations where the blood supply is interrupted. This is most commonly seen in femoral neck fractures where the presence of a necrotic femoral head is an indication for insertion of a metal prosthesis.

DISEASES OF JOINTS

CONGENITAL

There are several diseases in which the underlying defect is a biochemical abnormality of connective tissue. In the so-called Marfan's syndrome, patients are tall and thin with excessive length of arms and legs and loose-jointedness. There is subluxation of the lens of the eye and weakness and dilatation of the aorta. The Ehlers-Danlos syndrome is characterized clinically by fragility and hypoelasticity of the skin and loose-jointedness. Osteogenesis imperfecta is a disease the cause of which falls into the same category; it was discussed in the section on bone. In pseudoxanthoma elasticum, there is a premature breakdown of collagen fibers resulting in lax, redundant skin, angioid streaks in the ocular fundi which can go on to proliferative changes interfering with vision, early changes of arteriosclerosis with calcification of blood vessels, and a tendency to bleed from various sites—gastrointestinal, uterine, urinary, nasal, and subarachnoid. The Hurler syndrome shows skeletal malformations, stiff joints, disease of the heart valves, deafness, enlarged liver and spleen, clouding of the cornea, and impairment of intellect. All of these diseases may occur in varying degrees of severity and often come to the attention of the physician because of musculoskeletal symptoms. Rehabilitation workers will see these patients generally as adolescents with educational, social, and vocational problems.

There are a variety of congenital deformities involving the bones and joints, some severe, some minor. In the following, the more common will be discussed. Congenital dislocation of the hip is caused by the acetabulum being too shallow to contain the head of the femur, which slips up and back. If the condition is recognized early, the hip may be reduced and immobilized in the abducted or frogleg position. In this way, the small infant will reform the acetabulum, and a good result may be expected. If the condition is not recognized, a characteristic waddling gait appears when the child begins to walk. The older the child, the more difficult the reduction; at times surgical revision of the acetabulum may be necessary to maintain the femoral head in proper position.

Congenital *talipes equinovarus,* or clubfoot, consists of varying degrees of four elements of deformity: flexion of the ankle, inversion of the foot, abduction of the forefoot, and medial rotation of the tibia. In the early case this is a deformity of soft tissue only, and treatment, consisting of manipulating the foot into the proper position and maintaining this position with appropriate splints, is always easy and successful. In cases where this early program has not been carried out, operative intervention may be necessary to correct the deformity.

Cervical rib and the *scalenus syndrome* are discussed together since the symptoms are similar, caused by pressure on nerves and vessels as they emerge from the base of the neck. Nerve symptoms are sensory, consisting of weakness and atrophy of muscles in the hand. Vessel symptoms consist usually only of a dusky discoloration of the hand, but if severe, gangrene of the fingers may appear secondary to obstruction of blood flow. When the symptoms are mild, postural exercises may provide relief; when severe, surgical removal of the extra rib or section of the scalenus anticus muscle may be necessary to relieve the pressure.

The spine is subject to many congenital variations, some serious, some of no consequence. The articular facets that join the vetebrae to each other may be oriented in many different ways, some of which are not entirely sound mechanically and make the spine susceptible to various sprains and strains. *Spondylolisthesis* is a condition in which the neural arch is not complete—that is, the anterior and posterior parts of the vertebra are not joined together, so that the anterior half tends to slide forward. Depending on the severity of the condition, treatment may be conservative, with exercises and a corset, or operative, producing fusion of the spine. Just as extra ribs may grow on the lowest cervical or the highest lumbar vertebra, so the lowest lumbar vertebra may become part of the sacrum in that the transverse processes form joints with the ilium. In opposite fashion, the first sacral vertebra may have all the characteristics of a lumbar vertebra.

A wide range of variation is possible which, as mentioned above, causes symptoms when not mechanically sound.

Scoliosis, or lateral curvature of the spine, can be divided into two general categories: (1) functional, which is within the normal range of motion of the spine; it is due to abnormal postural habits and can be corrected voluntarily by the child; and (2) structural, in which there is an actual deformity of the spine and ribs. The vertebral column rotates toward the convex side of the curve as well as bending laterally. The cause of this type is completely unknown. It occurs in children, coming on generally at about the age of five or six, and may be mild or rapidly progressive. Treatment consists of exercises, corrective jackets, and if the deformity is severe, spinal fusion.

Spina bifida is a congenital gap in the vertebral column through which the contents of the spinal canal may be protruded. This, like so many other congenital defects, may occur in all grades of severity, ranging from a bony defect in the spine causing no symptoms and only seen incidentally on x-ray, to an extensive myelomeningocele where the spinal cord and its coverings are on the surface of the back, a situation incompatible with life.

Many less common congenital deformities of the limbs have their origin in growth abnormalities of the limb buds in the embryo; among these are absence of various parts of the limbs, bifid fingers, webbed fingers, short neck or webbed neck, and dislocation of the knees. These defects often occur in combination with one another; occasionally extensive surgical reconstruction and use of prosthetic devices are required.

TRAUMA

A wide variety of joints are subject to dislocation caused by trauma. In most instances, the trauma must be serious; often there are associated fractures. There are two exceptions to this general statement—dislocation of the shoulder and dislocation of the patella. Dislocation of the shoulder may be accomplished without the application of great force; once the joint has dislocated, it is subject to recurrent dislocation with less force required each time. This is a disease of young adults who find that after a number of these episodes the shoulder may be reduced without help. The uncertainty that such a disability causes in a young, active individual makes it generally advisable to correct the lesion surgically, which can be done easily with assurance of a good result. The second dislocation of a habitual and recurrent nature is that of the patella, which slides laterally out of its groove between the femoral condyles, causing the patient, usually a young woman, to fall to the ground. Initially the treatment is conservative—a firm bandage or knee cage and exercises for the quadriceps. If the condition persists, there are several types of operative procedures that give good results.

Another general type of injury is tendon rupture. The so-called mallet finger results when the end of the finger is struck, by a ball, for instance, forcibly flexed, and the extensor tendon detached from its insertion in the distal phalanx. Often a bit of bone is pulled away by the tendon. Treatment is conservative—immobilization in plaster with the finger extended. The biceps tendons are occasionally ruptured, more often at the shoulder than at the elbow, and treatment is operative. The extensor tendon of the thumb is rarely ruptured at the wrist secondary to fracture in this area. During powerful contraction of the anterior thigh muscles or quadriceps, rupture may occur above, through the middle of, or below the patella. Operative repair is always indicated. The most common injury of this type is rupture of the Achilles tendon, an accident of middle life seen commonly in tennis or badminton players. As with injuries about the knee, treatment is surgical and should be prompt.

There is a category of conditions called internal derangement of the knee, generally secondary to trauma, which includes rupture of the medial ligaments, fracture of the tibial spine, rupture of the cruciate ligaments, loose bodies in the joint due to a variety of causes, injury to the patellar fat pad, and injury to the semilunar cartilages or menisci.

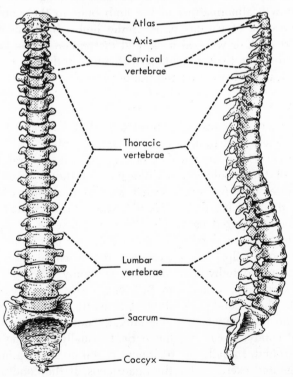

Atlas
Axis
Cervical vertebrae
Thoracic vertebrae
Lumbar vertebrae
Sacrum
Coccyx

Figure 4. The vertebral column—posterior and lateral views.

The last, which is by far the most common, is usually related to athletic injury in which the lower leg is twisted outward with the knee flexed. This is followed by pain and swelling of the knee, often with locking of the joint in the flexed position. The significance of this injury is that healing of the torn cartilage does not readily occur, and the loose segment tends to slip between the opposing surfaces of the femur and tibia, causing recurrent locking of the joint. Should this situation develop, the cartilage may be readily removed surgically.

The spine is susceptible to a wide variety of trauma. The major injuries producing fractures of different types have been discussed in a previous section. Also discussed previously were several congenital conditions that weaken the mechanical integrity of the spine. Minor trauma which produces various strains and sprains of the joints of the spinal column is exceedingly common, and back pain as the symptom is one of man's most frequent complaints. The spine as originally developed in vertebrate creatures is very nicely adapted to its purpose—namely, a flexible compression member the position of which is controlled by muscle groups alternately contracting and relaxing on all four sides.

The quadripedal gait provides no unusual problems in terms of adaptation. However, when man assumed the upright bipedal posture it was necessary that the lower end of the spine be bent backward at an angle of about 45 degrees (the normal lumbar lordosis) and that compensatory curves (the dorsal kyphosis, the cervical lordosis) make their appearance so that balance might be achieved. In addition to producing a mechanism that was slightly awkward mechanically, this new arrangement added gravity (the weight of the upper part of the body) as a compression force on the spine. The problem of balancing the upper half of the body on the pelvis and of balancing the head on the shoulders is very nicely handled by a delicate system of neuromuscular reflexes in which information about the relative positions of the different joints and the tension on different ligaments and tendons is sent to the spinal cord over proprioceptive sensory nerves. From there, after some computation, the necessary commands are sent back to the muscles over motor nerves, causing some to contract and some to relax, thereby keeping the head and body balanced on the flexible spinal column. Strains and sprains of the joints of the spine that would be considered minor if they occurred in an ankle, for instance, cause symptoms all out of proportion to their severity, since the very delicate neuromuscular reflexes are upset, and marked spasm and inhibition of different muscle groups supervene. These in themselves are painful and disabling. Oftentimes the trauma necessary is minimal, such as sneezing or rolling over in bed.

Poor posture can predispose to backstrain, the joints of the spine being held in inappropriate mechanical relationship by muscles that are

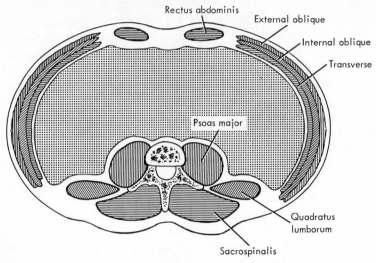

Rectus abdominis

External oblique

Internal oblique

Transverse

Psoas major

Quadratus lumborum

Sacrospinalis

Figure 5. Transverse section of the body at the level of the abdomen showing the muscle groups that maintain the upright posture.

slack. Chronic low back pain can often be improved by exercises aimed at strengthening certain groups of muscles that hold the spine erect.

Protrusion or rupture of an intervertebral disc is caused by a weakening of the strong fibrous ring that forms the outer wall of the disc, and protrusion through this ring, or *annulus fibrosus*, of the gelatinous material forming the inner structure of the disc, the *nucleus pulposus*. When this occurs, nerve roots from the spinal cord are compressed where they leave the spinal canal, and symptoms are produced in the distribution of the nerves. This condition is most often seen in the lower lumbar spine. The nerve affected is the sciatic, hence the name *sciatica*, referring to the symptom of pain in the posterior thigh and calf with radiation to the buttock and to the lateral aspect of the lower leg and foot. Associated may be sensory symptoms of numbness or tingling and muscle symptoms of weakness. On examination, straight leg raising may be limited, reflexes in the leg may be lessened, and muscle bulk may be reduced. Symptoms and signs vary with the extent of the protrusion and the level in the spine at which it is located. In severe cases, there may be paralysis of the lower extremities and interference with the function of the bowel and bladder.

All cases of sciatica are not caused by intervertebral disc rupture. Strains and sprains of certain areas in the spinal column will produce pain radiating into a limb. Because of this, the introduction of a radiopaque liquid into the spinal canal, for a *myelogram*, is often helpful in outlining the disc protrusion by x-ray. Treatment is either conservative or operative. It is estimated that approximately half of the cases will recover over the course of a few months to a year on a regimen of rest, bed board, heat, exercises, and sedation. In these cases, apparently the protruded section of disc is lacking in proper blood supply and is gradually absorbed. If this does not prove to be the case, and especially if there is evidence of loss of nerve function, the treatment of choice is operative, removal of the disc. Whether this is combined with a spinal fusion depends on evidence for stability of the spine determined by history, physical examination, and at the operating table. The results of surgery in the straightforward case are excellent.

Low back pain as a general complaint presents the physician with an extremely difficult problem to diagnose and treat. There are many causes of this symptom; a great number of them have their origin in obscure abnormalities in function, with little or nothing that can be made out anatomically. Two additional considerations should be noted: back pain and the disability caused therefrom are frequently magnified for psychological reasons, and the problem of compensation for injury often enters the picture. With these intertwined factors to untangle, one can easily understand the difficulties often encountered. The rehabilitation center will see many cases of this sort, and for obvious reasons the more complicated patients will be included.

Myositis ossificans occurs as a complication of trauma to muscles. It is most frequently related to fractures and dislocations about the elbow, or injuries affecting the anterior and medial thigh muscles. The condition consists of metaplastic production of bone in scar. Under the microscope the tissue consists of a random mixture of bone, cartilage, muscle, and connective tissue. Symptoms consist of pain and swelling which recur two to three weeks after the pain and swelling of the original injury have subsided. After several months the pain subsides, and the swelling becomes more firm as the metaplastic tissue becomes increasingly ossified. In the early stages the most difficult and important lesion to differentiate is bone sarcoma; the x-ray appearance and even the pathological appearance may be similar. Regarding treatment, the less that is done to the early lesion of myositis ossificans the better. Most cases will, after a period of time, show a marked tendency to regress; therefore biopsy, operative removal, and physical therapy should be avoided. Excision of the mass may be considered when it has become stationary by x-ray examination, but then only if it is unusually large or is causing great limitation of motion.

Volkmann's ischemic contracture, which may follow fractures about the elbow joint, is caused by injury to the principal artery of the arm with spasm and resulting loss of blood supply to the muscles of the forearm. The symptoms appear within 24 hours after the injury and consist of a cold, swollen cyanotic, functionless hand with prominent pain in the forearm and often numbness of the fingers. The damage has been done within two days. Subsequently, the muscles of the forearm become fibrosed, and flexion deformity of the wrist and fingers gradually appears. The condition may occur in varying degrees of severity from minimal contraction of the fingers to marked changes with involvement of the median and ulnar nerves, partial anesthesia, paralysis of the small muscles of the hand, and trophic ulceration. Early treatment is extremely important, the goal being to restore adequate circulation before irreparable damage is done. All constricting bandages should be removed, Novocaine block of the cervical sympathetic vasoconstrictor nerves should be carried out, and if these measures do not produce improvement, direct surgical exposure of the involved segment of vessel with removal of perivascular sympathetic nerves may be done. Open reduction of the fracture to produce the best possible alignment of fragments should also be considered at this point. Treatment of the fully developed stage depends on its severity; manipulation, splints, physical therapy, or operative intervention to lengthen muscles and to free nerves may be carried out.

ARTHRITIS DUE TO KNOWN INFECTIOUS AGENT

The term *arthritis* means simply inflammation of a joint, and there are, as one might expect, many causes. When infection with a specific bacterium produces arthritis, the clinical picture is usually that of single joint involvement, either acute or chronic, depending on the nature of the organism. The streptococcus, gonococcus, pneumococcus, staphylococcus, produce an acute arthritis with pain, swelling, and heat in the joint, and fever and malaise in the patient. A more chronic low-grade infection is caused by the tubercle bacillus and rarely certain fungi. All such cases are emergencies, since prompt and proper diagnosis and treatment may stop the infection before appreciable tissue damage has taken place. Diagnosis is made by aspirating fluid from the joint and identifying the offending organism. When this is done the appropriate antibiotic may be given, readily bringing the infection under control. In the days before antibiotics it was often necessary to drain the joint surgically; as a result the healing process could be very prolonged. This is still the situation in infections that have been neglected.

In the preceding paragraph we have been speaking about the hematogenous or blood-borne infection as it occurs naturally. In recent years, arthritis of various types has been treated by injecting cortisone-type drugs directly into the joints. On occasion, bacteria, principally staphylococci, have been inadvertently introduced, resulting in sepsis. Treatment is based on the same principles as in naturally occurring infection.

RHEUMATOID ARTHRITIS

Rheumatoid arthritis may be defined as a chronic relapsing disease of unknown cause characterized by inflammation in multiple joints. It is also known as *atrophic arthritis, proliferative arthritis,* and *nonspecific polyarthritis.* Of all the rheumatic diseases it causes the most man-hours of disability, not because of severe cases being so common, but because of the lifelong duration of symptoms once the disease is firmly established.

The etiological factors may be divided generally into two groups, those having to do with the individual afflicted by the disease, the so-called intrinsic factors, and the environmental or extrinsic factors. The average age at onset is in the neighborhood of 40 years. The great majority of cases begin between ages 25 and 55. Cases have begun in infancy or in the ninth decade. Women are affected more frequently than men in a ratio of about 2 to 1. Hereditary or constitutional factors have long been suspected, since there is the occasional family in which multiple cases occur. This concept has received support recently from studies that showed that asymptomatic family members presented laboratory abnormalities characteristic of the disease. Body build and endocrine imbalance have been suggested, but not proved. A popular theory recently has been that of autoimmunity, a state in which the individual is sensitive or allergic to components of his own tissues. Undoubtedly, when the cause is discovered, it will turn out to be a simple chemical reaction in the body, since there are several situations clinically in which it is apparent that the inflammatory process is very quickly reversible.

Extrinsic factors have been postulated, but likewise never proved. Extensive search has been made of occult infection with many tonsils and teeth removed in hopes of eradicating a focus. Environmental factors such as cold and dampness certainly can exacerbate symptoms, but probably have little to do with activity of the disease. Poor housing, overcrowding, impaired nutritional state, and inferior social status have all been implicated, but more detailed study has shown the disease to be equally prevalent in the well-to-do. For many years, attention has been called to the frequency with which a history of excessive physical effort or of emotional strain has preceded the onset of rheumatoid arthritis. Studies of controlled series have shown that stressful situations occur as frequently in the normal population, but this does not necessarily diminish the importance of stress as an inciting agent. It can be compared to pulling the trigger of a gun.

Pathologically, the essential change consists of an inflammation in connective tissue that is in no way unusual except that it contains areas that have the appearance of fibrin and are therefore called fibrinoid degeneration. This seems to be the basic change, although in early lesions and with severe involvement, inflammation of small blood vessels is seen, so-called *vasculitis.* The joints contain more connective tissue proportionately than other areas of the body, and it is in the joints that the inflammatory process is most intense. There are other factors responsible for localizing the disease, however, since it is rather common to find certain joints involved while the symmetrical joints on the other side of the body are free. If the disease progresses, inflammatory and proliferative changes increase. Inflammatory tissue overgrows the cartilage, which is eroded and may actually be entirely destroyed. It also appears in the ends of the bone adjacent to the joints, causing decalcification and actual bone destruction. If the disease continues unchecked, fibrous or even bony fusion or ankylosis may appear. On the other hand, the involved joint and its neighboring bone may be completely destroyed—reduced to a mass of scar tissue. Lesions occur elsewhere than in the joint. The subcutaneous nodule is characteristic of the severe form of the disease. It consists of an area of necrosis, or dead tissue, surrounded by proliferating and inflammatory tissue located over bony prominences, the elbows, the knees, and the back of the head. Tiny lesions are often present in muscle and along the course of nerves, and on occasion lesions occur in many organs of the body.

Clinically the disease can present a most protean appearance. The symptoms and signs related to the joints are pain, swelling, stiffness, muscle wasting, limitation of motion, and deformity. The general symptoms and signs are fatigue, malaise, insomnia, agitation, depression, anorexia, weight loss, chills, sweats, fever, and anemia. These can occur in all combinations and in all grades of severity. The typical case shows symmetrical involvement of small joints of hands and wrists, feet and ankles, the knees, and perhaps the elbows and shoulders. The disease may appear in different forms, however, and even after the passage of many years the classical picture does not always become manifest. Systemic symptoms such as high fever may dominate the picture with minimal joint symptoms and signs. Only one joint may be involved. The occasional patient whose disease begins in the typical way enjoys a complete spontaneous remission which may last for years, even a lifetime. Commonly, patients have symptoms and laboratory abnormalities only with no abnormal physical findings.

There are several important variants of the clinical picture described above, and at the present time there is some question whether these constitute different diseases. Rheumatoid arthritis involving the spine—rheumatoid spondylitis or Marie-Strümpell spondylitis—is a disease of men in the ratio of 10 to 1. Severe cases progress to complete fusion of the spine; about half the time the hips and/or shoulders are affected. Other peripheral joints are involved less frequently. The rheumatoid arthritis associated with psoriasis generally presents a different pattern. The joint involvement on the whole tends to be more asymmetrical, and the rheumatoid factor, the abnormal protein in the blood that is responsible for the latex fixation and other agglutinating tests, is generally not present. Rheumatoid arthritis of children presents the same wide range of involvement as in the adult, except that rheumatoid nodules rarely develop and the rheumatoid factor is usually absent from the blood.

The course of these different patterns of disease through the years may be markedly different. At one end of the spectrum is the rapidly advancing malignant form of the disease in which the patient dies of fever and inanition within a year of onset. Starting with this same pattern, the disease may then quiet down and continue at a relatively low level of activity for years. The pattern is frequently seen in which there is an initial period of disease activity lasting anywhere up to several years, followed by a very gratifying improvement, which in turn is followed by a recrudescence of symptoms that continue subsequently. On the whole, the course of well-established disease is intermittently but gradually and inexorably progressive over the years. At the other end of the spectrum, rheumatoid arthritis may be a very mild disease with, for instance, only minor involvement of finger joints throughout the patient's life. The chief quality the physician or rehabilitation worker must deal with in regard to this disease is unpredictability. A certain degree of equanimity must be developed in the face of this problem. There is no point in arguing with the patient who believes that his arthritis was cured by six lemons taken each day before breakfast, particularly when this advice was given by an elderly aunt from California. Conversely, there is, in general, a tendency for rheumatoid arthritis to remit, and if one can only maintain an optimistic viewpoint, often the natural course of the disease will break in the patient's favor.

We do not yet have available a drug or other method of treatment whereby positive control of the disease can be achieved. Lesser measures must therefore be used which through experience have proven to be helpful although perhaps not curative; thus there is often what appears to be a certain amount of experimentation with different drugs and programs.

Treatment may be divided into several categories. The first is a conservative regimen consisting of rest, heat, physical therapy, and aspirin. The aim of this program is to support the patient physically and psychologically in expectation of a remission. The anti-inflammatory drugs are aspirin and its chemical relative, phenylbutazone and related drugs, and the various types of corticosteroid medication such as cortisone and prednisone. The last are, of course, by far the most effective but also have the greatest toxic potential. Two other types of medication are available: the aminoquinolines (chloroquine and hydroxychloroquine) used originally against malaria, and the various chemical compounds that incorporate gold. The drugs in both these groups work more slowly and have a more prolonged action once the effect is achieved.

Orthopedic treatment includes the prevention or correction of deformities by the use of plaster casts, traction, or other mechanical devices. The joints may at times be manipulated with the patient under anesthesia, and improved range of motion will result. On the other hand, when scar tissue is too heavy or when cartilage and bone destruction are present, various reconstructive surgical procedures may be carried out. The success of these different maneuvers depends basically on two factors—the activity of the inflammatory process and the vigor with which the patient carries out the postoperative physical therapy program. If the disease is quiescent, a good operative result may be expected. However, continued inflammation with its attendant scarring and tissue destruction may leave the patient in a worse position functionally than in the preoperative state. It takes a great deal of fortitude for a patient to exercise a painful joint following an operation, but this is essential, since to a great extent the function of a joint depends on the strength of the muscles that control it, and muscle strength is developed only through exercise.

The rehabilitation worker's equanimity will be sorely tried by the patient with rheumatoid arthritis. The uncertain course of the disease, the slow pace of treatment, and the intertwined psychological difficulties, which seem to be almost universally present, make therapy a difficult exercise at best. These is a certain satisfaction to be gained, however, from dealing with the problem that no one else can handle, and the occasional success is very gratifying.

DEGENERATIVE JOINT DISEASE

The term *degenerative joint disease* emphasizes a certain aspect of the condition; the other terms used—*hypertrophic arthritis* and *osteoarthritis*—emphasize other aspects. These are as follows: In all individuals there are certain degenerative changes that take place in articular cartilage. They first appear in childhood and gradually increase in frequency and severity as the years go by. These have been designated degenerative joint disease. Similar changes occur in the joints of individuals in middle age associated with evidences of abnormality in joint tissue other than cartilage. At times there may be actual inflammation of the ligaments and synovia. This is the aspect of the condition that suggests the use of the term arthritis, meaning specifically inflammation in a joint. These cases present a very interesting dilemma: how much is inflammation; how much is degeneration; what is the relationship to rheumatoid or true inflammatory arthritis? Certain aspects of the disease are clearly related to "wear and tear." This is particularly apparent in joints that have been damaged—for instance, congenital dislocation of the hip, reduced in satisfactory fashion, but still not perfect anatomically; these joints may become the sites of premature degenerative joint disease. Heredity clearly plays a role. Degenerative joint disease of the distal interphalangeal joints of the fingers (Heberden's nodes) is ten times more common in women than in men and is inherited as a sex-influenced characteristic dominant in the female and recessive in the male.

Pathologically, the cartilage becomes yellow, opaque, and less elastic. Fissures appear in its surface, and later there are chipping and pitting. In this way the cartilage is gradually destroyed. Secondarily, the bone under the cartilage becomes more dense, a process known as eburnation, and bony excrescences called osteophytes or spurs develop in the ligaments around the joint margins.

Weight-bearing joints are chiefly involved—knees, hips, lumbar spine, and cervical spine. Notable exceptions to this rule are the carpometacarpal joints of the thumbs and the distal interphalangeal joints of the fingers. Interestingly, the disease is almost universal in persons over the age of 50, and only a small proportion present symptoms, pain, stiffness, and limited mobility. Errors of overdiagnosis are frequently made, particularly in relation to the spine; before labeling the condition arthritis, one should look carefully for other causes in patients with low back pain.

While this is an annoying and often uncomfortable disease, it does not produce the crippling found in rheumatoid arthritis. Conservative measures—rest, physical therapy, and analgesia—usually suffice. Traumatic influences should be minimized. The weight should be reduced if obesity is present. Back supports, cervical collars, neck traction, may be used for the spine. Often crutches or a cane will help the patient with lower extremity involvement. Intra-articular hydrocortisone is temporarily beneficial, and in the caes with severe involvement, reconstructive orthopedic surgery offers a good result.

The disease generally occurs in older people. When one does encounter this diagnosis in a younger individual it is well to be on the lookout for other factors such as congenital conditions, old injuries, and other diseases. One should also look for psychological problems as the basic cause for referral. The joint condition may simply be a diagnosis of convenience.

GOUT

The disease *gout* was set apart as an entity very early in recorded medical history because of two rather dramatic clinical features, the tophus and the acute self-limited attack of arthritis. The tophus is a subcutaneous deposit of uric acid that occurs usually on the elbows, knees, back of the hands, and feet. It signifies that an excess of uric acid in the system is precipitating in the tissues. Deposits also occur in the joints and in the kidneys, but, of course, cannot be seen in these locations. This excess uric acid (hyperuricemia) can easily be demonstrated in the blood chemically. The condition is familial; in fact, studies of families have shown that hyperuricemia is prevalent in asymptomatic relatives of gouty patients.

The attack of arthritis is particularly dramatic because when severe it can be indistinguishable from a septic joint—heat, redness, swelling, severe pain, immobility, and a sick febrile patient. Then instead of going on to destruction of the joint as would occur with infection, the whole process subsides over the course of two to four weeks, leaving no trace. Gout is a disease that can vary greatly in severity: an individual may have only one attack in his entire life or attacks may be frequent with progressive severe destruction of joints. In general, during the early phases of the disease the attacks clear completely, but as the years go by, a chronic phase develops, joint damage becomes manifest, and symptoms do not clear following each attack.

This is a condition affecting men in a ratio of about 20 to 1. There is a definite familial incidence. Diet and intake of alcoholic beverages, once felt to be important, are no longer considered so. Trauma of all sorts, including burns, operations, and excessive unaccustomed physical exercise, may set off an attack.

Treatment may be divided into two phases. There is a group of drugs that encourage excretion of uric acid by the kidney, probenecid being the one most commonly used; administration of these over a prolonged period will reduce the amount of uric acid in the body. It is felt that the number of attacks of gouty arthritis will also be reduced, although this is more difficult to determine, since attacks are apt to occur in an irregular fashion. These drugs have no effect on the acute attack of gouty arthritis; at times attacks may become more prevalent for a few months following initiation of therapy. Colchicine, on the other hand, is the classic drug for treating the attack. It has no effect on the uric acid in the body, but if symptoms are recognized and if treatment is initiated early, the attack may be halted within 24 to 48 hours. Its side effects—nausea, vomiting, and diarrhea—make it a difficult drug to use; in recent years phenylbutazone, equally effective in controlling symptoms, has become the drug of choice. Most patients with gout are little disabled by the disease, so that the rehabilitation worker will see only the occasional severely involved case or the case in which the difficulties are primarily psychological.

MISCELLANEOUS

The term *collagen disease* is applied to a group of conditions in which the most important feature is an inflammatory process involving connective tissue. Connective tissue is the fibrous supporting tissue of the body, and collagen is one of its constituents. Pathologically, these diseases are characterized by so-called fibrinoid degeneration of collagen. The collagen appears under the microscope similar to the fibrin of a blood clot. There is also inflammation of small vessels—vasculitis. Included in the group are rheumatoid arthritis, rheumatic fever, polyarteritis nodosa, disseminated lupus erythematosus, scleroderma, and dermatomyositis. Rheumatoid arthritis and rheumatic fever are discussed separately. The other four will be dealt with in this section. It is interesting to note that serum sickness, the reaction that follows the administraion of diphtheria or tetanus antitoxin, both of which are made from horse serum, shows many of the pathological features of these diseases. This is one of the bits of evidence on which are based the theories of hypersensitivity and autoimmunization as causes for the collagen diseases. No definite conclusions have been reached.

In *polyarteritis nodosa* the inflammation occurs in the walls of small and medium-sized arteries. The symptoms and findings depend on the location of the arteries involved and are caused by obstruction of these vessels with death of the tissue beyond the obstruction. The course of the disease varies from complete spontaneous remission to rapid demise. Effective treatment is limited to the cortisone-type drugs.

Disseminated lupus erythematosus likewise presents an extremely varied picture. The classic case is a young woman with intermittent fever, joint pains, a characteristic skin rash, anemia, low white cell count, and evidence of kidney damage. The finding of abnormal white blood cells, referred to as LE cells, is typical. Cortisone-type drugs in large doses suppress the symptoms and findings but do not cure the condition. In general, one should be conservative with regard to their use, since in many cases the disease remits spontaneously.

Scleroderma, as the name suggests, is characterized by fibrous scarring of the skin and of the internal organs—lungs, heart, kidneys, and digestive tract. Again, the course of the disease is variable. Cases with minimal involvement may go on for years; the disease may at times regress. Death is attributable to the cardiac, pulmonary, and renal lesions.

Dermatomyositis is similar in many ways to the other diseases in the group. It is set apart mainly by involvement of muscles. Clinically the muscles are tender, weak, and atrophied. Pathologically, there are varying degrees of inflammation and destruction. It is important to realize that these diseases are not clear-cut entities. One often sees cases in which features of several can be easily recognized. Prognosis in general must be guarded; rehabilitation procedures should be governed accordingly.

Hemophilia is a disease characterized by abnormal clotting of the blood; it is mentioned in this discussion because bleeding may occur episodically into the joints. The bleeding occurs acutely with minimal trauma; if this happens many times, "arthritic" changes—hyperplasia of the synovia and erosion of the cartilage—occur. This is a condition of children and young adults that may present rehabilitation problems related to education and work.

Psoriasis, a circumscribed, scaly skin rash, occurs in approximately 5 per cent of patients with rheumatoid arthritis, a higher incidence than could be accounted for on the basis of chance. Although there is some question as to whether the joint involvement is qualitatively or quantitatively different when psoriasis is present, all observers agree that subcutaneous nodules are notably absent, and the serological reactions for rheumatoid factor are rarely positive. Problems of therapy and prognosis are similar to those in rheumatoid arthritis without psoriasis. The skin lesion does not often call for rehabilitative efforts.

Rheumatic fever is a complication of beta streptococcal infection, most commonly occurring in the upper respiratory tract. One to two weeks after the acute infection, the patient notes the onset of malaise, fever, and arthralgias; occasionally arthritis or rashes may be noted. In childhood, symptoms of cardiac involvement appear. It is said that rheumatic fever licks the joints but bites the heart. The arthritis of rheumatic fever is not serious; it is self-limited, causing no damage to the joints. Its symptoms respond well to aspirin. Inflammation and subsequent scarring of the muscle and valves of the heart produce the disability in this disease, which is discussed elsewhere. It is mentioned here since in the adult patient rheumatic fever is often seen as arthritis without carditis; hence the heart involvement is not helpful as a differential point, the diagnosis being established by laboratory test.

Reiter's syndrome consists of the combination of urethritis, conjunctivitis, and arthritis with at times diarrhea and various rashes. The cause of this condition is unknown. Evidence suggests a relationship to infection with pleuropneumonia organisms or the dysentery bacillus. It tends to be a disease of young adult white males. The urethritis appears first, then the conjunctivitis and arthritis. The arthritis which usually persists the longest, may be present for over a year. Fever, a skin rash that glories in the name of *keratoderma blennorrhagica*, ulcerations of the penis, ulcerations in the mouth, and inflammation of the bladder, all occur in the more severely involved cases. This is a disease with a well-marked tendency to remit, the individual attack lasting up to one to two years. Interestingly in these cases there is no permanent joint damage. However, there is a tendency for the disease to recur, even after a period of years. After several recurrences it is apt to become chronic, blending gradually into what is indistinguishable from chronic rheumatoid arthritis.

Reflex sympathetic dystrophy, also known as the *shoulder-hand syn-*

drome, is a peculiar dysfunction of the autonomic nervous system supplying an extremity in which there is pain and limited motion of the shoulder, and pain and swelling of the hand. This progresses to limited motion in the hand, atrophy of muscles, and a characteristic decalcification of bone known as *Sudeck's atrophy*. This pattern of symptoms may follow an injury to the extremity, a myocardial infarct, or disease of the spine or shoulder. If recognized early, Novocain block of the cervical sympathetic nerves can result in complete cure. At a later stage, block provides only partial relief, and long periods of physical therapy may be necessary to restore mobility and strength.

Bursitis means to the patient an attack of pain and limitation of motion of the shoulder. To the physician it means inflammation in any one of a good many bursae in the body. A bursa is a sac filled with fluid between tissues that move in relationship to each other. The bursae most commonly involved are the subacromial of the shoulder, the supratrochanteric of the hip, and the Achilles in the heel. Superficial bursae (between bony prominences and skin) most often involved are the olecranon at the elbow and prepatellar at the knee. The pathogenesis is obscure. In fact, it is not entirely clear whether involvement in these different areas is on the same basis. The shoulder is by far the most common site of involvement; here the basic disease appears to be related to the tendon of the supraspinatus muscle, which traverses the floor of the subacromial bursa. Injury to the tendon produces inflammation, the acute symptoms of pain, and limitation of motion of the joint. In addition, degenerative changes may take place in the tendon and deposits of calcium appear. These two situations may bear no relationship to each other, since the latter process may on occasion be completely asymptomatic. However, as a rule there are minor pain and stiffness in the shoulder, and the area is more subject to injury, with resulting severe symptoms as noted.

Adhesive capsulitis, or "frozen shoulder," is distinguished from bursitis by a more insidious onset and a more chronic course with, as a rule, less pain. There is some speculation as to whether this is an entirely different disease, especially since a majority of recently studied cases showed small amounts of rheumatoid factor in the blood, suggesting a relationship with rheumatoid arthritis.

Treatment of the acute attack of bursitis consists of rest, immobilization, analgesia, and physical therapy. The condition is usually self-limited, clearing within a week or two. Local injection of cortisone-type drugs often provides prompt relief. X-ray therapy, although frequently used, has never been proven effective. Surgical removal of calcific deposits may be carried out for persistent disabling symptoms. Whatever other types of treatment are used, physical therapy for range of motion and muscle strength is extremely important.

There are several conditions in which an inflammation of unknown cause occurs in relation to certain tendons, ligaments, and tissues. These are not serious diseases but may be recurrent, chronic, and troublesome, thereby requiring rehabilitation services.

In *Dupuytren's contracture*, inflammation involves tissues in the palm of the hand, the palmar fascia. This results, over the course of years, in scarring and flexion contracture of the fingers, most commonly the fifth and fourth, which eventually may be pulled down to the palm. Treatment in the early stages consists of physical therapy; in the later stages it is surgical.

"Trigger finger" is caused by a similar unknown type of low-grade inflammation which causes narrowing or stenosis of the tendon sheaths in the palm of the hand. When the finger is extended, resistance is encountered until a certain point is reached where it gives way and motion is free. Treatment is conservative; the condition usually clears spontaneously.

Stenosing tendovaginitis at the radial styloid, or *de Quervain's disease*, is a similar process affecting the long abductor and short extensor tendons of the thumb on the lateral side of the wrist. The main clinical feature is pain aggravated by certain motions of the thumb and wrist which would tend to put tension on these tendons. The condition may necessitate surgical release of the constricted tendon.

A ganglion is a cystic swelling in the neighborhood of a joint or tendon sheath. It occurs most commonly over the dorsum of the wrist or of the foot or on the medial aspect of the knee. The cyst, made up of one or many cavities, contains a clear jellylike material or a thick mucinous fluid. It does not communicate with the joint. The old-fashioned treatment is to rupture the ganglion by hitting it with the family Bible, but there are many alternatives to this, including surgical excision.

Lateral humeral epicondylitis, or "tennis elbow," is a painful inflammation of unknown cause occurring over the lateral aspect of the elbow at the origin of the extensor muscles of the forearm. It responds promptly to local injection of hydrocortisone.

Diseases of the feet are many and varied; their causes are generally obscure. In some instances, congenital variation in bone structure appears to be important. In others, there appears to be congenital lack of tone in certain muscles, the tibial group for instance, which produces a flatfoot deformity. It is clear that deformity may occur secondary to certain neuromuscular diseases such as poliomyelitis, but this is a rare cause of a common condition. The role played by various rheumatic or inflammatory diseases is not clear. As an example, spastic flatfoot is often a well-recognized part of otherwise typical rheumatoid arthritis. Faulty footwear and inappropriate postural habits are often implicated. There are many people with flat longitudinal arches (from the heel to the base of the great toe). If the condition is asymptomatic, it is best to withhold treatment. However, foot exercises to strengthen the muscles that maintain the arch, and arch supports of various types which go in the shoe, are standard treatment. In severe cases especially with the so-called spastic flatfoot, operation may occasionally be undertaken.

The metatarsals and toes are subject to several conditions. Lateral deviation of the great toe, or *hallux valgus*, commonly occurs associated with an enlarged bursa and/or corn, and/or callus, over its medial aspect. This is known as a bunion. Treatment may be conservative with exercises and adjustments in the shoes, or operative with a variety of procedures available.

Hallux valgus is often associated with flattening of the transverse arch, which extends across the ball of the foot, so that the calluses on the sole instead of being under the first and fifth metatarsal heads are under the second, third, or fourth. As a variation on this condition, the digital nerves between the toes may be irritated, resulting in the occasional development of neuromas in this area. Treatment is usually conservative with exercises and arch supports.

Another associated feature is known as hammer toe, or cockup deformity of the toe. This consists of dorsiflexion of the proximal phalanx, plantar flexion of the second phalanx, and either flexion or extension of the distal phalanx. Painful corns may develop on the tops and the ends of the toes. Again, treatment may be conservative, with exercises and plaster strapping, or operative.

Hallux rigidus is a condition of unknown cause in which the metatarsophalangeal joint at the base of the great toe becomes stiff, dorsiflexion particularly being limited. In severe cases, all movement of the joint may be abolished. Various adjustments may be made in the shoes, or surgical resection of a segment of the joint may be carried out.

"March foot" or "fracture" consists of deposits of osteoid tissue about the shafts of the metatarsals. Minor trauma may produce fracture in the area of deposit. The condition is related to continuous trauma of slight degree, as in the marching of soldiers, and is probably similar to myositis ossificans. Treatment consists of cessation of trauma and immobilization in plaster if a fracture has taken place.

There are a variety of ill-defined painful conditions of the heel variously described as *tendonitis, bursitis,* or *fibrositis,* which, when severe can lead to osteophytes or spurs on the heel bone, or os calcis. Treatment generally should be conservative, since the acute painful phase of symptomatology is often self-limited.

NEOPLASMS

Tumors of joints generally fall into three categories: *pigmented villonodular synovitis, chondromatosis* and other benign tumors, and *synovial sarcoma.* All of these tumors enter the differential diagnostic problem of chronic monoarticular arthritis. Occasionally the benign tumor may cause the clinical picture of internal derangement of the knee. Pigmented villonodular synovitis appears under the microscope halfway between an inflammatory process and a tumor. It occurs mainly in the knee joint and is cured by local excision. These tumors also occur in bursae and tendon sheaths where they occasionally show giant cells, and hence are called giant cell tumors. Chondromatosis shows multiple areas of metaplastic cartilage and bone growth within the synovial tissue. The condition is cured by complete excision. Other benign tumors originate in blood vessels, (hemangioma) or are composed of fibrous of fatty tissue (fibroma, lipoma). Synovial sarcoma is notable in that it metastasizes early; the only hope of cure lies in early radical surgery. Radiation is not effective.

DISEASES OF MUSCLE

Since the function of muscle is so intimately related to the function of the nervous system, it is often difficult to distinguish clinically the exact locus of the disease when the patient's chief complaint is weakness. In the diseases described below, characteristic patterns do develop as these conditions progress, and if the pattern is not forthcoming one should look for disease elsewhere than in muscle. Examination under the microscope of tissue obtained at biopsy is often helpful.

PROGRESSIVE MUSCULAR DYSTROPHY

The cause of progressive muscular dystrophy is unknown but is presumably related to the genetic deficiency or abnormality of some metabolic process resulting in degeneration of muscle fibers and their replacement by fibrous and fatty tissue. Once initiated, the process is slowly progressive until often the entire muscle is replaced by fat and fibrous scar. The disease occurs in a variety of patterns. The childhood type occurs mainly in boys; its onset is noted before the age of six. The clinical picture is initially one of weakness. There may be enlargement of certain muscles, so-called pseudohypertrophy, but as the disease progresses muscle atrophy supervenes. With this may come contractions and deformity of the trunk and limbs. The heart muscle is also involved, and congestive heart failure may be part of the picture. In general, the condition is not compatible with survival to adult life; hence this illness will be rarely encountered in the rehabilitation setting. On the other hand, the fascioscapulohumeral type comes on most commonly when the patient is in his teens. As the name suggests, the chief involvement is in the muscles of the face and of the shoulder girdle. Atrophy of muscles in the lower leg appears early; muscles of the body show no changes until late. There are marked variations in severity. Involvement may be so minimal that the patient is unaware of any disability. At the other end of the spectrum the patient may be incapacitated before the age of 20. Complications are the same as in the childhood type but become incapacitating only very late in life, if at all. Treatment is entirely unsatisfactory, but the patient should be encouraged to be as active as possible; a rehabilitation program is helpful.

MYOTONIC DYSTROPHY

The onset of *myotonic dystrophy* usually takes place in early adult life. However, the myotonia may precede the other signs of the disease by many years. *Myotonia* is the inability to relax a muscle normally after its contraction. Often the patient has difficulty letting go when he shakes hands. The *dystrophy* consists of weakness and loss of strength in muscles in a pattern somewhat different from what has been previously described; chiefly involved are the muscles of the face and neck. Also both male and female patients develop progressive loss of hair in the frontal region of the scalp. Testicular atrophy develops in men. Other parts of the disease pattern consist of fine subcapsular opacities in the lens of the eye, premature cataracts of the more usual type, and nonspecific inflammation of the conjunctivas and eyelids. The picture of the disease presented by the patient may be extremely variable; its course is generally slowly progressive. Diagnosis may be difficult in the early stages, since myotonia, the most prominent sign, occurs in several neurological diseases and in two other muscle disease, both of which carry a good prognosis. The myotonia in all these muscle diseases responds to quinine, but no treatment is helpful for the other muscle symptom.

MYASTHENIA GRAVIS

Myasthenia gravis is characterized by easy fatigability and weakness of muscles. The muscles first involved are those about the face and neck. The patient may have difficulty keeping his eyes open or difficulty swallowing because of weakness of the muscles of the throat. The fatigability is of a characteristic sort in that the first few contractions of a muscle are normal, but then as use of the muscle continues, fatigue and weakness rapidly appear only to disappear again after a short period of rest. Eventually involvement may be extensive, and respiratory insufficiency may appear. Remissions and relapses of the disease occur in an unpredictable fashion even after many months. There are several drugs that give very excellent results in the condition, the most important being neostigmine, the only drawback of which is its short duration of action. Frequent doses must be taken. The mechanism of action of these drugs is not entirely clear, but has to do with potentiating the effect of acetylcholine at the nerve-muscle junction. Much has been written in recent years about the relationship of the thymus gland to this disease. It has been excised in many cases with good results. However, because of the unpredictability of natural remissions, the relatively few examples of marked improvement following operation, and the danger to the patient—oxygen, respirators, intravenously administered neostigmine—thymectomy cannot be recommended as a routine precedure.

FAMILIAL PERIODIC PARALYSIS

Familial periodic paralysis is a rare disorder occurring in certain families. The patients are normal except for striking episodes of muscular weakness averaging a few hours to a few days in duration. It is most frequently seen in early adult life. The level of serum potassium drops during an attack, and since the potassium does not appear in the urine, it presumably goes into the cells of the body. Diagnosis may be a difficult problem. There are other conditions associated with weakness and a low serum potassium, but these are not basically muscle diseases. There is no known treatment except for the administration of potassium during attacks.

MISCELLANEOUS

Among the diseases discussed in the preceding sections, the most significant symptom has been weakness. The patient describing weakness may mean many things; it is important to determine initially what the term signifies. Faintness suggests heart, brain, or circulatory disease. The lack of energy or lassitude frequently described, difficult to evaluate, is probably most often due to psychological disturbance. However, anemia of any origin, obscure chronic infection such as tuberculosis or brucellosis, collagen disease such as subacute rheumatic fever or rheumatoid arthritis, and endocrine disorder such as hyperthyroidism or hypothyroidism, diabetes, hypopituitarism (Simmonds' disease) and hypoadrenalism (Addison's disease) may all be responsible for this symptom. Actual loss of muscle strength means serious disorder of neuromuscular function if such causes as senility and prolonged confinement to bed are ruled out.

Diagnosis is established when study of the patient is completed. The rehabilitation worker does not as a rule have to contend with this problem, but in cases where the diagnosis has been established, he will frequently have to identify, separate, and deal with symptoms of psychological origin in this category.

BIBLIOGRAPHY

Anderson, W. A. D. *Pathology*, 4th ed. St. Louis: The C. V. Mosby Co., 1961.

Best, C. H., and N. B. Taylor. *The Physiological Basis of Medical Practice.* Baltimore: The Williams & Wilkins Co., 1961.

Gray, H. *Anatomy of the Human Body,* 27th ed. Goss, C. M., ed. Philadelphia: Lea & Febiger, 1959.

Harrison, T. R. *et al.,* eds. *Principles of Internal Medicine.* New York: McGraw-Hill Book Co., 1962.

Hollander, J. L., ed. *Arthritis and Allied Conditions: A Textbook of Rheumatology.* Philadelphia: Lea & Febiger, 1960.

Jaffe, H. L. *Tumors and Tumorous Conditions of the Bones and Joints.* Philadelphia: Lea & Febiger, 1958.

Short, C. L., W. Gauer, and W. E. Reynolds. *Rheumatoid Arthritis.* Cambridge: Harvard University Press, 1957.

Turek, S. L. *Orthopaedics, Principles and Their Application.* Philadelphia: J. B. Lippincott Co., 1959.

V

DISORDERS OF THE GASTROINTESTINAL SYSTEM

The gastrointestinal tract takes the great variety of foods we eat and transforms them into a relatively few simple constituents, some of which are then selectively absorbed into the blood. The tract consists of two portions. The first is an elongate tube comprising the mouth, pharynx, esophagus, stomach, small intestine, and large intestine (colon), in series, each area representing a portion of the tube with specialized structure and function. The unit as a whole serves to propel swallowed food from the mouth to anus, to add to it various chemical substances that digest or break down food to absorbable form, and to absorb selectively from this digestive mixture into the blood those materials useful to the body. Certain other materials of which the body seeks to dispose may be excreted from the blood into the hollow portion (lumen) of the intestine and passed downward to be excreted in the feces, together with other nonabsorbed materials.

The second portion of the gastrointestinal tract consists of two organs connected to the small intestine by ducts—the liver (with the gallbladder) and the pancreas. These two organs have digestive functions, for they secrete and introduce into the small intestine via their respective ducts materials that aid in the breakdown and absorption of foods. Certain other important functions may be termed nondigestive. The liver is an important organ in the regulation of the metabolism (that is, the breakdown and synthesis) of sugars, fats, and protein within the body. In addition, the liver extracts certain products from the blood and excretes them into the small intestine via the bile. The pancreas, too, has nondigestive metabolic functions. Certain portions of the gland

By HERBERT L. COOPER, M.D. Assistant in Medicine, Massachusetts Memorial Hospital; Instructor in Medicine, Boston University School of Medicine, Boston, Massachusetts.

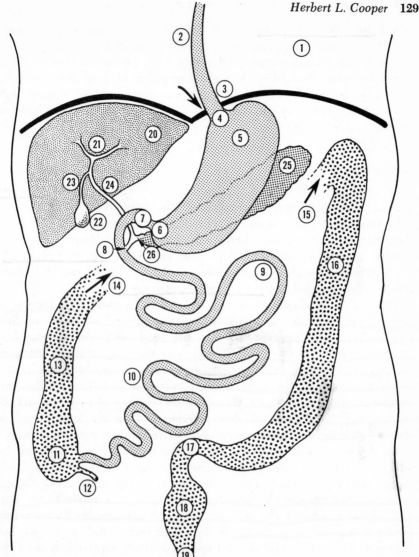

Figure 6. Schematic representation of the gastrointestinal tract. *1.* Chest (heart and lungs not shown). *2.* Esophagus. *3.* Left diaphragm (arrow indicates esophageal hiatus). *4.* Gastroesophageal junction (shown open as during a swallow). *5.* Stomach. *6.* Pylorus. *7.* Duodenum (first portion called the duodenal cap). *8.* Ampulla of Vater. *9.* Jejunum (second portion of small intestine). *10.* Ileum. *11.* Cecum (first portion of the colon; the transverse colon is omitted to simplify the diagram. Arrows indicate the direction of flow of colonic contents). *12.* Appendix. *13.* Ascending colon. *14* and *15.* Beginning and end of the transverse portion of the colon. *16.* Descending colon. *17.* Sigmoid colon. *18.* Rectum. *19.* Anus. *20.* Liver. *21.* Liver bile ducts. *22.* Gallbladder. *23.* Cystic duct. *24.* Common bile duct. *25.* Pancreas. *26.* Pancreatic duct. The remaining abdominal organs (spleen, kidneys, etc.), not discussed in this chapter, are not shown.

called *islets of Langerhans* secrete the hormone insulin into the blood and thus regulate sugar, fat, and amino acid metabolism.

Diseases of such a complicated system may produce a host of signs, symptoms, and disabilities. We shall consider each of the areas individually, briefly discuss its structure and normal function, and then consider its most frequent disorders, their manifestations, methods of diagnosis, and management.

ESOPHAGUS

As food is swallowed, it passes from the mouth to the *pharynx* (throat) and then into the esophagus. The latter is a flattened, muscular tube lined with mucous membrane, which passes downward from the pharynx through the chest and enters the abdomen through a narrow opening in the left diaphragm called the *esophageal hiatus*. After passing through the hiatus, the esophagus empties into the stomach at a point called the *gastroesophageal junction*.

The act of swallowing sets in motion an automatic sequence of extraordinary complex and coordinated muscular contractions of lips, tongue, face, and pharynx, so that the food or liquid is propelled from the mouth to the pharynx and into the esophagus. A wave of muscular contraction, called *peristalsis*, sweeps down the length of the esophagus, pushing the mass of food before it and through the gastroesophageal junction into the stomach. Except during the act of swallowing, the gastroesophageal junction is normally kept closed so that acid stomach contents cannot regurgitate into the esophagus, which is lined with a membrane intolerant to such acid. The mechanism by which the hollow of the stomach and esophagus are kept from freely communicating except during swallowing is poorly understood, though numerous theories are offered in explanation. It may relate to the passage of the esophagus through the narrow diaphragmatic hiatus before joining the stomach, pinching off the lower end of the esophagus, but it is probably more complicated. Pressure measurements taken from the interior of the lower esophagus have indicated a zone of high pressure, called the *lower esophageal sphincter*, which relaxes and opens only during a swallow, permitting the passage of food into the stomach. The normal location of this closing mechanism (sphincter) near the diaphragmatic hiatus, with the gastroesophageal junction below the hiatus, seems important in preventing reflux of stomach contents into the esophagus. As we shall see, derangements of these anatomical relations may result in freer communication between the interior of stomach and esophagus.

Disorders of the esophagus may be of many types: first, motor abnormalities—that is, disorders of peristalsis in which food is not pushed through the esophagus rapidly; second, disorders that permit acid stomach juice to enter the esophagus and damage its lining; and third, diseases that obstruct the lumen of the esophagus, producing obstruction to the path of swallowed materials. Several neurological disorders such as myasthenia gravis and bulbar poliomyelitis can interfere with swallowing. In these instances, the patient may be unable to move the food from mouth to pharynx and into the esophagus. These disorders are discussed elsewhere.

MOTOR DISORDERS

ACHALASIA (CARDIOSPASM). This disorder, of unknown cause, produces two abnormalities of esophageal function. First, the orderly, progressive waves of muscular contraction (peristalsis) that normally sweep a swallow of food through the esophagus into the stomach do not occur. Rather, a number of disorderly nonpropulsive contractions may occur, producing a mixing and churning of the contents, but not orderly clearing of the lumen. Second, the lower esophageal sphincter does not open normally to permit the passage of food into the stomach. The disorder is a chronic one, causing difficulty in swallowing, called *dysphagia.* The patient may actually regurgitate the portion of swallowed material that fails to get through to his stomach.

The diagnosis of this and many other gastrointestinal disorders involves the use of the x-ray. Since the gastrointestinal tract is not readily visible on regular x-ray pictures or on fluoroscopy, some material visible under x-ray is swallowed by the patient. As this material progresses down the tract, its course may be followed fluoroscopically and with x-ray pictures. The material, barium sulfate, is given in a drink the consistency of a malted (barium meal), and the entire procedure is called a gastrointestinal (GI) series. Not only can the outline of esophagus, stomach, and small intestine be followed by such a procedure, but their motor function can also be evaluated.

Thus, the abnormality of peristalsis and the failure of relaxation of the lower esophageal sphincter in achalasia can be seen on fluoroscopy following a swallow of barium sulfate. Measurements of the pressure within the esophagus are also useful in diagnosis. In a specific diagnostic test the drug Mecholyl is injected, producing temporary accentuation of the motor abnormality.

Little can be done to improve the organization or force of peristalsis in this condition. Treatment is directed at trying to dilate or open the lower end of the esophagus so that swallowed material that gets to this area may pass through more easily. The dilation may be accomplished by stretching from within, using a balloon, or by a surgical procedure.

DIFFUSE SPASM. In this motor disorder, as in achalasia, normal esophageal peristalsis is replaced by nonpropulsive spasmodic contractions. Here, however, the lower esophageal sphincter usually opens normally. Patients with this disorder complain not only of difficulty in swallowing, but sometimes of chest pain as well, the latter due to particularly strong spasms of the esophagus. As the disorder here is one of peristalsis and not of any narrowing of the esophagus, the stretching measures employed in achalasia are not applicable. Though medicines may be tried, no completely satisfactory treatment is presently available.

HIATUS HERNIA

As we have seen, the junction of esophagus and stomach lies below the diaphragm; the stomach thus normally lies wholly within the abdomen. In certain patients, a portion of the stomach protrudes or herniates through the diaphragmatic hiatus into the chest. The incidence of this condition increases with age, and it is often completely without symptoms. In certain patients, however, this abnormal position of the stomach and gastroesophageal junction permits abnormally free communication between the hollow of the stomach and esophagus. Strong acid- and enzyme-containing stomach juices may then enter the esophagus and damage its sensitive lining, a condition called _peptic esophagitis._ This may be felt by the patient as a burning sensation behind the breastbone—heartburn. Medically, one can treat the symptom of heartburn by giving antacids, which neutralize the stomach acid. Hence, when stomach contents do reflux into the esophagus, they will do less damage. Patients are told not to lie down following a meal, for in this position reflux of stomach juices into the esophagus is obviously more likely. If these measures fail, and particularly if more severe difficulties develop, surgical correction of the hernia with placement of the entire stomach back below the diaphragm into the abdomen may be done.

STRICTURE

Patients who have suffered with peptic esophagitis for prolonged periods may develop a scarring of the esophagus, so that its hollow becomes progressively more narrow, impeding the passage of food. This condition, called a _stricture,_ may be treated by stretching the esophagus from within with tubes passed through the mouth or may require surgical correction with removal of the narrow area. Such stricture may also be produced following the drinking of certain caustics such as lye, usually taken in suicidal attempts by adults or accidentally by children.

VARICES

Brief mention will be made here of a disorder of the esophagus actually caused by chronic liver disease. In this condition, the tiny

veins that normally lie just beneath the lining membrane of the esophagus become enlarged, engorged, and tortuous, appearing rather wormlike and similar to varicose veins of the legs. These enlarged esophageal
veins, called *varices*, are of great concern, for they may rupture,
producing massive bleeding into the esophagus with vomiting of blood
(hematemesis). Unless rapidly treated, this may be fatal.

CANCER

The general problem of neoplasms is discussed elsewhere in the text.
Cancer of the esophagus characteristically produces progressive difficulty in swallowing, for the tumor gradually occludes the lumen. The
treatment is either radiotherapy or surgical removal. Patients who
have cancers that are too advanced for successful treatment by these
means and who are unable to swallow may need *gastrostomy*. In
this surgical procedure, a permanent opening is made between the
interior of the stomach and the abdominal skin. Feeding solutions may
be directly introduced through the opening into the stomach, and the
patient may thus be fed even though totally unable to swallow. Considerable encouragement and assistance are necessary from those surrounding the patient with a gastrostomy in order that he may
successfully adjust to it. Once accustomed to this, many patients are
able to introduce the feeding solutions themselves.

STOMACH AND DUODENUM

Having traversed the esophagus, swallowed material enters the stomach, a pouchlike and distensible portion of the gastrointestinal tract.
Though the food has been partially broken down by chewing before
being swallowed and has been partially exposed to certain enzymes in
the saliva, it is in the stomach that significant digestion really begins.
The lining membrane of the stomach secretes two materials of digestive
importance, pepsin and hydrochloric acid. The pepsin (actually secreted
into the hollow of the stomach as a precursor, pepsinogen, which is
then converted to the active pepsin) is a potent enzyme which begins
the breakdown of dietary protein to smaller fragements. Pepsin works
best in an acid environment, and thus the hydrochloric acid enhances
its activity. The food remains in the stomach, is churned and mixed
with the acid, pepsin, and other secretions (for example, mucus), and
is then slowly emptied by peristalsis through the pyloric canal into
the duodenum, the first portion of the small intestine.

Hydrochloric acid is secreted by specialized cells (parietal cells)
located in the lining of the upper two-thirds of the stomach. These
cells secrete in response to several stimuli. Certain nerves to the stomach (the *vagi*) may stimulate secretion, both while the patient is fasting
and in response to the smell and taste of food. Acid is also secreted

in response to the presence of food in the stomach. In this situation, the presence of certain types of foods in the lower portion of the stomach (the antrum) will cause the release of a hormone (gastrin) which stimulates the parietal cells in the upper two-thirds of the stomach to secrete acid.

In considering the stomach's digestive function one cannot help but be impressed by a most extraordinary fact. The stomach secretes an acid—pepsin juice—which readily digests meat and other dietary proteins. If this juice refluxes into the esophagus it may cause severe damage. Yet, the interior lining of the stomach, always exposed to the juice, is not normally damaged by it. Why is it too not digested away by this potent acid-enzyme solution? What protects the mucous membrane lining the stomach from destruction by its own secretions? Some investigators feel that the mucus secreted by the stomach lining coats it and protects it. The answer, however, probably is more complex. The question is of more than academic interest, for in peptic ulcer, one of the commonest disorders of the stomach and duodenum, this resistance of the lining is overcome by the forces of digestion, the membrane is breached, and ulcer results.

One additional secretion of the stomach lining deserves mention before preceeding to the discussion of gastric (stomach) and duodenal disorders. *Intrinsic factor,* secreted in small amounts by the mucous membrane of the stomach, combines with dietary vitamin B_{12} and is essential to its subsequent absorption. Absence of intrinsic factor results in deficient vitamin B_{12} absorption, which in turn can produce defects in red cell production (*pernicious anemia*) and certain neurological disorders (*combined system disease*).

PEPTIC ULCER

In this disorder a small portion of the lining of the stomach or duodenum (the first portion of the small intestine) is eroded away, presumably because its resistance is overcome by the peptic-acid gastric juice. A punched-out crater called an *ulcer* is produced. The patient complains of upper abdominal distress, often relieved by food, though sometime provoked by eating. Some ulcers may bleed, producing vomiting of blood (hematemesis) or the passage of altered dark blood in the stools (melena). Peptic ulcers may also perforate through the entire lining of the stomach wall or duodenum sometimes producing peritonitis—inflammation of the lining of the abdomen. A third complication occurs when the ulcer is in the portion of the stomach near the pylorus or in the duodenum itself. Such ulcers, because of inflammation or scarring, may obstruct the outlet of the stomach. The patient will then suffer from persistent vomiting.

Despite volumes of investigation, the precise cause of peptic ulcer (gastric or duodenal) is still not known. It is clear that benign peptic ulcer of stomach or duodenum occurs only in patients whose stomachs can secrete acid. Not every patient who has an ulcer, however, secretes an excess of acid. Some investigators have felt that personality and environment play a role in causing ulcer or in precipitating recurrences. Though some patients with peptic ulcer are indeed very "high-strung" people and others work under particularly stressful circumstances, neither of these conditions applies to every ulcer patient. Despite much evidence in animal studies to indicate precisely that stress can produce ulcer, there is no unequivocal body of data to indicate the role of the emotions in the genesis of peptic ulcer in humans. In certain patients the relation between emotional stress and attacks of ulcer pain may be clear enough. In such people, and in ulcer patients in general, rest and relaxation seem helpful in getting ulcers to heal. Any more sweeping decision regarding the role of personality and emotions in this disorder must be withheld pending further investigation.

Peptic ulcer is diagnosed from the patient's history, the rhythm of the pain often being characteristic. The diagnosis is confirmed with a "GI series," the x-ray of the stomach and duodenum with barium sulfate contrast material. Since acid is so important in these disorders, the physician will want to find out how much the patient produces. This is done by having the patient swallow a small soft plastic or rubber tube, which is then passed into the stomach, from which a sample of juice is withdrawn for analysis.

The cornerstone of peptic ulcer treatment is the neutralization of stomach acid, accomplished by giving food and antacid medication hourly through the day and several times through the night. Some physicians prescribe soft, bland diets (milk, cheese, soups) for their ulcer patients during the early stages of treatment. Others feel that the type of food is of less importance in treatment than great frequency in feeding. The latter group would allow a liberal diet with hourly feedings between meals, omitting only alcohol, coffee, and spicy foods. Medicines called *anticholinergics,* which decrease the acid secretion and the motility of the stomach, are also used. Rest and sedation can be helpful.

Patients with duodenal ulcer may be treated at home or in the hospital, as their circumstances and their doctor's desires dictate. Gastric ulcer is usually treated in the hospital, for in this disorder it is particularly important that the medical regimen be carefully followed and the patient get adequate rest. Should a gastric ulcer fail to heal after a course of such treatment, surgery may be indicated. Those gastric ulcers which seem to heal on medical treatment must be followed up with repeat GI series to be sure that healing is complete.

The indications for surgery in ulcer disease will not be discussed here in any detail. Suffice it to say that in addition to those patients who need surgery because of the complications of ulcer outlined before, certain patients experience recurrence of ulcer or failure of the original ulcer to heal. It is not always clear whether the patient or his ulcer is intractable to healing—that is, whether the patient is following the treatment prescribed and his ulcer is not responding, or the patient is in fact failing to follow his doctor's instructions because he cannot or will not do so and is thus not improving. The advice and assistance of the social worker are often of great importance in this situation. It is necessary to determine whether or not the patient's home environment and his job will indeed permit him to follow his medical regimen. Can he actually take hourly antacids? Is his job so stressful that it might be contributing to his troubles? In the latter case, hospitalization or rest at home might be indicated until the ulcer has healed, with consideration later of a change of job.

Treatment of the complications of ulcer—bleeding, perforation, and obstruction—requires hospitalization and will not be further discussed here.

ACUTE GASTRITIS

This disorder, a diffuse inflammation of the stomach lining, may be provoked by the ingestion of large amounts of irritating material such as alcohol. There may be very superficial erosions of the stomach lining which may result in massive bleeding, requiring transfusion and sometimes surgery. In the more common, milder variety, the complaint is of indigestion or upper abdominal distress, perhaps with some nausea or vomiting. Though antacids and diet may be used, the crucial feature of treatment is elimination of the irritating material. In the case of alcohol, this may be very troublesome. The problem of the rehabilitation of the alcoholic patient is a difficult one and is raised in this section on the gastrointestinal tract because so many of the ill effects of chronic excess alcohol ingestion are manifested in this system. Acute gastritis, pancreatitis, and cirrhosis may all be associated with alcoholism. The social and economic problems of such patients in addition to their other medical (for example, neurological and nutritional) difficulties provide an even larger dimension to the problem of rehabilitating the chronic alcoholic. Such patients present not only strictly medical problems but also a challenge to society's resources. Further reference to this will be made later in the chapter.

CHRONIC GASTRITIS

In contrast to the relatively well defined entity, acute gastritis, the disorders lumped together under "chronic gastritis" are much less clearly delineated. Since medical literature is presently replete with systems of reclassification and criteria for diagnosis of these disorders, no attempt at an outline of their features or management would be appropriate here. One particular entity is, however, fairly well accepted. *Chronic atrophic gastritis,* a disorder in which the lining membrane of the stomach is atrophied or flattened, is seen in pernicious anemia. The mucosa fails to secrete not only acid and pepsin, but intrinsic factor as well. It will be remembered that intrinsic factor is essential to vitamin B_{12} absorption from the intestine. Failing to absorb this vitamin normally, these patients develop severe anemia and neurological disorders. Both the anemia and, if treated early, the neurological disorder, may be prevented and even cured by the monthly injection of vitamin B_{12}. This treatment must be continued throughout the patient's lifetime. The contribution of physical medicine and physical therapy to those patients whose neurological disorder is not completely reversible is discussed in another chapter.

NEOPLASMS

The commonest malignancy of the stomach is carcinoma. Although declining in frequency over the past few years, gastric cancer remains a significant problem. Its manifestations may be many, ranging from abdominal distress to the massive vomiting of blood. Its treatment is primarily surgical with attempt at removal of the stomach and tumor intact.

GASTRECTOMY

Removal of the entire stomach, *total gastrectomy,* is most often performed in patients with stomach cancer. *Partial gastrectomy,* or removal of part of the stomach, may be performed on certain patients with duodenal or gastric ulcer. The purposes of gastric surgery in ulcer may be surmised from the section on gastric physiology and ulcer. One attempts to eliminate acid secretion by one or more of the following procedures: (1) removal of the lower one-third of the stomach, thus eliminating the site of production of gastrin, the hormone that stimulates acid secretion; (2) removal, in addition, of varying amounts of the upper two-thirds of the stomach, thus removing some of the parietal cells which secrete the acid; (3) cutting of the vagus nerves (*vagotomy*) which normally stimulate acid secretion; (4) *pyloroplasty*—surgical widening of the pyloric canal to allow rapid emptying of acid from the stomach.

Following removal of a portion of the stomach, the surgeon has a number of ways of reconnecting (anastomosing) the cut ends of stomach and intestine to restore continuity of the gastrointestinal tract. In gastric ulcer, the ulcer is usually removed with the portion of the stomach taken out. In duodenal ulcer, one or more of the outlined procedures having been performed, the ulcer may actually be left in place. If the surgeon has been successful in completely eliminating acid secretion by the stomach, the ulcer will heal and will not recur.

The benefits of gastric surgery in removing ulcers or in treating cancer are evident. Accompanying these benefits certain difficulties, of course, might be expected, resulting from the removal of an important portion of the gastrointestinal tract. Following a meal, the stomach normally acts as a reservoir, emptying its contents gradually into the small intestine. Most of the surgical procedures outlined, particularly those which remove all or part of the stomach or widen its outlet into the intestine, interfere with its reservoir function. As a result, a meal may be rapidly emptied or "dumped" in its entirety from the stomach into the small intestine. In this disturbance, called *the dumping syndrome,* the patient experiences weakness, dizziness, palpitations (rapid heart action), and abdominal discomfort following a heavy meal. One attempts to treat such patients with frequent small feedings rather than large meals, avoiding liquids with meals and avoiding simple sugars as much as possible, for these seem to accentuate the symptoms. The patient is asked to lie down after each meal. This removes the force of gravity and reduces the rate of dumping of gastric contents into the intestine.

In addition to the dumping syndrome, which can usually be controlled with the measures described, several other sequelae to gastric surgery are seen. Some patients lose weight and may fail to regain their preoperative levels. Providing they stabilize at an acceptable weight postoperatively, this is in itself of no consequence. Some gastrectomy patients have diarrhea following meals, perhaps also due to the rapid dumping of large amounts of food into the intestine. Such loose bowel movements can usually be controlled with the measures outlined and the addition of certain medications. A very few patients with dumping will fail to respond to therapy, and these, as well as a few others whose digestive and absorptive mechanisms have been severely deranged as a result of the surgery, may require additional medical therapy or surgery.

Varying amounts of readjustment of diet and eating habits are required following gastric surgery. Those who must make such adjustments usually accomplish them without difficulty, but they may require assistance. The post gastrectomy patient, however, can usually return to a normal sort of activity following convalescence. The proper diet and the opportunity to lie down following meals for those with dumping must be available. Patients who have *total* gastrectomy (and who present the most severe forms of dumping syndrome) cannot absorb vitamin B_{12} properly, since they cannot secrete intrinsic factor. They therefore require injections of B_{12} for the rest of their lives.

SMALL INTESTINE

Having left the stomach, the digestive mixture enters the small intestine. This organ, a tube of about 10 to 18 feet in length (depending upon the method of measurement), is somewhat arbitrarily divided into three parts: *duodenum, jejunum, and ileum*. The surface area of its mucous membrane lining is greatly increased by two features. First, it is thrown into folds. Second, under microscopic examination, the lining is made up of minute, fingerlike projections (villi) containing capillaries and lymphatic vessels and covered with a single layer of specialized epithelial cells. The greatly increased area is important in absorption.

In the *duodenum,* or first portion of the small intestine, the partially digested mixture of food and stomach juice becomes mixed with the secretions of the pancreas and liver, introduced through ducts of these organs. In the more alkaline environment of the small intestine, pepsin is less active than in the stomach. Other enzymes, however, which work optimally in such an environment, appear here. Pancreatic juice contains enzymes capable of breaking down carbohydrate, fat, and protein to simpler constituents. The bile contributes chemical substances that help fatty materials to dissolve, aiding in their digestion and their absorption. The cells of the lining membrane of the small intestine themselves contain enzymes active in digestion. This mixture of food, enzymes, and additional materials supplied by the liver, pancreas, and small intestine is churned by segmental contractions of the bowel and propelled down the length of the intestine by waves of peristalsis. Digestion meanwhile proceeds not only within the lumen of the intestine but on its inner surface as well. Extremely high power microscopic examination of the cells lining the intestine indicates yet another anatomical feature. That surface of the lining cells of the mucous membrane which faces the lumen of the intestine is made up of a "brush border"—that is, a series of many minute bristlelike projections from the tip of the cell. Final digestion of some portions of the diet may take place on this brush border or perhaps within the cell itself.

Of further interest is the fact that not only is food digested to simpler absorbable constituents, but the proteins of the digestive secretions of the liver, pancreas, and small bowel are themselves digested in the lumen of the intestine after they have contributed to the digestion of foods. Accordingly, the intestine not only absorbs for the body the vital nutrients in our diet, but digests and reclaims for resynthesis and reuse some of the secretions of the gastrointestinal tract itself— a highly efficient and economical arrangement.

Although we have discussed digestion and will now discuss absorption, it should be clear that both processes take place simultaneously. For some materials, particularly those which are digested within the cells of the mucous membrane linings, the two processes might in fact be considered as one. In any case, as the digestive mixture progresses down the small intestine, absorption takes place. This absorption is a function of the specialized epithelial cells lining the lumen of the bowel. Some transfer of nutrients and water takes place by simple diffusion from intestinal lumen to capillaries across the lining cells of the bowel. Of greater interest, and perhaps of greater significance, is the active and specific transport of selected materials from the intestinal lumen into the blood, performed by intestinal cells, utilizing metabolic energy. Because the nature of the process and its specificity are a source of tremendous interest to physiologists, a great deal of study is presently being done in this area. It is becoming clear that certain materials are absorbed in certain specific areas of the small intestine; glucose, for example, is principally absorbed in the jejunum, while vitamin B_{12} is absorbed in the ileum.

Following passage through duodenum, jejunum, and ileum, the liquid intestinal contents are delivered to the cecum. It remains for the large intestine to reclaim for the body most of the water from this mixture, thus dehydrating the material to the solid consistency of normal stool.

The blood supply to the large and small intestine comes from the arterial branches of the aorta. As we shall see in our discussion of the liver, the drainage of venous blood (containing absorbed materials) from the bowel is unique. In contrast to the veins of other organs of the body which drain into the superior or inferior vena cava and then to the heart, the intestinal veins combine to form the portal vein, which then goes to the liver. Only after the blood from the intestine has passed through the liver does it enter the inferior vena cava and go to the heart. The liver then, of all the organs of the body, is first exposed to the blood from the small and large intestine, and hence gets first opportunity to extract absorbed materials from it. The lymph vessels also drain the small and large bowel. These channels (lacteals), which lie adjacent to the capillaries in the villi, eventually unite to form a larger vessel called the thoracic duct, which drains into the venous system in the chest. This pathway of absorption does not pass through the liver.

REGIONAL ENTERITIS

Patients with this disorder present one of the most challenging problems in gastroenterology. The youth of those affected (most patients are in their twenties and thirties when the disease is first diagnosed), the chronicity of the disorder, and its often unpredictable course over many years contribute to this challenge.

The disease, thought to begin in the lymph channels draining the small intestine, results in a great swelling and inflammation (edema) of the wall of the small bowel, which may progress to a scarring and narrowing of its lumen. Adjacent loops of bowel may become matted together by the inflammation, with kinking of the bowel. Perforation of the intestinal wall with abscess formation and fistulas (tracts leading from bowel to bowel or bowel to skin) may result. In some patients, scarring or kinking of the matted areas of bowel or inflammation may cause permanent or temporary obstruction to the flow of intestinal contents. The disease usually involves one or more segments of the small bowel (thus *regional* enteritis) rather than its entire length. The terminal small intestine or ileum is most frequently affected, hence the name *regional ileitis.*

The diagnosis is suggested by the patient's history and physical examination and confirmed by a gastrointestinal x-ray series. Patients with regional enteritis may present a wide spectrum of illness. Some, thought to have acute enteritis, recover following a single attack and are well thereafter. Most present recurrent disease. Some patients with mild disease may experience only intermittent flare-ups of the disorder with abdominal pain, diarrhea, and fever and may be treated at home or in the hospital. Months or years of well-being may follow such episodes. Other patients have more persistent difficulty, with chronic diarrhea and abdominal distress. Still other have a progressive course, with flare-ups of increasing frequency and development over several years of one or more of the complications of the disease—intestinal obstruction, fistulas, abscess formation, and compromise of the intestinal absorptive function producing weight loss and anemia.

Treatment is both medical and surgical; rest, nutritious diet, vitamin supplements, antibiotics, and the cortisone family of drugs are used. Transfusions of blood may be necessary in cases of severe disease. When obstruction, abscess, or fistulas are a problem, surgery may be performed to remove an area of disease or to short-circuit the bowel, bypassing the diseased area. Successful surgery, though usually not permanently curative, may provide a remission of symptoms for years.

The physician and those helping to care for the patient with regional enteritis should have as their aim the achievement of the most normal life possible for him. For those with mild disease, a normal vocational and recreational life is possible. Others may be capable of this sort of life as well, interrupted occasionally by exacerbations of the disease. The latter group, who may require hospitalization and surgery at the time of a flare-up, may still lead normal lives for months and years between attacks.

The rehabilitation of those with severe disease is more of a problem. Those with moderate disease, which leaves them less than well but still able to be employed or care for their homes, must be helped to do the best they can. Help in maintaining a home for the housewife or retaining a job that is not too taxing for the breadwinner is essential to such patients, who must not be allowed to become invalids.

A life of less than perfect health is life nonetheless, and may be a useful, satisfying, and rewarding one. A few unfortunate patients with extremely severe disease will suffer a progressive downhill course despite maximal medical and surgical help.

NONTROPICAL SPRUE

In this disorder the small intestinal lining cells fail to absorb the products of digestion normally. Accordingly, the patient loses weight, fails to absorb vitamins and other vital foodstuffs, and passes an excess of valuable nutrients in the feces, a condition called _malabsorption_. The most evident of the materials lost in the stool, fat, gives the excreta a greasy appearance. The patient may fail to appreciate that he is ill for some time, for the only manifestation of the disorder may be insidious weight loss and diarrhea. Later, however, diarrhea, evidence of vitamin deficiency, and anemia may lead him to seek medical aid. Incidentally, it is thought that adult _nontropical sprue_ is the same disease as _celiac disease_ of childhood.

Sprue is diagnosed by demonstrating defective absorption of a number of substances. Increased fat and nitrogen in the stool may be measured chemically after collecting the feces passed over a one- to three-day period. The absorption of certain test sugars (for example, xylose) fed to the patient may be measured. Blood levels of certain substances may also help in evaluating absorption. Finally, biopsy of the small intestinal lining may be obtained for microscopic examination. This procedure is performed by passing a tube through the patient's mouth down into the stomach and into the small intestine. A tiny piece of the lining of this organ is then obtained by suction. The patient feels no pain and usually experiences little discomfort during the procedure. In nontropical sprue, microscopic examination of the specimen demonstrates villi that are blunted and flattened, rather than normally fingerlike.

The treatment of nontropical sprue is extremely rewarding to patients and physicians if carefully carried out. It was discovered in Holland following World War II that sprue patients who stopped eating wheat improved greatly. Further study indicated that the injurious material in wheat is contained in the _gluten_ fraction. Complete elimination of this material from the diet of nontropical sprue patients produces remarkable return to well-being. The rehabilitation problem in this disorder, then, consists of helping the patient to obtain a gluten-free diet and encouraging him to follow it permanently. Supplemental vitamins are also of importance.

For intelligent and cooperative patients who take all of their meals at home and have sufficient funds to accomplish the diet, there is little difficulty. Those lacking these advantages need help. Not only must bread, cereals, and cakes containing wheat, rye, barley, and oat flour be strictly avoided, but a variety of other foods—for example, certain candies, syrups, and beverages that contain added wheat—must also be eliminated. To be effective, the diet must be strictly followed, with careful reading of labels on packaged foods to be sure they contain no added wheat. Patients who must take their meals at work or in restaurants experience some difficulty in knowing how their meals are prepared. All patients with sprue thus require instruction for proper diet. Some will require further assistance in accomplishing this diet.

HERNIA AND INTESTINAL OBSTRUCTION

Hernia, an abnormal protrusion of tissue through a natural or abnormal opening, can occur in various areas of the abdomen. *Femoral* and *inguinal hernias*, which occur in the groin, are among the most common. Elective surgical correction of such protrusions is the indicated treatment if the patient's general health permits. Uncorrected not only are they a source of disability (lifting and heavy work will increase their size), but they present an additional risk. The contents of the hernia may become irreducible—that is, the protrusion may become fixed. The blood supply of its contents may be compromised, or if intestine is involved, intestinal obstruction may result, sometimes requiring emergency surgery.

Intestinal obstruction may result from other disorders as well. Regional enteritis which narrows the small intestinal lumen has been mentioned. Patients who have had one or more abdominal operations may acquire *adhesions*—that is, strands of scar tissue in the abdomen around which loops of intestine may bend or kink producing obstruction to the flow of digestive mixture. Such episodes may be treated with an intestinal tube and suction until they subside, but may require surgery.

TUMORS

Cancer of the small intestine is quite uncommon. Much more frequent are *polyps*, benign clublike protrusions into the lumen from the intestinal lining. Such polyps may be multiple, and in some cases are familial. Often asymptomatic, they may occasionally bleed or produce obstruction. Another tumor of the small intestine, *carcinoid*, often arises in the appendix, a wormlike outpouching of the cecum, the first portion of the colon. Lymphatic tumors (lymphomas) of the small bowel are also seen.

COLON

Following its passage through the small bowel, the digestive mixture enters the colon. The latter organ begins as the cecum in the right lower portion of the abdomen then proceeds up and across to the left side where it descends again to the left lower abdomen. Here, called the sigmoid colon because of its "s" shape, it descends into the pelvis, becomes continuous with the rectum, and empties to the outside via the anus. The lining of the colon is an epithelial cell membrane which grossly and microscopically is thrown into folds. The areas between the bases of the folds are called the crypts.

The important products of digestion having been absorbed during passage through the small bowel, it remains for the colon to remove water and certain electrolytes (sodium and chloride) from the digestive mixture, thus producing the solid stool. This water and electrolyte absorptive function of the colon's lining membrane is of great importance in the body's conservation of these materials. The colonic mucosa also transfers potassium into the lumen of the bowel, for excretion in the stool.

The colon normally contains an important bacterial population which breaks down certain substances in the bowel contents and synthesizes others. A large proportion of the fecal mass is in fact bacteria. The colonic contents become progressively dehydrated as they traverse the colon and finally reach the rectum. Distention of the rectum by this material produces the desire to evacuate the bowel; the rectal sphincter permits postponement of this function and thus permits fecal continence.

INFECTIONS

As noted, there is normally a bacterial population in the colon. These are nonpathogenic—that is, they do not produce disease in this situation. Certain other bacteria, however, may infect the large intestine and produce illness. Most notable among these are members of the *salmonella* group, of which the typhoid bacillus is a member, and the *shigella* group, which produce bacillary dysentery. While these organisms may produce quite a severe illness with diarrhea, abdominal cramps, and fever, they can usually be treated medically. Certain patients, either following a known salmonella infection or without clinical history of such infection, continue to harbor salmonella organisms and pass them in their stools. Such people, called "carriers," represent a public health hazard. Though they are themselves without symptoms, they may transmit salmonella infection to others who may become quite ill. It is of importance that they do not engage in food-handling occupations, for in this sort of work they present the greatest hazard to the public. Attempts to eliminate the carrier state include antibiotic treatment and sometimes removal of the gallbladder where salmonella may be harbored.

The colon may also be infected by a type of protozoa, an ameba, which may produce not only an acute diarrheal illness, *amebic dysentery* but chronic diarrhea as well. Upon occasion, it may infect the liver. Medical treatment with a variety of drugs is available to eradicate the ameba.

DIVERTICULOSIS

Small outpouchings of the colon, particularly of the sigmoid area, called *diverticula,* occur frequently in middle and older age groups. Most often they produce no difficulty, in which case the condition is called *diverticulosis.* On occasion, the diverticula become inflamed, with spasm and narrowing of the colon, a condition called *diverticulitis.* The patient may experience lower abdominal pain, change in bowel habits, sometime fever, and even bleeding. Diagnosis is made with a barium enema, a procedure by which a suspension of barium sulfate is given by enema and x-rays are taken of the colon, which is thus outlined. Before such a procedure can be performed, the colon must be cleansed of feces by enemas.

Though medical treatment will usually control an episode of diverticulitis, recurrent attacks may require surgical removal of involved areas of colon. Sometimes this can be done in a single operation, with removal of the diseased segment of the colon and reconnection (anastomosis) of the cut ends to restore continuity. In other cases a procedure in two or more stages may be required. In such a situation the surgeon may first wish to divert the fecal stream from the diseased area of colon before removing it at a later date. This diversion is accomplished with a *colostomy,* an opening made between the hollow of a segment of colon preceding the diseased area, and the skin. Feces passing down the colon then empty to the exterior on the abdominal wall rather than passing down the remainder of the colon through the area of diverticulitis. At a subsequent date, with removal of the inflamed segment, the colostomy is surgically closed and the continuity of the bowel restored. The patient may then once again have evacuations by the rectum and anus. The colostomy that is sometimes performed on patients with diverticulitis is thus a temporary one; its management will be discussed later. (Also see Figures 30 and 31.)

ULCERATIVE COLITIS

In our discussion of the small intestine we noted that one disorder, regional enteritis, offered a particularly challenging problem in patient management and rehabilitation. The same must be said of ulcerative colitis. It is a chronic, recurrent disorder of unknown cause with highest incidence in the young adult. The pathological process begins in the depths of the mucous membrane lining the large intestine, in the areas called the crypts. Small abscesses form, and as the disorder progresses, a rather diffuse inflammation of the mucous membrane occurs. Ulcerations may develop and varying areas of the colonic lining may be left shaggy and bleeding.

The patient usually complains of abdominal cramps with recurrent or chronic diarrhea, occasionally of constipation. The passage of red blood, pus, or mucus through the rectum is common. In one form of the disease in which only the rectal portion of the colon is involved, _proctitis,_ the complaint may be of purulent bloody discharge without diarrhea. The patient may have recurrent acute flare-ups of the disease with fever, which may require hospitalization interspersed between months or years of relative well-being. Some patients will experience a more persistent disease with daily diarrhea and/or rectal discharge containing pus or blood. In the most severe cases, severe hemorrhage or perforation of the colon may occur.

The history of diarrhea and rectal discharge suggests the diagnosis. _Sigmoidoscopy,_ in which an illuminated metal tube is passed through the anus into the rectum and sigmoid colon, will reveal the diseased mucous membrane. An examination of the upper reaches of the colon is performed with a barium enema.

The frequency and urgency of bowel movements can often be controlled with the use of medications taken orally. If the disease is more severe or "active" with fever or much bleeding, or if the diarrhea cannot be controlled with milder medications, hospitalization and use of antibiotics and the cortisone family of drugs may be indicated. For reasons that are not clear (perhaps the freedom from home and vocational stresses) hospitalization and rest _per se_ are very helpful in the treatment of ulcerative colitis. In patients whose disease cannot be controlled with medicines and occasional hospitalization, and who are either acutely or chronically ill or severely disabled, surgery must be considered. A total colectomy, surgical removal of the entire colon and rectum with construction of an ileostomy, is performed. In this procedure, following the removal of the colon, an opening is made between the lumen of the ileum and the abdominal skin, so the ileal contents drain through the hole onto the exterior abdominal wall, where they are collected in a rubber appliance.

Though surgical treatment of regional enteritis is not infrequently followed by recurrence of the disease elsewhere in the small intestine (for one may not remove the entire small bowel) surgical removal of the colon cures ulcerative colitis (for the entire colon may be removed). Management of the patients with total colectomy and ileostomy is discussed later.

Some surgeons, in dealing with the ulcerative colitis patient whose rectum is not diseased, will leave the rectum and anus in place, removing the remainder of the large intestine and making a temporary ileostomy. They will later attempt to connect the ileum to the rectum in order to allow bowel evacuation through the anus.

One group of disorders that seems to be midway between ulcerative colitis and regional enteritis deserves mention. In this disease or diseases called *ileocolitis*, both the small bowel and the colon are inflamed. Whether such patients have ulcerative colitis involving the small intestine or regional enteritis involving the colon is not clear. Their treatment is similar to that outlined for patients with regional enteritis.

The disability associated with ulcerative colitis varies from little in those patients with mild disease which flares up infrequently, to quite severe in those with more extensive, more active disease. The decision as to when the disease is so bad, either acutely or chronically, as to warrant surgery is often difficult. The surgery that cures the colitis produces an ileostomy. Thus, the patient must have had sufficient troubles from his colitis to make him accept the adjustment required in this procedure. The majority of ulcerative colitis patients are managed medically without colectomy. Good diet, medications, adequate rest, are important. For some a job that is very stressful or does not allow them access to toilet facilities may need to be changed. The patient with recurrent episodes of the disease must have an employer willing to tolerate absences from work.

Probably more has been written about the emotional and personality characteristics of ulcerative colitis patients than any other group of patients with gastrointestinal disease. Such patients are often described as passive-aggressive, highly demanding people. There is, however, no solid body of evidence to prove any universal personality type in ulcerative colitis. In any case, recurrent abdominal cramps, fecal urgency, and diarrhea are likely to upset the equanimity of most patients, and one must beware of confusing the influence of personality on disease and the effects of disease on personality. Much work needs to be done in this area before the contributions of emotions in the genesis of colitis are clear. However, in this disorder as in others, sympathetic, encouraging, helpful attendants greatly aid in the patient's management.

TUMORS

Benign tumors of the colon, polyps, described above, are frequently seen and may be observed on a barium enema or through a sigmoidoscope, depending upon their location. Polyps occasionally bleed, causing the patient to pass red blood through the rectum. Because some types of polyps are thought to give rise to malignancy, they require surgical removal when discovered. Others are considered to have no malignant potential and hence are of less concern. When the physician wishes to be sure about which type he is dealing with, he may take a biopsy of the polyp. If it lies low enough in the colon, this may be accomplished through a sigmoidoscope.

Cancer of the large intestine is one of the most common gastrointestinal neoplasms. The majority of such cancers occur in the lower portion of the colon and are visible through a sigmoidoscope. Diagnosis may be made through such an instrument, or if the neoplasm rises higher in the colon, a barium enema may demonstrate it. The patient with a cancer of the colon may experience a change of bowel habits or bleeding through the rectum. Tumors arising high in the colon, particularly in the cecum, characteristically have a more insidious onset and may be discovered only after the patient has lost considerable blood.

Cancers deemed potentially curable are treated surgically with removal of the tumor, the adjacent colon, and the regional lymph nodes. When possible, the cut edges of the colon are approximated, restoring the continuity of the bowel. When this is impossible, or when the rectum or anus must be removed in resecting the tumor, a permanent colostomy may need to be performed as part of the operation.

COLOSTOMY AND ILEOSTOMY

Several of the disorders we have discussed may be treated surgically with either a temporary or permanent colostomy or ileostomy. The adjustment required by a patient whose fecal stream empties onto the abdominal wall rather than through the rectum is obviously considerable. Yet, when properly trained, such patients may lead normal lives, with their friends and associates unaware of this abnormality.

A colostomy appears as a pouting rosette of red tissue, the mucous membrane of the colon, on the lower abdominal wall. In the center of the rosette is a small opening, which is the actual lumen of the colon and the point through which feces exit. For some weeks following the healing of a colostomy site the colon will empty rather unpredictably, making it necessary for the patient to wear a colostomy appliance. Such appliances consist of a ring and a plastic or rubber bag to contain the expelled fecal drainage. A belt may be worn around the waist attached to the apparatus to further support it. The bag-ring arrangement is such that the fecal material is sealed off from the remainder of the abdominal wall and thus produces little odor. Some appliances permit a changing and replacement of the bag without removing the ring, thus allowing the ring to remain cemented in place for one or more days.

The patient whose colostomy is a temporary one (for example for diverticulitis), and is thus closed following definitive surgery for the primary disease, may proceed no further than the stage of management described, with periodic emptying of the colostomy bag and recementing of the retaining ring. The patient whose colostomy is left functioning more permanently will note a gradual thickening of the discharge. Since the intestinal contents pass through at least a portion of the colon before emptying into the colostomy, it is expected that some water will have been removed by the colonic mucosa. Hence the discharge will be quite thick, and eventually even formed. Further, with training and adjustment of diet, the patient will usually be able to have one or two predictably regular daily movements through the colostomy. Most patients perform a daily irrigation or enema with warm water through the abdominal opening with prompt drainage of the day's excreta via a bag into the toilet. The patient with such a well-functioning colostomy need wear over the opening only a plastic-covered gauze pad held in place with a lightweight belt, for the colostomy will not drain during the remainder of the day. Some patients will continue to wear a bag and ring arrangement with daily emptying. No fecal drainage should occur, of course, through the anus of the patient whose entire colon has been removed.

Success in achieving this admirable adjustment depends mostly on the patient's desire to do so and on the efforts of those caring for him to train and assist him. Prior to surgery, the patient must understand something of what awaits him. Afterward, sympathetic help, sometimes utilizing the aid of another patient who has successfully managed a colostomy, is important. Certain groups of patients however, present special problems.

1. Although the housewife who spends most of her time at home can tolerate occasional accidents with leakage of colostomy drainage, those who must work away from home accept such incidents with less equanimity. The latter group must have readily available toilet facilities at work to manage the colostomy in its early stages. Later, the daily movements or irrigations may be managed in the early morning or evening at home; leakage is then less often a problem.

2. The elderly or debilitated patient who cannot manage the changing of the bag or the irrigations needs nursing help to do so. Either the visiting nurse service or the aid of someone living with the patient must be arranged for him. Above all, the patient with a colostomy should understand that once trained, the colostomy *per se* will not interfere with normal activities. Such a patient may seek any sort of job and engage in any sort of recreation, including swimming.

The ileostomy patient presents a somewhat different problem. Though the ileal drainage does thicken, it remains always liquid, in contrast to the formed fecal material ejected from the mature colostomy. This is so because the intestinal contents draining from an ileostomy have never been exposed to the dehydrating function of the mucous membrane of the colon. Further, in contrast to the regular daily emptying of the colostomy which can often be achieved, the ileostomy will empty out in spurts during the day. Finally, the liquid ileostomy drainage tends to be somewhat irritating to the skin of the abdominal wall, and special care must be taken to protect such skin from being damaged.

The opening of the ileostomy on the skin of the abdomen appears similar to that described for the colostomy—a raised rosette of pink or red intestinal mucous membrane, in the center of which opens the lumen or hollow of the bowel. During the postoperative period, the ileostomy *stoma* (mouth) will be kept covered with a disposable plastic bag and ring arrangement. Later, the patient comes to use a more permanent appliance. This apparatus, also cemented to the skin around the ileostomy stoma, and supported by a belt around the waist, needs to be replaced and recemented every three to seven days. The rubber bag may be opened and drained into the toilet several times daily while it remains cemented in place and may then be closed off again. Materials are available (for example, karaya gum) which, when applied to the skin around the ileostomy before cementing the bag on, prevent irritation. Proper diet and regular eating habits may decrease the amount of drainage and thicken its consistency somewhat. Ileostomy patients must, however, accept the presence of the ileostomy appliance and bag with periodic emptying and replacement. Aside from this, they need experience no other limitation of activity. Organizations such as QT and the Ileoptomists, made up of patients who have ileostomies and colostomies, offer much help to others who have had these procedures. Their members compile and share information about the management of ileostomy and colostomy that might not otherwise be available.

Liver

The liver, the largest gland in the body, performs a multitude of complex and essential functions. It is classically considered a portion of the gastrointestinal system for three reasons. First, embryologically it arises as an outgrowth of the intestinal tract. Second, it secretes a fluid, bile, into the intestine that is vital to normal absorptive function. Third, the venous blood of the small and large intestine normally drains via the portal vein into the liver. Though much involved in the digestive and absorptive process, the liver has other nondigestive functions related to carbohydrate, fat, and protein metabolism.

Lying in the right upper portion of the abdomen just beneath the right diaphragm, the liver is a large smooth-surfaced organ. Microscopically, it is made up of plates of cuboidal polygonal cells called hepatic parenchymal cells. The blood supply of the liver is from the portal vein and hepatic artery. These vessels enter at an area called the hilus and divide into progressively smaller branches which ramify in the substance of the liver. Finally, the blood from the two sources mixes and is distributed to the parenchymal cells through minute microscopic channels called sinusoids, which run throughout the organ. As the plates of hepatic parenchymal cells are but one cell thick, each cell has ready access to the blood in the sinusoids. Between the blood in the sinusoids and the parenchymal cells is yet another type of structure, the Kupffer cell. These elongate cells are also found elsewhere in the body and serve to remove certain materials from the blood. The blood passing through the sinusoids eventually drains into progressively larger channels called the venules, which form the larger hepatic veins. These veins empty into the inferior vena cava, which drains to the right side of the heart.

The bile, formed by the hepatic parenchymal cells, is secreted into small spaces within the liver called cholangioles, and drains into progressively larger biliary ductules. The direction of biliary drainage is directly opposite to the blood flow, so the biliary ductules run along the small branches of the hepatic artery and portal vein. Such areas of the branches of the two vessels and one or more branches of the biliary ductule are called portal triads. The ductules eventually unite to form the hepatic ducts; these join to form the *common bile duct,* which leaves the liver at the point of entry of the hepatic artery and portal vein. The common bile duct drains into the small intestine through an opening called the ampulla of Vater. A small branch of the common bile duct, called the cystic duct, leads to the *gallbladder.* This latter structure is a sac or a bag connected to the common bile duct and serves to concentrate and store bile. When it contracts in response to the simulus of a fatty meal, it empties it contents into the common bile duct and thence into the small bowel.

No attempt can be made in as brief a discussion as this even to list completely the functions of the liver. What follows is merely a summary, with a few examples of the part the liver plays in metabolism and digestion.

The hepatic parenchymal cells extract a number of substances from the blood in the hepatic sinusoids, change them chemically, and transfer them across the cell and into the bile. Such substances (for example, bilirubin) then pass via the biliary channels into the intestine. For molecules such as bilirubin this is purely a means of disposal of waste product. Another group of substances, bile acids, are excreted into the bile by the liver and serve a useful function when they reach the intestine. They are important in aiding digestion and absorption of fat. The liver chemically alters a number of materials in the blood (both naturally occurring in the body, and drugs), thus inactivating them. Ammonia, for example, which is formed in the intestine by bacteria, is absorbed, reaches the liver via the portal vein, and is there converted to another compound, urea. Certain medications, for example, barbiturates, are inactivated in the liver.

The liver manufactures a number of compounds. It is, for example, the sole source of a most important plasma protein, albumin, and synthesizes other plasma proteins as well. Glucose is stored in the liver in the form of glycogen and can be released into the circulating blood when the blood glucose level falls, thus providing this important chemical source of energy to the brain. The liver also plays a vital role in the breakdown and synthesis of fatty compounds.

VIRAL HEPATITIS

Two types of acute inflammatory disease of the liver believed due to viral infection are recognized. One, _serum hepatitis,_ is transmitted by blood transfusion from a hepatitis carrier or injection with improperly sterilized needles containing the infectious agent. _Infectious hepatitis,_ in contrast, is transmitted by food or water contaminated with the infectious agent. Contaminated shellfish have, of late, been recognized as prominent sources of human infectious hepatitis. In these diseases, following an incubation period (which for serum hepatitis may be several months), the patient classically develops nonspecific symptoms of feeling ill and loss of appetite followed by jaundice. The latter sign, a yellow coloration to the skin and eyes, is a prominent manifestation of a number of liver diseases. It will be remembered that the liver normally extracts the yellow material bilirubin from the blood and excretes it into the bile. In disorders where the liver or biliary passages are damaged, this function is not adequately performed, and the yellow bilirubin accumulates in the blood, producing jaundice. Some of the excess pigment may also be excreted by the kidneys, giving a dark color to the urine. The failure of normal amounts of bilirubin to reach the intestine may also result in a lightening of the color of the stool in hepatitis, for the bile pigments are thought responsible for the normal dark brown color of feces.

Patients with hepatitis are usually treated in the hospital. Physicians' opinions about the length of time the patient should be at rest vary. Most agree that so long as the patient feels quite ill, he should be at rest. Some feel that the patient may get out of bed as soon as he feels able. Others keep the patient at bed rest until the blood tests of liver function are nearly normal.

Milder forms of either type of hepatitis are recognized by doing chemical tests of the patient's blood. Such patients may have only mild symptoms or none at all, and need not be jaundiced. Chemical tests on the blood, called _liver function tests,_ are useful in the diagnosis of hepatitis in the jaundiced patient as well.

Only the blood of the patient with serum hepatitis can transmit the infection, and this only if injected into another person. Accordingly, needles and syringes used on such patients should be especially carefully sterilized, and their blood samples should not be handled by anybody with an open wound. Further, patients who have had hepatitis are never acceptable thereafter as blood donors. Save for these precautions, serum hepatitis patients are not isolated. In contrast, patients with infectious hepatitis, at least during the acute illness, excrete the infectious agent in their stools. Suitable precautions must therefore be taken to see that fecal-oral transmission of the infection to others attending the patient does not occur. The patient's blood too is infectious.

The usual course of serum or infectious hepatitis is complete recovery following rest and treatment with nutritious diet. The patient usually is hospitalized for several weeks. The period of convalescence following discharge from the hospital varies, but may involve limitation of heavy activity for a number of months. Following such convalescence and once pronounced well, the patient need not observe any further restrictions. A few less fortunate patients do not heal their infections so rapidly and continue to have persistent low-grade infection in their livers, called *chronic hepatitis.* These people may need a more prolonged, and occasionally permanent, restriction of heavy activity, depending upon how they feel and the severity of their disease. In addition to a nutritious diet, the cortisone family of drugs may be used in treatment. These patients, too, with treatment and rest may heal. It is thought that a small group of patients with long-continued chronic hepatitis that does not heal progress to a stage of permanent liver damage and scarring called *cirrhosis.*

CIRRHOSIS

Cirrhosis of the liver designates a group of chronic diseases in which there is destruction of liver parenchymal cells, some regeneration of nodules of new liver cells, the laying down of scar tissue, and inflammation within the liver. Several causes and types of cirrhosis are recognized, the relative frequency of each varying with the location of the population under study. Certain general characteristics of this cirrhotic process apply to each of the types and will be discussed first.

The manifestations of cirrhosis may be considered in three groups: those caused by progressive destruction of the liver cells; those produced by increased pressure in the portal vein which often accompanies cirrhosis; and those caused by a combination of liver destruction and increased portal vein pressure. As an example of the first group we might list jaundice. The diseased liver in cirrhosis as in hepatitis fails to remove bilirubin completely from the blood. Accordingly, the yellow material accumulates in the body and causes the skin and eyes to appear yellow. Other less specific manifestations of the failing liver include loss of appetite, weakness, and easy fatigability.

The regenerating nodules of liver cells in cirrhosis compress the small branches of the portal vein within the liver, thus producing a rise in the pressure within the portal vein. If this pressure is transmitted back to the smaller veins that connect to the portal vein, these vessels may become progressively enlarged and tortuous. Examples of such veins are the large vessels sometimes seen on the abdominal wall of the cirrhotic patient and, of much greater importance, *esophageal varices*. The latter, as mentioned in the section on the esophagus, are the veins just beneath the mucous membrane lining of the lower esophagus. Normally tiny, they eventually drain into the portal vein. When back pressure in the portal vein builds up in cirrhosis and is transmitted to these veins, they may become dilated, tortuous, and thin-walled. The possibility of spontaneous rupture of such vessels with massive gastrointestinal hemorrhage is a danger in cirrhotic patients.

Finally, let us consider a third group of manifestations of cirrhosis: those caused by combined liver cell failure and portal vein hypertension. The liver, as has been noted, is the source of the body's plasma albumin. It is the plasma albumin that exerts the osmotic pressure necessary to keep the plasma from leaking out of the capillaries into the tissues. Accordingly, in cirrhotic patients with a low serum albumin, edema or swelling of the tissues, usually of the legs, may result. When a lowered serum albumin is combined with a high pressure in the portal vein, fluid leaks from vessels into the abdominal cavity. Such fluid, called *ascites*, results in a progressive enlargement and distention of the abdomen.

Certain neurological and mental abnormalities are seen in cirrhotic patients with severe liver damage (which is often combined with portal hypertension). These may range from mild personality changes to deep coma and may occur spontaneously in severe liver disease or may be provoked by gastrointestinal bleeding, a high protein diet, infection, or certain drugs. Much investigation is presently under way to establish the cause of this neurological-psychiatric disorder (called *hepatic coma* or *hepatic encephalopathy*), which may come and go and may be quite disabling. It may be that the liver fails to detoxify some material arising in the gastrointestinal tract (for example, ammonia), and this material accumulating in the blood and brain results in the changes described.

LAENNEC'S (PORTAL) CIRRHOSIS. In this disorder, areas of parenchymal cell destruction, inflammation, and scarring surround the portal triads of the liver. The liver cells regenerate, forming small nodules giving the surface of the organ a hobnail appearance. Despite this regeneration, however, the net effect is loss of normal liver cell function. The signs and symptoms of the disease are those described for cirrhosis in general. They range from the finding of a large liver in an asymptomatic patient to jaundice, ascites, and coma in the severely ill patient. The diagnosis may be confirmed with the aid of liver function tests and chemical analyses done on the patient's blood and urine which enable the liver disease to be characterized. Liver biopsy, in which a small piece of liver is removed with a needle, may also be helpful.

The course, treatment, rehabilitation, and prognosis of the patient with Laennec's cirrhosis are best considered together. The principle cause, though by no means the only one, is alcoholism. Whether alcohol itself damages the liver when taken in excess, or whether the poor diet that accompanies alcoholism is the cause of defect, is not clear. It may be that both alcohol and a protein-poor diet are important in causing cirrhosis and in producing the accumulation of fat in the liver which is thought to be an early stage of this process.

At least some of the liver changes in Laennec's cirrhosis can be treated and improved with good diet, high in protein and vitamins, and avoidance of alcohol. The accomplishment of such a regimen in the alcoholic is no mean feat. It requires that the patient be willing to give up drinking and be able to obtain the diet prescribed. Vigorous effort and support by the family and the physician, with the aid of social agencies in the case of the indigent patient, are necessary. Many alcoholic patients are very resistant to giving up drinking, and their treatment is extremely frustrating, for no medication can really replace the regimen prescribed. Organizations such as Alcoholics Anonymous, made up of people who have been cured of alcoholism, can serve a unique function for such patients. Older members try to help new candidates to abandon alcohol, and with the mutual support and companionship offered by such groups, success may be achieved.

Patients with mild forms of Laennec's cirrhosis, if properly treated, may be capable of reasonably normal activity. Those with more severe disease may have varying disability. Those with jaundice or ascites or varieties of hepatic encephalopathy are the most severely disabled and may require chronic hospitalization. Manifestations such as ascites, jaundice, and bleeding esophageal varices are extremely serious prognostic signs. Prolonged hospitalization may be required for such patients. Ascites may be treated with a variety of medications called *diuretics*, but usually a diet low in salt is required as well. Such a diet, with low salt, bread, and milk, and the medications to decrease fluid are often fairly expensive, and the low-income patient may need financial assistance to maintain them. Occasionally a *paracentesis*, removal of ascites by a needle tap of the abdomen, may be necessary.

The patient who has recovered from hemorrhage of esophageal varices and who is deemed a good operative risk may undergo a *portacaval shunt*. In this procedure, the portal vein is surgically connected to the inferior vena cava, so that the back pressure from the cirrhotic liver is relieved, and the varices may then disappear. A prolonged period of convalescence may be required after such surgery. No general statement can be made about the work ability of patients with Laennec's cirrhosis, for this obviously depends upon the severity of the disease in each patient.

Some patients with Laennec's (portal) cirrhosis have no history of alcoholism or poor diet, and the cause of their disease is not known. The dietary treatment and diuretic medications discussed are used here as well.

POSTHEPATIC CIRRHOSIS. This variety of hepatic disease is thought to be the result of a chronic inflammation in the liver, perhaps starting with a viral hepatitis many years in the past. Such an acute episode may have been recognized at the time, for it may have produced jaundice, or it may have been undetected. Patients with posthepatic cirrhosis are said to have larger nodules of regenerating liver cells than those in Laennec's cirrhosis, and their clinical course differs in certain ways. In general, however, the complications, manifestations, and management of both types of disease are similar, with signs and symptoms due to loss of normal liver tissue and portal hypertension. Although in dealing with the patient with posthepatic cirrhosis the doctor is not necessarily faced with the problem of alcoholism, neither does he have any evident cause of the disease which he might try to eliminate.

BILIARY CIRRHOSIS. *Primary biliary cirrhosis* occurs most frequently in women and characteristically causes years of intermittent jaundice and itching. During this time the patient feels otherwise quite well, for it is only after years have elapsed that liver function further deteriorates. Patients with this disorder in its earlier forms therefore may be capable of full and active lives, providing they can adjust to the discomfort of the itching and the social problems that may be presented by the jaundice. Much of what has been said about the manifestations of other types of cirrhosis applies to primary biliary cirrhosis in its later stages.

Following prolonged obstruction to the biliary tree, for example, by stricture or gallstones, secondary damage to the liver may occur. This damage, called *secondary biliary cirrhosis,* may be in some measure reversible with prompt surgical relief of the obstruction.

OTHER TYPES OF CIRRHOSIS. Chronic disease of the liver which has some of the characteristics of cirrhosis is seen in at least two other disorders. In *Wilson's disease,* a familial metabolic disorder, copper is deposited in the brain and liver, producing neurological disorders and chronic liver disease. In *hemochromatosis,* for reasons not clear, iron is deposited in the liver, pancreas, and skin, producing cirrhosis, diabetes, and skin pigmentation. In both these disorders, treatment consists of trying to remove medically the excess metal deposits. There is some evidence that early diagnosis is important in each of these diseases, for medical attempts at prevention of the copper or iron deposition may prevent subsequent organ damage.

DISEASES OF THE BILIARY TRACT

Stones in the gallbladder and biliary tract (*cholelithiasis*) occur with increasing frequency as age increases, but are seen in young people as well. Many patients have no symptoms from them, while others may have manifestations of pain or obstruction with jaundice due to such stones. Acute attacks of inflammation of the gallbladder (*acute cholecystitis*) may occur. Surgical removal of the diseased gallbladder and stones is usually advised in those who have had biliary symptoms and who present a good operative risk.

The diagnosis of gallstones is made by history and confirmed by x-ray. Some stones contain calcium and are visible on a plain x-ray of the abdomen. More frequently, however, stones do not show up on such films and an additional special x-ray study, called an *oral chole-cystogram,* is necessary to demonstrate them. The night before such a test the patient swallows several tablets of a dye that is opaque to x-ray. During the night this dye is absorbed from the intestine and is excreted by the liver into the biliary system. The gallbladder concentrates the dye and thus appears opaque on x-ray the following morning. Stones may be seen as radiolucent defects within the gallbladder with such a technique. A fat-containing drink is then given, in response to which the normal gallbladder contracts and empties the dye into the common bile duct, from whence it flows into the small intestine. This process may be seen on fluoroscopy. Patients with *chronic cholecystitis* (chronic inflammation of the gallbladder), with or without gallstones, may fail to concentrate the dye in the gallbladder. Such failure to visualize this organ is of diagnostic importance.

BILIARY OBSTRUCTION

Obstruction to the flow of bile down the biliary tract produces jaundice, presumably because of regurgitation of bilirubin back into the blood from the biliary system. Such obstruction may be due to gallstones, to scarring of the common bile duct (stricture), or to cancer of biliary ducts, the ampulla of Vater, or the pancreas. Cancer of the ampulla causes obstruction at the point the common bile duct enters the intestine. The head of the pancreas lies in close proximity to the common bile duct just before it enters the intestine. Accordingly, pancreatic cancer can obstruct the duct and produce jaundice. Neoplasms of pancreas and ampulla are treated surgically when deemed resectable. As noted, prolonged biliary obstruction (usually due to gallstones or stricture) can cause liver damage (secondary biliary cirrhosis) if left uncorrected.

Pancreas

This gland is a flattened elongate structure lying horizontally in the upper abdomen behind the abdominal lining (peritoneum). It thus lies behind the stomach against tissues of the back. The head of the pancreas is a somewhat rounded portion of the gland which lies adjacent to the duodenum.

Microscopically, the pancreas consists of two types of structures. First, there are the *acini,* a group of cells that manufacture the digestive enzymes and secrete them via the pancreatic ducts into the small bowel. Scattered throughout the pancreas are other groups of cells called the *islets of Langerhans*, which do not communicate with the duct system. The islets secrete insulin and perhaps another hormone into the blood.

Stimulation of the cells of the acini to secrete digestive enzymes and fluid comes from several sources. In response to acid in the upper small intestine, the mucous membrane of the duodenum liberates two hormones, pancreozymin and secretin, into the blood. Pancreozymin stimulates the secretion of the pancreatic enzymes by the cells of the acini, and secretin causes the release of bicarbonate-rich liquid from the acinar cells. Another stimulus to pancreatic secretion comes from the vagus nerves.

Diseases that damage the acini and thus influence their enzyme output will produce failure of normal digestion of carbohydrate, protein, and fat. *Pancreatitis, cancer,* and *cystic fibrosis* of the pancreas are examples of such disorders. Failure of normal function of the islets results in insulin deficiency and diabetes. Pancreatitis and cancer can do this. However, in most patients with diabetes the basic reason for the insulin deficiency is not clear, but seems genetically determined.

PANCREATITIS

Two major types of inflammatory disease of the pancreas are recognized. The first, *acute pancreatitis,* produces one or more acute episodes of severe abdominal pain, fever, and sometimes shock, requiring intensive hospital care. This type of disorder will not be further discussed here. The second variety is more chronic, producing recurrent abdominal pain over many years and progressive destruction of the pancreas, without the episodes of shock and fever characteristic of acute pancreatitis. Such *chronic relapsing pancreatitis* is in some patients familial, in others it is associated with gallstones, and in some with hyperactivity of the parathyroid glands. In some, no cause can be found. However, a large group of patients with pancreatitis are found to be heavy drinkers of alcohol, and it is felt that in these cases the alcohol is in some way related to the pancreatic damage. In some of these patients, progressive destruction of the pancreas may occur without pain.

With progressive destruction of both major types of structures in the pancreas, diabetes, malabsorption, and maldigestion occur. Patients wth chronic pancreatitis may have fatty or greasy stools similar to those seen in sprue, but, of course, for a different reason. In pancreatic disease, maldigestion due to loss of pancreatic enzymes produces malabsorption. In sprue, intestinal malabsorption is the primary abnormality.

The characteristic history of the pain of pancreatitis combined with certain x-ray findings in the abdomen (calcification in the area of the pancreas), evidence of malabsorption of foods, and diabetes mellitus (demonstrated by measurement of blood and urine sugar; enables the physician to make the diagnosis.

The aims in therapy of chronic relapsing pancreatitis are threefold: (1) control of diabetes, (2) correction of maldigestion and thus improvement of absorption, and (3) control of pain. In the case of the alcoholic, the additional effort must be made to eliminate alcohol in order to prevent further attacks of pain and further damage to the pancreas. Treatment of the diabetes mellitus is with insulin and diet, and will be discussed in another chapter. Pancreatic enzyme replacement with powders or capsules containing pancreatic extract, taken with meals, will improve digestion and absorption. The control of pain is often the most troublesome part of treatment. For some, episodes of pain are infrequent and can be controlled with medicines. Those with more frequent or even daily pain have a much greater problem. The chronic use of strong analgesics is unsatisfactory, for not only are they addicting, but they often become progressively less effective. It is this group of patients with pancreatitis, those with chronic, persistent, or frequent pain, who suffer most. Their ability to work or even enjoy their lives may be severely limited. It is for such patients that a variety of operations that attempt to either improve drainage from the pancreas or actually remove the pancreas are performed.

Those patients who have had total removal of the pancreas (*pancreatectomy*) for pain obviously must be maintained on pancreatic extract with meals and insulin. Certain complications of pancreatitis (cysts or abscesses) may also require surgical treatment.

PANCREATIC CANCER

One of the most insidious of gastrointestinal neoplasms, cancer of the pancreas is treated surgically when deemed resectable. Sometimes producing abdominal pain, the neoplasm may destroy a significant portion of the pancreas, producing maldigestion and malabsorption. The management of the patient who has had a pancreatectomy for such a cancer is identical with that of the patient with pancreatitis who has has a similar operation.

Certain cancers of the pancreas rise from the islets of Langerhans. Such neoplasms may actually produce insulin, in which case they are called *functioning islet cell tumors*. This excessive and inappropriate secretion of insulin produces a lowering of the blood sugar, which may cause the patient to feel sweaty or actually faint. Surgical removal of these tumors is the proper treatment. The occurrence of islet tumors and intractable peptic ulcers is called the Zollinger-Ellison syndrome.

CYSTIC FIBROSIS OF THE PANCREAS

Brief mention will be made of this disease, which is actually a disorder of several glands throughout the body. Beginning in childhood and genetically determined, it produces chronic and recurrent pulmonary infections (bronchitis and pneumonia), destruction of the acinar portion of the pancreas, and excess salt excretion in the sweat. Pancreatic extract replacement therapy and antibiotic treatment of the pulmonary infections are permitting more and more of these patients to reach adulthood. Many hospitalizations may be required for such children, both before the diagnosis is made and subsequently from the pulmonary disorder. Long-term antibiotic treatment and pancreatic extract therapy are expensive to maintain, and the families of such patients with borderline incomes may require assistance.

FUNCTIONAL GASTROINTESTINAL DISORDERS

This ill-defined group of disorders is included largely because the diagnostic term "functional" is so often used by physicians. In its strictest sense, a functional disorder is one in which function (usually the motility of the gastrointestinal tract) is abnormal. Such abnormal function may or may not be apparent on x-ray examination or chemical tests, but is quite apparent to the patient who experiences a variety of abdominal pains and abnormalities of bowel habits (diarrhea and/or constipation). An example of such a functional disorder is the *irritable colon* or *spastic colon syndrome*, sometimes called *mucous colitis*. Recurrent episodes of diarrhea or constipation with abdominal pain are characteristic. No abnormality, save for spasticity of the colon, is apparent on x-ray or sigmoidoscopy. Management of such patients with anticholinergic drugs and tranquilizers or sedatives is usually helpful. A large number of variants of this *irritable bowel* syndrome are seen but are not discussed here because they are usually troublesome rather than debilitating.

The designation "functional disorder" is also used by some physicians to indicate a symptom or symptoms the cause of which cannot be found but which are thought to be psychoneurotic. Such patients may have no objective evidence of disease, but nonetheless have symptoms, usually abdominal discomfort, which seems real enough to them. A whole host of disorders are probably included in this group, many of which are due to abnormal motor function and some of which may be of emotional origin. Little more can be said of these patients because of the diverse nature of the disorders. The conditions may range from mild discomfort to more troublesome bowel distress. They do not usually produce real debility.

Throughout the chapter reference has been made to possible emotional causes of gastrointestinal disease—for example, peptic ulcer and ulcerative colitis. Although it is personally felt that no clear case has yet been made that any specific gastrointestinal disorder is invariably caused by a specific emotional disorder, it seems clear that emotional factors surely play a crucial role in a variety of gastrointestinal disorders, be they causal or contributory. It remains for further investigation to determine the nature and importance of such contributions. A most fruitful area for the investigation of emotional factors in gastrointestinal disease, however, would surely be the so-called functional disorders.

BIBLIOGRAPHY

Cecil, Russell L., Robert F. Loeb, *et. al.* *Textbook of Medicine,* 11th ed. Philadelphia: W. B. Saunders Co., 1963.

Davenport, Horace W. *Physiology of the Digestive Tract.* Chicago: Yearbook Publishers, Inc., 1961.

Harrison, Tinsley R., *et al.* *Principles of Internal Medicine,* 4th ed. New York: McGraw-Hill Book Co., 1962.

VI

DISEASES OF THE KIDNEY

Since the most obvious function of the kidney is to make urine, it is usually thought of as primarily an excretory organ. However, the most significant activities of the kidney relate to regulation of the volume and composition of the body fluids, particularly the blood plasma and other extracellular fluids. In addition, the kidney is involved, in a manner as yet ill-defined, in the regulation of other bodily functions, such as blood pressure and red blood cell formation. Future investigations will undoubtedly uncover additional regulatory and metabolic activities of the kidney. Because of the multiplicity of excretory, regulatory, and metabolic functions performed by the normal kidney, the clinical features of kidney disease are varied and involve subtle or gross derangements in virtually all other organ systems.

ANATOMY AND NORMAL PHYSIOLOGY

The kidneys, which together weigh approximately 300 gm in man, are two flattened, lima-bean–shaped organs that lie just beneath the diaphragm on either side of the spine (vertebral column). Approximately two million nephrons, each made up of a filtering portion, the _glomerulus_, attached to an elongated, convoluted _tubule_, are the anatomical and functional units of the kidney. Blood enters the kidney via the renal artery and is distributed through a series of successively smaller arterial connections to the glomeruli. Each glomerulus is a specialized filtering device in which blood, enclosed in thin-walled

By Norman G. Levinsky, M.D. Assistant Professor of Medicine, Boston University School of Medicine; Physician-in-Charge, Boston University Renal Service, Boston City Hospital, Boston, Massachusetts.

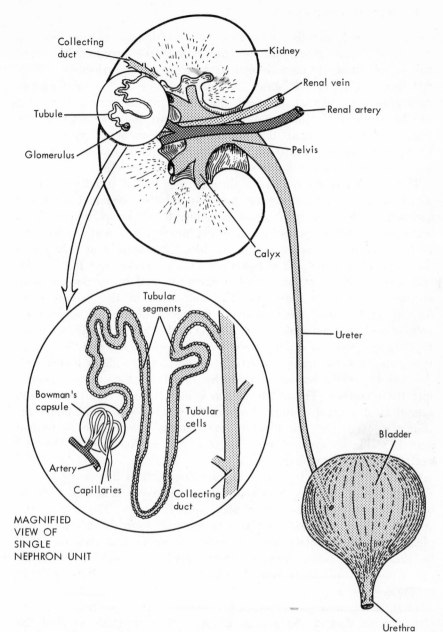

Figure 7. Diagram of the kidney and lower urinary tract. The kidney is shown in cut section. The insert shows an expanded view of a single nephron unit.

capillaries, is brought into intimate contact with a thin capsular structure (Bowman's capsule), which represents the expanded end of an individual nephron. All components of the blood, with the exception of

163

the largest, such as cells (red cells or white cells) and plasma proteins, pass through the glomerular membranes into the nephron. The total volume of filtrate formed in normal humans is approximately 150 to 200 liters daily. This is some 25 times as large as the total plasma volume in man, so that, in effect, the entire plasma volume is filtered by the kidneys 25 times a day. It is obvious that the bulk of the water and other materials that are normal components of plasma must be returned to the circulation; otherwise, the entire volume of plasma and other extracellular fluids would rapidly be depleted.

The glomerular filtrate passes through a series of tubular segments which carry out this reabsorptive function and other essential regulatory activities of the kidney. Normal components of the plasma—such as water, salts (sodium, potassium, chloride, bicarbonate), amino acids, and glucose—are transferred back into the blood by the tubular cells lining the nephron segments. These reabsorptive processes are individually regulated, both by intrinsic renal mechanisms and by extrinsic control mechanisms such as hormones. The net result of the various reabsorptive and control mechanisms is the reconstitution of the normal volume and concentration of the plasma and other extracellular fluids. For example, when a surfeit of sodium is present in the diet, the excess is excreted into the urine; conversely, when dietary sodium is deficient, the kidney avidly reabsorbs into the blood all the sodium filtered into the glomeruli. The ability of the kidney to vary reabsorption and excretion of normal plasma components within very wide limits accounts in large part for the fact that plasma composition in normal man is stable in spite of wide shifts in the composition of the diet and in bodily metabolism.

Some materials can be added to the urine without first being filtered through the glomerulus. Surrounding each nephron is a rich network of tiny blood vessels, the peritubular capillary plexus. The cells of the several nephron segments can secrete material from the blood in this plexus into the tubular urine. A wide variety of materials can thus be excreted, including normal bodily constituents such as potassium and a number of drugs and chemicals that seemingly have little in common.

Thus, as the urine passes down the nephron, its composition is greatly altered from that of the plasma filtrate which originally entered the glomerulus. Materials to be conserved, such as sodium and water, have been reabsorbed by tubular activity. Waste products filtered from the blood, such as urea, have become concentrated in the urine. In addition, certain materials, such as potassium, have been secreted into the urine. Urine from the individual nephrons drains into a collecting system within the kidney. Urine collected from each kidney enters the renal pelvis, the expanded upper portion of the ureter, a muscular tube that connects the kidney with the urinary bladder. Storage of urine within the bladder and release via the urethra at convenient times is effected by bladder wall musculature and outlet (sphincter) muscles around the urethra. Voiding is coordinated and controlled both by local nerves and by the central nervous system (spinal cord and brain).

CLINICAL INVESTIGATION OF KIDNEY FUNCTION

A great number of techniques have been used to evaluate the anatomical integrity and functional capacity of the kidney in man. Only a few of the principal methods will be described briefly.

PROTEINURIA

As mentioned above, the normal glomerulus does not permit large molecules such as plasma proteins to enter the urine. The presence of protein in the urine (proteinuria), therefore, is a sign of abnormal kidney function and is, in fact, one of the commonest means by which renal disease is discovered. Proteins can be detected readily by precipitating them as a visible cloud with various chemical agents or with heat. Normal urine contains less than 0.1 gram of protein per day, an amount too small to be detected by routine laboratory methods. Any increase in protein excretion above this amount is nearly always evidence of underlying renal disease. However, the amount of protein excreted is not correlated with the severity or prognosis of the disease process.

In occasional instances, proteinuria occurs only when the patient is in the upright position and disappears during recumbency. This condition, *postural or orthostatic proteinuria,* is in the majority of children and adolescents a benign disorder that disappears before age 18 or 20. In adults, postural proteinuria may also be benign, but since it is in the majority of cases a manifestation of renal disease, it cannot be dismissed without complete studies to evaluate its significance. Continuous proteinuria at any age is always a sign of renal disease.

SEDIMENT

Cells and casts are the principal elements in the urinary sediment. The cells that may be seen include white cells, red cells, and tissue (epithelial) cells from the kidney and lower urinary tract. Casts, which are formed in renal tubules that are damaged or in which urine flow is slow, are composed either of coagulated protein (hyaline casts) or of white, red, or tubular cells that have been compressed together (cellular casts). Occasional white cells, red cells, or hyaline casts may be found in normal urine; any increase in the numbers of these elements or the presence of any number of cellular casts is always abnormal. A careful microscopic examination of the urinary sediment is part of the initial work-up of any patient with suspected renal disease and often directs attention toward the proper diagnosis immediately. For example, the appearance of white cell casts in the urine indicates that inflammation, most commonly due to bacterial infection, is taking place in the kidney. Similarly, the presence of red cell casts in the urine is a sign of glomerular damage, permitting red cells, normally retained within the glomerular capillaries, to escape into the tubules. Although the nature of the sediment is an important clue to the type of disease present, it gives no information about the severity of renal involvement.

KIDNEY FUNCTION TESTS

The severity of renal disease is usually evaluated by several simple kidney function tests. The rate of filtration into the glomeruli can be estimated for clinical purposes by measuring the plasma levels of urea, creatinine, or "nonprotein nitrogen." Each of these nitrogenous waste products is excreted by filtration; when glomerular filtration is reduced, their plasma levels increase. The functional progress of acute and chronic renal disease is commonly followed by repeated measurements of plasma urea or creatinine. The tests most commonly used in the clinic to evaluate tubular function measure ability to concentrate the urine or to excrete a red dye known as PSP (phenolsulfonphthalein). When the filtration rate is substantially reduced, tubular function is always decreased as well. In addition, tests of tubular functions sometimes demonstrate subtle degrees of renal damage before the filtration rate has decreased.

X-RAY EXAMINATIONS

Certain anatomical features of kidney disease can be visualized by appropriate radiographic (x-ray) studies. A technique frequently employed is the intravenous pyelogram; in this procedure, an iodine-containing dye that is opaque to x-rays is injected intravenously, and a succession of films is taken at appropriate timed intervals. The dye is seen within the largest collecting ducts (calyces), the renal pelvis, the ureters, and the bladder. The size of the kidneys can be determined, and the concentration of dye serves as an indirect test of kidney function. Stones or obstruction to urine flow can be seen. A variety of specialized radiographic techniques, such as renal angiography and laminography, permit visualization of structures not seen by routine pyelography and are occasionally necessary to investigate complicated problems.

BIOPSY

In recent years, renal biopsy has become a safe and painless procedure that does not require surgery or general anesthesia. A special needle is introduced through the locally anesthetized skin into the kidney, and a minute amount of tissue is withdrawn for microscopic examination. Study of biopsy specimens is occasionally the only method that will establish a specific diagnosis in renal disease and is often helpful in determining whether certain types of treatment are likely to be beneficial.

CLINICAL FEATURES OF KIDNEY DISEASE

Many patients with kidney disease have no manifest symptoms during part or all of their illness. In such individuals, the presence of kidney disease can be appreciated only through special clinical or laboratory examinations. However, most patients develop symptoms and physical findings characteristic either of a particular type of functional damage or of a specific disease entity.

UREMIA

When kidney function is markedly reduced by an acute or chronic disease, a group of clinical manifestations known as *uremia* gradually appears. Although the blood level of nitrogenous waste products such as urea or creatinine is used as an index of the severity of renal failure, no single compound causes the total picture of uremia. Undoubtedly, a variety of factors, including failure to excrete waste products, inability to maintain the normal volume, composition, and acidity of plasma and other extracellular fluids, malnutrition, hypertension, and anemia are all involved. It must be emphasized that uremia is not specific to any single renal disease but is rather the general result of renal failure, however produced. The earliest symptom of uremia is often lassitude, with gradual decrease in vigor, strength, and mental alertness over a period of weeks, months, or even many years. Bizarre and irrational behavior may occur. Neuromuscular manifestations such as twitching, pains in the extremities, muscle cramps, and convulsions may be prominent. Among the most unpleasant symptoms are those relating to the gastrointestinal tract. Loss of appetite is the rule and is often accompanied by nausea, vomiting, or diarrhea. When prolonged, these symptoms may give rise to progressive malnutrition. Almost all patients with uremia develop anemia, which, when severe, is probably responsible in part for the weakness and general debility. High blood pressure (hypertension) and heart failure are common finding in patients with uremia and result in headaches, difficulty in breathing, and edema. In children, a prominent feature is interference with normal growth and development.

EDEMA

Excess fluid is a common finding at several stages in the development of renal disease. Edema collects under the skin, especially that of the lower extremities, and in body cavities, such as the chest and abdomen. Fluid retention occurs in acute renal disease and in advanced chronic renal disease because salt and water excretion by the damaged kidney is inadequate. It also occurs in the *nephrotic syndrome*, a stage in several types of renal disease in which plasma protein is deficient (see section on nephrotic syndrome). Edema under the skin is merely unattractive and uncomfortable; in the chest (pulmonary edema, pleural effusion), it may seriously compromise breathing.

HYPERTENSION

High blood pressure, as already noted, is common in chronic uremia. It also may occur in some types of acute renal disease, such as glomerulonephritis, and in certain forms of chronic renal disease, such as pyelonephritis, before uremia is present. A complete explanation for the frequency of hypertension in renal disease is not known, but release by the damaged kidney of excessive amounts of angiotensin, which causes blood vessels to undergo narrowing, undoubtedly plays a role. Since hypertension itself can cause renal disease, a vicious circle may occur in which renal disease causes hypertension, which in turn aggravates the underlying disease. In addition, hypertension may lead to heart failure, which also affects kidney function adversely. Thus, the advent of hypertension in chronic renal disease often results in rapid deterioration of the clinical course. Fortunately, potent antihypertensive drugs which can arrest this unhappy sequence of events have become available in the past few years.

SPECIFIC DISEASES OF THE KIDNEY

GLOMERULONEPHRITIS

Renal disease in which inflammation of the glomeruli is the initial and principal lesion is known as glomerulonephritis; both acute and chronic forms are recognized. In the majority of instances, acute glomerulonephritis begins one to three weeks after infections with streptococci, usually in the respiratory tract (for example, a "strep throat"). Certain types of streptococci, such as type 12, seem to be particularly likely to cause renal damage. During epidemics due to this or similar types of streptococci, 10 or 20 per cent of those infected may develop signs of renal injury. Although the exact cause of the renal damage is not known, much evidence suggests that an autoimmune mechanism is involved. In other words, the streptococcus initiates some change in the kidney of susceptible or "allergic" individuals which results in a self-perpetuating inflammation that continues long after the infecting organism is gone.

Acute glomerulonephritis may be so mild it is clinically asymptomatic and can be detected only by microscopic examination of the urine, or it may be fulminating, with rapid progression to uremia and death. It is most common in children and in young adults but may occur at any age, even in the seventh and eighth decades. The patient first notices red or brown urine (blood in the urine, hematuria), puffiness of the face or eyelids, swelling of the ankles (edema), headache, malaise, weakness, or a decrease in urinary output. Physical examination in moderately severe cases often reveals hypertension and edema. Urinalysis suggests or confirms the clinical diagnosis when red cell casts, red cells, and protein are found. Evidence of active streptococcal infection may be found on physical examination or by culture of the throat, but more commonly only indirect laboratory evidence of a previous infection is obtained (elevated antistreptococcal antibodies in the patient's blood).

If the nephritis is severe, the symptom complex of uremia may rapidly appear and death may occur in days, weeks, or months from hypertension and its complications, congestive heart failure, or superimposed infection. In the vast majority of instances, however, the symptoms disappear more or less rapidly, and the patient returns to normal health within a matter of weeks or at most a few months. No specific treatment for acute glomerulonephritis is known; each manifestation of renal failure is treated individually. Since the streptococcal infection is the initiating event in most patients, it is common practice to administer penicillin for ten days to eradicate possible persistent streptococcal infection. It should be emphasized, however, that the inflammatory process in the kidneys, once begun, is independent of the streptococcal initiating agent. The value of bed rest in the treatment of acute glomerulonephritis is unproven, but most experts in renal disease consider it highly desirable for patients with active nephritis to remain more or less completely at rest. Since in most cases acute nephritis heals completely within a matter of weeks, disruption of personal and family life is relatively minimal. In a few individuals, however, active nephritis may persist for many months. Since healing is possible after as much as a year of activity, the disease must be considered acute nephritis during this entire period; hence, prolonged bed rest may theoretically be beneficial. Such prolonged absence from work or school is obviously psychologically and socially extremely undesirable. Therefore, after several weeks of continuing active nephritis many physicians test the effects of moderate exertion. If restricted activity does not adversely affect the urinary sediment or kidney function, cautious increase in activity may be permitted.

Complete healing eventually occurs in more than 95 per cent of children who develop acute glomerulonephritis; in adults, the prognosis is less favorable. Nephritis is healed when the sediment is normal, proteinuria is absent, and there is no evidence of functional impairment. Complete healing usually occurs within six months, and is rare after one year. When acute nephritis has healed completely, the kidneys are entirely normal; they are not especially susceptible to other renal disease, nor do they have a "low reserve." Therefore, a patient with healed acute glomerulonephritis can return to an entirely normal life.

In occasional children and in up to 50 per cent of adults, signs of active disease, such as excretion of casts and proteinuria, persist beyond one year. Since it is then very unlikely that complete healing will ever occur, the disease is at this point designated *chronic glomerulonephritis.* When the only findings are proteinuria and an abnormal urinary sediment, the disease is said to be in the latent phase. The latent phase of chronic nephritis varies greatly in length, from several months to many years; a rare patient may survive for decades. At some point in the latent phase, a minority of patients develop the *nephrotic syndrome,* characterized by massive proteinuria and edema. Eventually, all patients develop progressive renal failure, and the clinical picture becomes that of uremia. Survival for more than a few years after renal insufficiency develops is unusual.

Because the course of latent nephritis is very variable, it is important that statements regarding prognosis be as honestly optimistic as is possible. Patients with latent disease have no symptoms and require no medication or special diets. There is no evidence that bed rest is beneficial, and activity need not be restricted. Periodic examinations, including laboratory tests of renal function, are required. When uremia supervenes, the patient usually limits himself to moderate or minimal activity because of weakness and lassitude. However, occasional patients can continue to work even with advanced uremia, almost until the time of death. No restriction of activity is desirable beyond that imposed by the patient's symptoms. It is often necessary to modify the diet by restriction of salt and protein. Medication may be required for relief of symptoms such as nausea or itching or for treatment of associated problems such as hypertension or congestive heart failure. Patients adapt well to the slowly progressive anemia of uremia and rarely require transfusions. As uremia becomes advanced, multiple hospital admissions for treatment of symptoms and complications are often necessary. The psychological, social, and family problems attendant on the prolonged but inexorable progress of the uremic phase of chronic glomerulonephritis are enormous and require the most skillful management.

The clinical and pathological picture of chronic glomerulonephritis also occurs in many patients in whom there is no evidence for preceding acute nephritis. In these patients, the disease may begin with the insidious onset of a nephrotic phase or with the symptoms of hypertension or early uremia. Many experts believe that the present diagnosis of chronic glomerulonephritis may include a number of diseases of different origin. More precise separation of the causes of chronic glomerulonephritis will undoubtedly improve treatment and prevention in the future. At present, there is little practical difference in the course and prognosis of patients with chronic glomerulonephritis that begins after well-recognized acute glomerulonephritis ("type 1") and that which begins insidiously ("type 2").

THE NEPHROTIC SYNDROME

When profuse proteinuria continues for some time, a group of findings known as the *nephrotic syndrome* develops. When fully developed, the nephrotic syndrome is characterized by (1) profuse proteinuria (albuminuria), (2) diminished serum albumin (protein) levels, (3) increase in blood fats (hyperlipemia), and (4) edema. Heavy proteinuria is the *sine qua non* of the nephrotic syndrome. However, the intensity of the other clinical manifestations may vary greatly from time to time during the course of the patient's illness, depending on various factors which modify the degree of proteinuria and its effects on the patient. Since a number of disease entities can cause massive proteinuria, the presence of a nephrotic syndrome by no means establishes a definitive diagnosis. The pathological feature common to all these entities is diffuse damage to glomerular basement membranes. This interferes with the selective filtering function of the glomeruli, so that large protein molecules, normally retained within the glomerular blood vessels, pass more or less freely into the tubular urine.

In a minority of cases, the nephrotic syndrome is caused by a specific disease. The most common specific causes are diabetic glomerulosclerosis, disseminated lupus erythematosis (which involves many organs in addition to the kidneys), obstruction to the renal venous circulation (renal vein thrombosis), and amyloidosis (a disease of unknown cause in which abnormal material is deposited in various tissues including the kidneys). In cases due to specific diseases such as these, it is obvious that the course and prognosis of the nephrotic syndrome will be, in great measure, that of the underlying disease.

In the majority of cases, the cause of the nephrotic syndrome is unknown (idiopathic). Idiopathic nephrotic syndrome is also known as *membranous glomerulonephritis* or, in children, as *lipoid nephrosis*. It is not clear whether the adult and childhood forms are variants of the same disease process or are causally distinct diseases with similar clinical and pathological features. In children, lipoid nephrosis can occur at any age from birth onward but is most common between one and six. There are no reliable data on the relative frequency at various ages in adults, but cases have been observed from early adult life to late old age.

In general, the nephrotic syndrome begins clinically with the insidious onset of edema, noted most frequently in the face (puffy eyelids) or in the ankles. In more severe cases, subcutaneous edema may be massive, and fluid may collect in the various body cavities as well. The patient usually notices no change in his urine, although occasionally some reduction in volume may occur. Although blood pressure is most frequently normal initially, moderate degrees of hypertension occasionally occur even at the onset of the illness. The patient often is relatively asymptomatic, but sometimes malaise and weakness are present.

The course and prognosis of idiopathic nephrotic syndrome are somewhat different in children and in adults. In children, the course is one of edema with exacerbations and remissions progressing over a period of one to several years. Intercurrent infection is common in children and before the availability of antibiotics was a major cause of death. At present, deaths from infection are rare and most children survive for at least several years. In one-third to one-half of children, the disease eventually heals completely. The others gradually develop the picture of progressive uremia and die from this cause. In adults, there seems to be a tendency for the prognosis to become worse with increasing age at the onset of the disease. Although there may be temporary remissions, more than three-quarters of adults with idiopathic nephrotic syndrome die of uremia.

Treatment has recently undergone a radical change, because corticosteriods such as cortisone will induce a prompt remission of edema and proteinuria in the majority of children and in a substantial minority of adults. The schedule of administration varies as to detail; in general, patients initially are treated for several weeks with high doses of steroids. If a remission results, treatment is usually continued for several months, and in occasional instances, indefinitely. Although not without risk, the use of steroids has become widespread because relief of symptoms is often dramatic, especially in children. It is not known, however, whether steroids alter prognosis or prevent progression of the disease toward uremia and death. In patients who for various reasons are not suitable for treatment with steroids, or who fail to respond, diuretics may be given to relieve edema. The use of diuretics often obviates the need for rigidly salt-restricted diets, thereby encouraging adequate intake. Since large amounts of protein are lost in the urine, a nutritious diet including sufficient protein is highly desirable. Patients are encouraged to maintain full activity unless they are symptomatic or grossly edematous. When progressive renal insufficiency develops, the management and prognosis become that of chronic uremia.

PYELONEPHRITIS AND OTHER URINARY TRACT INFECTIONS

A great variety of bacterial species may infect the kidney (pyelonephritis) and lower urinary tract. Pyelonephritis is undoubtedly the commonest of renal diseases. It occurs in both sexes and throughout life, but it is much more common in women and girls than in males. The short length of the urethra (which connects the bladder to the genitalia) in females is probably a factor in the frequency of urinary tract infection in female infants, in young girls, and in adult women, particularly during pregnancy. Since diabetics are prone to infection, it is not surprising that acute and chronic pyelonephritis are common in patients with diabetes. Catheters or other instruments introduced into the urinary tract often initiate infection. When flow in the urinary tract is obstructed, as by congenital anomalies, an enlarged prostate gland, or stones, infection is common.

Acute pyelonephritis usually begins with fever, chills, and pain in the flank; the urine may become cloudy. White cells are seen on microscopic examination of the urine, and bacteriological study demonstrates large numbers of bacteria. Symptoms are usually severe enough so that the patient seeks medical advice and characteristic enough so that diagnosis is easy. In the great majority of cases of acute uncomplicated pyelonephritis, treatment for about two weeks with antibiotics or sulfonamides is successful. However, careful follow-up is required to establish that the infecting organism has been eradicated permanently.

In some patients, acute pyelonephritis does not heal completely and becomes chronic. Chronic pyelonephritis also occurs in a large number of patients who have not had clear-cut episodes of acute infection. Unfortunately, symptoms are often absent in patients with chronic pyelonephritis, although pain on urination or pyuria (urine cloudy with white cells) may occur. The first manifestation of chronic pyelonephritis, therefore, may be the insidious onset of the symptoms of uremia. Diagnosis is established by microscopic examination of the urine for white cells and white cell casts, by bacteriological cultures to identify the infecting organisms, and by characteristic changes visible by radiological studies (pyelography).

Chronic pyelonephritis is often a relatively indolent disease and is compatible with a life-span of many years. On the other hand, more rapid progression may occur, particularly if complicating hypertension develops, as is often the case. Treatment begins with a search for surgically correctable complicating factors, such as obstruction due to hypertrophy of the prostate gland or a congenital anomaly. Specific treatment with appropriate antibiotics is usually attempted, but more than three-quarters of patients with chronic pyelonephritis cannot be cured. In these patients, the picture is one of slow development of hypertension or renal insufficiency over a period of several years, and the clinical picture eventually becomes that of chronic uremia.

NEPHROSCLEROSIS

Most patients with high blood pressure, whatever the cause, develop degenerative changes in the kidneys known as *arteriolar nephrosclerosis*. However, in the large majority of cases, death from cardiac or cerebral complications occurs before nephrosclerosis becomes of clinical significance. Thus, proteinuria and changes in urinary sediment may persist for many years without symptoms referable to kidney failure, although kidney function tests may indicate that moderate renal insufficiency is present. In about 10 per cent of patients with benign hypertension, slowly developing uremia may be the cause of death. In a few patients with very severe ("malignant") hypertension, the course of nephrosclerosis is greatly accelerated, and clinical manifestations of uremia may develop in a few weeks or months. There is no specific treatment for nephrosclerosis itself, but successful reduction of blood pressure by antihypertensive drugs undoubtedly slows or stops the course of malignant nephrosclerosis and probably is similarly effective in benign nephrosclerosis.

VASCULAR DISEASES OF THE KIDNEY

With advancing age, renal arteries and their subdivisions usually become narrowed by arteriosclerotic changes; pathologically, atrophic nephrons become increasingly common. Although special kidney function tests demonstrate that renal blood flow and glomerular filtration decrease progressively, the loss of function with increasing age is too small to be clinically significant.

Occasionally, obstruction of blood flow to all or part of a kidney seriously compromises function or results in complete destruction (infarction). This may occur slowly, for example, by gradual growth of plaques (arteriosclerosis) in the arterial wall, or suddenly when a blood clot (embolus) lodges in a renal artery. Sudden arterial obstruction usually causes pain and bloody urine (hematuria), whereas slow obstruction is most often silent, being recognized in retrospect when a nonfunctioning kidney is demonstated. Arterial obstruction of any kind may result in sudden hypertension, often of great severity. In many cases, this type of hypertension disappears permanently after surgery on the affected artery or kidney. Recently, a number of procedures, such as renal angiography (x-rays of renal arteries) and split function tests (Howard test), have been devised to facilitate recognition of hypertension caused by renal vascular disease.

THE KIDNEY IN DIABETES MELLITUS

At least three forms of renal disease, which often occur in combination, are common complications of diabetes. *Nephrosclerosis* begins earlier and is apparently more frequent in diabetics than in the general population. *Pyelonephritis* is common, often severe, and difficult to eradicate in diabetic patients. More than half of the reported cases of *papillary necrosis,* a fulminating form of pyelonephritis which rapidly destroys kidney tissue and is usually fatal, have been in diabetic patients.

One form of renal disease, *diabetic glomerulosclerosis,* is unique to diabetics. It is not clear whether this is a complication of poorly controlled diabetes, or whether it is an inherent part of the diabetic state. Since kidney biopsies in very early diabetes frequently demonstrate the presence of glomerulosclerosis, many investigators are now leaning toward the latter view. The lesions are characterized pathologically by the deposition of an abnormal material of unknown composition around the glomerular capillary loops. In early cases, the disease is without clinical manifestations, and diagnosis can be made only by biopsy. As it becomes more severe, proteinuria appears, and renal insufficiency and hypertension may follow. The proteinuria is occasionally very heavy, leading to the development of a nephrotic syndrome. Once well established, clinically significant diabetic glomerulosclerosis usually leads to uremia in a few years. "Diabetic kidney disease," a compound of glomerulosclerosis, pyelonephritis, and nephrosclerosis, is a frequent cause of death in diabetes. No treatment for diabetic glomerulosclerosis is known.

RENAL DISEASE IN PREGNANCY

Acute urinary tract infections, including pyelonephritis, are common during pregnancy. In addition to clinically evident disease, asymptomatic infection is found in a surprisingly high proportion of pregnant women if routine urine cultures are done. The significance of asymptomatic infection is only now beginning to be explored, but preliminary information suggests that it may lead to pyelonephritis in the mother and to prematurity of the infant. Vigorous treatment with antibacterial agents is indicated, therefore, for both symptomatic and asymptomatic infection.

Toxemia is characterized by hypertension, proteinuria, and edema, beginning in the last three or four months of pregnancy. These findings together constitute *preeclampsia;* if convulsions or coma occurs, the term *eclampsia* is used. The cause of toxemia is unknown. Although preeclampsia is fairly common, occurring in perhaps one pregnancy in twenty, proper management should reduce the incidence of frank eclampsia virtually to the vanishing point. Treatment with diuretics to relieve edema and with antihypertensive drugs will usually control the manifestations of preeclampsia sufficiently well to permit the pregnancy to go to term. In more severe cases, hospitalization for intensive therapy, sedation, and bed rest may be required. If a remission cannot be achieved, it is usually necessary to terminate the pregnancy. Fetal mortality in patients with toxemia is increased. It is not known whether chronic hypertension or renal disease ever develops from toxemia.

Most physicians believe that it is medically undesirable for many patients with chronic renal disease to become pregnant. Renal insufficiency and hypertension often become worse during pregnancy, and the course of the renal disease may be accelerated downhill. Moreover, many patients do not deliver living infants. If the renal disease is latent, with no evidence of renal insufficiency or hypertension, prospects for mother and child are brighter. Because of the uncertain effects of pregnancy in any individual case, counseling about the desirability of pregnancy in women with renal disease is often difficult.

HEREDITARY FORMS OF RENAL DISEASE

Of a number of renal diseases in which hereditary or familial factors are known or suspected, two are especially noteworthy. In *polycystic kidney disease,* normal renal tissue is progressively replaced by fluid-filled sacs or cysts. The disease may first be noted in infancy, in which case survival beyond early childhood is unusual. In the adult form of the disease, which occurs in both men and women, the patient is usually asymptomatic for the first several decades of his life. He then notices abdominal or flank pain, or blood in the urine, or is found to have hypertension or an enlarged abdominal mass. X-ray examination usually is sufficient to establish the diagnosis of polycystic kidney disease. There is no specific treatment for this disorder, except that complications such as superimposed infection may be treated individually. The course and prognosis are quite variable, but most patients die of uremia in early middle age. Many instances are known in which the presence of polycystic kidney disease was compatible with a long and active life. The psychological and social implications of the discovery of this disease in one member of a family are enormous. Not only is the patient himself almost inevitably aware of the grave prognostic import of his disease, but problems such as the desirability of screening his relatives for the disease obviously arise. Approximately one-half of the children of a patient with polycystic disease will have the disease. Counseling about marriage in such circumstances obviously involves individual social and psychological considerations which cannot be generalized.

Another form of hereditary renal disease, *hereditary nephritis,* is a chronic disease often associated with nerve deafness. The disorder occurs in both sexes but seem to be clinically more severe in males. Although thus far only a handful of families with this disease have been described, further studies of the population will probably reveal a somewhat greater incidence. Males often first come to the attention of the physician with advanced uremia and rarely live beyond age 20 to 30. In females, although examination of the urine may reveal evidence of active renal disease, uremia usually does not develop and the life-span may be normal. There is no specific treatment for this form of renal disease.

A number of important *congenital anomalies* may occur in the kidneys and lower urinary tract. Of particular importance are those malformations which result in obstruction in the lower urinary tract. If sufficiently severe, the obstruction may lead to gradual atrophy and destruction of the kidneys with progressive uremia. Lesser degrees of obstruction are often significant because they increase the tendency for urinary tract infections such as pyelonephritis to develop. Diagnosis is established by x-ray studies or by direct urological examination. Since many of these congenital anomalies are amenable to specific surgical treatment, early detection is of considerable practical significance.

STONES

A number of normal and abnormal constitutents of urine precipitate out of solution under certain circumstances to form stones. Calcium stones may form because of increased calcium excretion, as in several disorders of calcium metabolism, or may develop without known cause. Uric acid, a metabolic waste product, may precipitate because of excess production. In rare instances, hereditary metabolic disorders such as *cystinuria* result in excessive excretion of normal metabolites or formation and excretion into the urine of abnormal metabolic products.

Stones are usually discovered when they give rise to pain, for example, if passing down the narrow ureter. Sometimes silent stones in the renal pelvis or the bladder are seen by chance on x-ray examination of the abdomen. Methods for prevention and treatment of each type of stone differ in detail. In general, patients are advised to drink large amounts of liquids so that the stone-forming material, diluted in a large urine volume, is more likely to stay in solution. Recurrences of some types of stones can be prevented by specific medication. Many small stones are passed spontaneously. When stones become large or are located at strategic places in the lower urinary tract and cause obstruction, surgical intervention may be necessary. Recurrent stones and superimposed infection are common, often requiring repeated hospitalizations and frequent surgery, with eventual renal insufficiency. On the other hand, some patients have only one or two stones in a lifetime and live out a normal and comfortable life-span.

ACUTE RENAL FAILURE (ACUTE TUBULAR NECROSIS)

In a great number of circumstances there may be sudden renal failure, resulting in diminished urine volume and rapidly developing uremia. The multiple causes include poisons such as mercury, wood alcohol, and antifreeze compounds (drunk in place of alcoholic beverages), and a number of factors that decrease renal blood supply, such as surgical shock, certain severe infections, severe heart attack (myocardial infarction). In each case, the kidney tubules are damaged and renal failure results. Acute tubular necrosis will heal completely in time, provided that the patient survives the effects of acute uremia. In many cases, careful management by routine methods will be sufficient to keep the patient alive until his kidneys regain normal function. Sometimes, the use of an "artificial kidney" or a similar device may be necessary to tide the patient over the period of acute renal failure. Once healing has occurred, there are no sequelae and no chronic damage results.

NEOPLASMS

Benign and malignant tumors may arise from any part of the genitourinary system. Malignant urinary tract tumors account for about 20 per cent of all malignancies in adults and children. In children, Wilms' tumor of the kidney (embryonal nephroma) is common, and in adults, renal carcinoma (hypernephroma) and bladder carcinoma are frequent. Although clinical features vary with the location and pathological nature of the tumor, in general blood in the urine, pain, weight loss, fever, and anemia may be expected. Diagnosis is confirmed by radiological and direct urological examination. When tumors are confined to the urological tract, surgery and radiation can effect a cure in a large minority of cases. Unfortunately, the first manifestations of renal tumors may be from metastases to other organs, and treatment then is only palliative.

TUBERCULOSIS

Urinary tract tuberculosis is common in patients with pulmonary or disseminated (miliary) tuberculosis. It also is frequently found as a primary lesion, without evidence of active tuberculosis elsewhere. Infection of the urinary tract is blood-borne. The kidneys are almost always involved and infection of the lower urinary tract is commonly associated. Renal tuberculosis may be silent clinically, or symptoms such as pain during voiding (dysuria) may result from infection of the bladder. Microscopic or grossly visible blood in the urine may be the first finding, or white cells may be seen on routine microscopic examination. Because of the relative lack of symptoms, renal tuberculosis may be far advanced before it is identified. Diagnosis is suspected from the presence of unexplained white or red cells in the urine and from changes on pyelograms and is confirmed by special bacteriological techniques. The use of modern antituberculous drugs has radically changed treatment and prognosis. At present, surgery and prolonged bed rest are rarely required. Most infections can be controlled by ambulatory drug treatment (isoniazid, streptomycin, PAS), which is continued for one or more years.

GENERAL CONSIDERATIONS IN CHRONIC RENAL DISEASE

It is a dismal fact that at present most common renal diseases cannot be cured. Available treatment is limited to correction of complications and mitigation of symptoms. Although the course of chronic renal disease may thereby be prolonged, it is directed inexorably toward uremia and death. Uremia usually progresses slowly and results in seemingly endless combinations of unpleasant symptoms. Since chronic renal diseases are common in early adult life, they are particularly distressing to the patient's relatives and disruptive of family life.

In recent years, much effort has been directed toward developing substitutes for sick kidneys. One approach has been *transplantation* of kidneys obtained from normal donors. When an identical twin is available to serve as a donor, successful transplants are the rule. Kidneys from all other donors, including close relatives, are usually destroyed (rejected) by the patient's immune mechanisms, and permanently successful transplants are the exception. Current work has suggested promising approaches to overcome these problems, but at this time transplantation, except between identical twins, is an experimental procedure.

Another avenue of approach to the problem of chronic uremia is the use of "artificial kidneys." Recent studies in a very limited number of patients have shown that it is possible to keep at least a few patients alive for months or years after their own kidneys have failed completely. Patients reported several times per week to a medical facility, where they are treated with an "artificial kidney." At present, a number of centers for chronic treatment of this type are being established throughout the country. How many patients will benefit from this treatment, for how long, and at what cost are all questions that will not be answered until experience accumulates over the next few years.

VII

DISORDERS OF THE ENDOCRINE GLANDS

The endocrine glands, or glands of internal secretion, are specialized structures which secrete specific substances called *hormones* directly into the blood stream. The hormones are chemically and functionally extremely diverse and are important factors in fetal differentiation, in mental and physical growth and development of the child and adolescent, in regulation of protein, fat, and carbohydrate metabolism, in adaptation to emergency and stress, in maintenance of the constancy of composition of the body fluids, and in many other functions. The endocrine gland "system" may be considered as regulating and integrating a variety of biological phenomena by humoral mechanisms.

THE ENDOCRINE GLANDS—ANATOMY AND PHYSIOLOGY

The endocrine glands include (1) the pituitary, which is composed of two embryologically and functionally distinct lobes, the anterior lobe and the posterior lobe; (2) the thyroid; (3) the parathyroid glands; (4) the adrenal (subdivided into the adrenal cortex and medulla); (5) the pancreas; (6) the gonads, consisting of the ovaries in the female and the testes in the male.

THE PITUITARY

The pituitary is a grape-sized structure, weighing about 500 milligrams, which lies in a bony cavity (the sella turcica) in the base of the skull. The anterior lobe of the pituitary is derived from ectodermal

By ISADORE N. ROSENBERG, M.D. Associate Professor of Medicine, Boston University School of Medicine; Physician-in-Chief, Sixth, Boston University, Medical Service, Boston City Hospital; Physician-in-Charge, Endocrine Laboratory, Fifth and Sixth, Boston University, Medical Services, Boston City Hospital, Boston, Massachusetts.

tissue of the roof of the mouth and is called the *adenohypophysis;* the posterior lobe is derived from neuroectoderm of the brain and is called the *neurohypophysis;* it is connected to the hypothalamic portion of the brain by the pituitary stalk. Portions of the hypothalamus may exert a regulatory action upon the adenohypophysis by nervous and humoral mechanisms transmitted via the pituitary stalk.

THE ADENOHYPOPHYSIS. The anterior pituitary is often called the master gland because of the multiplicity of its secretions and their essential role in the regulation of some of the other endocrine glands. The hormones produced by the anterior lobe are all peptides, being composed of chains of amino acids of varying length, which have the general properties of proteins. Some of these peptides have been purified and their structure elucidated. The hormones of the anterior lobe include (1) the thyroid-stimulating hormone (TSH); (2) the adreno-corticotropic hormone (ACTH); (3) the gonadotropic hormones, consisting of the follicle-stimulating hormone (FSH) and the luteinizing hormone (LH); (4) growth hormone (also called somatotrophin); (5) prolactin (also called luteotropin and mammotropin); and (6) the melanocyte-stimulating hormone (MSH).

The tropic hormones TSH, ACTH, FSH, and LH are necessary for the adequate functions of the specific target glands they stimulate— that is, the thyroid, the adrenal cortex, and the gonads. In the absence of the specific tropic hormone the target gland atrophies and its function ceases, while the administration by injection of appropriate preparations of TSH, ACTH, and the gonadotropins leads respectively to enhanced secretion by the thyroid gland, the adrenal cortex, and the gonads of their respective hormones. The action of FSH in the female is to stimulate the growth of the ovarian follicles which nurture the ovum and to promote the secretion by the follicle of estradiol, which has important effects on the uterus, vagina, and the female secondary sex characteristics; the action of LH, in combination with FSH, is to induce ovulation (that is, the extrusion of the ovum from the ovarian follicle so that it may be fertilized by spermatozoa) and the secretion by the ovary of progesterone, which prepares the uterine lining for reception of the fertilized ovum. In the male, FSH acts chiefly upon the seminiferous tubules of the testes, stimulating their growth and the development of spermatozoa, while the action of LH is to stimulate the endocrine cells of the testes (the Leydig cells) to secrete testosterone, the "male" hormone (androgens).

The control of the secretion of the thyroid, adrenal cortex, and the gonads is regulated by an ingenious negative feedback mechanism, whereby a slight rise in the secretion rate of the target gland leads to a decrease in the rate of release of the respective tropic hormone from the anterior pituitary, resulting in less stimulation of the target gland and hence a decrease in its secretion rate to its previous level. Thus, if the blood level of the major adrenocortical hormone, cortisol, should be increased above the normal range (for example, by the administration of cortisol tablets to the individual), there would be a prompt decrease in the quantity of ACTH released by the adenohypophysis; this would result in a decrease in the adrenal secretion of cortisol, until its blood level was restored. Conversely, if the adrenal secretion of cortisol were insufficient to maintain a normal blood level of cortisol (for example, because of diseased adrenal gland), the pituitary would secrete more ACTH, resulting in a greater degree of stimulation of the adrenal gland, until the plasma level of cortisol was restored. In general, a fall in the plasma level of the hormone produced by the target gland evokes a rise in the adenophypophysial release of the specific tropic hormone, and a rise in the plasma level leads to a fall in the release of the tropin. It is believed that the centers regulating the release of the tropic hormones in relation to the blood level of the target hormones are in the hypothalamus. It is possible for derangement of these centers to produce remarkable and inappropriate endocrine effects (see below).

The growth hormone of the adenohypophysis, which is essential for the growth of children and adolescents, is a protein which exerts a variety of metabolic effects. It acts upon body cells in general (hence the term somatotropin), increases the formation of body proteins, and accelerates the metabolism of fat. Although its most striking physiological effect is seen during the growth period, it is likely that its metabolic effects are of importance throughout life. The factors regulating the secretion of growth hormone are not well understood.

Prolactin is essential for lactation in the postpartum period; it acts upon the breast tissue to promote the secretion of milk. Prolactin appears to have an effect on the ovary after ovulation, in that it maintains the secretion of progesterone initiated by FSH and LH. The secretion of milk appears to be mediated by a neuroendocrine reflex, whereby the suckling stimulus to the breast initiates hypothalamic mechanisms leading to the release of prolactin from the adenohypophysis.

The melanocyte-stimulating hormone (MSH) controls the production of melanin pigment in certain pigment-producing cells (melanocytes) of the skin. Factors controlling MSH secretion are poorly understood. A decrease in MSH secretion leads to a lightening of skin color, while an increase leads to a brownish pigmentation.

THE NEUROHYPOPHYSIS. The posterior lobe of the pituitary is in close anatomical relationship to the anterior lobe. It is a reservoir for the two posterior lobe hormones, oxytocin and vasopressin, which are peptides containing eight amino acids each, and which are produced in the hypothalamus. Oxytocin is of importance in sustaining the flow of milk from the lactating breast and has a tonic effect on the uterine musculature at the time of parturition. Vasopressin, also called the antidiuretic hormone (ADH), plays an important role in the conservation of water; by permitting the formation of a more concentrated urine it enhances the ability of the kidney tubules to reabsorb water. Control of ADH secretion appears to depend upon certain hypothalamic centers (osmoregulators) which respond to changes in the state of hydration of the body fluids. When the concentration of water in body fluids is decreased (that is, when the body fluids are hypertonic, as in water deprivation or dehydration), the secretion of ADH is increased and water is conserved, instead of being excreted in the urine; on the other hand, when water is present in excess, as after excessive water drinking, overhydration of the body is prevented by the decreased secretion of ADH, permitting the elaboration by the kidneys of a very dilute urine and appropriate water losses.

THE THYROID

The thyroid gland is a shield-shaped structure weighing approximately 20 grams which lies in the neck closely applied to the front and sides of the upper part of the trachea. The thyroid concentrates inorganic iodide from the blood stream and synthesizes, stores, and secretes the thyroid hormones. The major secretory product is the iodine-containing amino acid thyroxin; small quantities of another iodinated amino acid, triiodothyronine, are also secreted. Thyroxin is transported in the circulation loosely bound to plasma proteins, and the plasma protein-bound iodine (PBI) concentration is a measure of the circulating thyroid hormone. Thyroxin has important metabolic functions; an adequate supply of the thyroid hormone is essential for normal rate of growth and development, maintenance of a normal rate of oxygen consumption and heat production, and for optimum function of the cardiovascular, gastrointestinal, and hematopoietic systems and of most other tissues. The secretion of thyroid hormone is regulated chiefly by pituitary TSH. The importance of adequate thyroid function to the organism can perhaps be most readily appreciated by studying the consequences of complete thyroidectomy (surgical removal of the thyroid gland) in young individuals; such persons are dwarfed, show mental and physical retardation, present a dull, lethargic puffy appearance, and have a subnormal body temperature. Thyroxin deficiency is characteristically reflected in a marked decrease in the *basal metabolic rate*, defined as the individual's rate of heat production while resting in the fasting state. Although one may increase the metabolic rate of thyroxin-deficient individuals by the administration of drugs such as dinitrophenol, the other manifestations of thyroxin deficiency do not improve, suggesting that the decreased calorigenesis (heat production) of thyroxin deficiency is not the cause of the other symptoms and signs.

THE PARATHYROID GLANDS

The parathyroids, generally four in number, are small structures, each weighing about 25 mg, which lie in the neck in the region of the thyroid, generally on the deep surface of the thyroid gland. They secrete a peptide hormone, parathormone, which is of prime importance in the regulation of the calcium concentration of the blood plasma and other body fluids. The primary effect of parathormone is to increase the concentration of ionic calcium in body fluids; this is accomplished primarily by its action on the bones, which leads to increased dissolution of bone with consequent liberation of bone mineral (largely calcium and phosphate) into the body fluids. Another effect of parathormone is to increase the urinary excretion of phosphate, this being accomplished by an effect on the kidney. States of parathormone excess are characterized by increased concentration of calcium and decreased concentration of phosphates in the blood plasma; parathyroid deficiency is characterized by decrease in the concentration of calcium and increase in the concentration of phosphate. The maintenance of the serum concentration within narrow limits is of great importance to the organism, since for normal neuromuscular activity, for normal cardiac function, for adequate skeletal maintenance, and for many other functions, a normal serum calcium concentration is essential. Decrease in serum calcium concentration below normal results in increased neuromuscular irritability, convulsions, and tetany (a sustained, inappropriately prolonged muscular contraction), while increase in serum calcium results in decreased neuromuscular excitability. The regulation of the calcium level in blood plasma and other body fluids is largely accomplished by variations in the secretion of parathormone. The control of parathyroid glandular secretion is not under pituitary control but is dependent largely upon the level of calcium in the plasma; an increase in serum calcium tends to decrease the secretion of parathormone, while a decrease in serum calcium leads to enhanced secretion of parathormone—that is, the change in the release rate of parathormone from the glands is in the direction that will restore toward normal the plasma calcium level.

THE ADRENAL GLANDS

The adrenal glands are two structures of triangular shape, whose combined weight is about 15 grams; each rests upon the upper pole of each kidney. The adrenal is really two glands, the outer, larger portion, the *adrenal cortex*, being embryologically, anatomically, and functionally distinct from the inner *medulla*. The adrenal cortex is derived from mesoderm and produces hormones that are steroids (substances having a chemical structure related to cholesterol), while the adrenal medulla is derived from neural tissue and its secretory products are catecholamines, related to the mediators of the sympathetic nervous system.

The adrenal cortex secretes two major steroid hormones, cortisol and aldosterone. Cortisol may produce a variety of metabolic effects, including *antianabolic,* (inhibiting protein synthesis from amino acids) and *gluconeogenic* (enhancing the conversion of proteins to glucose and raising the blood sugar level). In large quantities, cortisol is antiinflammatory, decreasing the normal defensive responses to injury. An important role of cortisol is its permissive role in a variety of homeostatic circulatory and metabolic phenomena; thus, when cortisol is deficient the organism cannot readily adapt to bleeding, injury, or stress by the usual adaptive mechanisms of reflex constriction of blood vessels. Appropriate excretion of a water load by the kidneys and mobilization of depot fat in response to fasting are similarly impaired in cortisol deficiency. Thus, the cortisol-deficient organism is peculiarly vulnerable to stress and cannot tolerate injury, food deprivation, vigorous muscular exercise, or serious illness without going into shock or dying.

Aldosterone is of importance in regulating the levels of sodium and potassium, and consequently the volume of body fluids, by controlling the renal excretion of these cations. Aldosterone promotes retention of sodium and excretion of potassium; in the absence of this steroid, bodily depletion of sodium occurs with associated potassium retention, and dehydration and circulatory collapse may result.

The adrenocortical secretion of cortisol is largely under control of anterior pituitary ACTH, by the negative feedback mechanism previously mentioned. Aldosterone secretion is not predominately under ACTH regulation, but its secretion is responsive to change in the volume and ionic composition of the body fluids and possibly to changes in the circulation to the kidneys.

Although small quantities of estrogen and androgen are secreted by the adrenal cortex, under normal circumstances these are of negligible physiological significance.

The adrenal medulla is really a specialized part of the autonomic nervous system, and hence it is not surprising that its main secretory products are epinephrine and norepinephrine, the latter being the substance produced by nerve fibers of the sympathetic nervous system, which innervates involuntary muscle of blood vessels, viscera, and glands. The major product of the adrenal medulla is epinephrine; a variety of circulatory metabolic responses, generally considered as useful adaptations to such situations as flight, combat, emergency, and stress, occur as a consequence of adrenal medullary secretion. Thus, the blood sugar is raised, the heart rate and blood pressure increase, the metabolic rate rises, the circulation to voluntary muscle improves. Secretion of the adrenal medulla is normally triggered by nervous impulses; there is no pituitary control of this part of the adrenal. Although the consequences of removal of the adrenal cortex are disastrous, the adrenal medulla is not essential, since many of its functions are shared by the autonomic nervous system.

THE GONADS

As mentioned previously, the ovaries and testes of the adult have both a gametogenic function (the production of ova and sperm) and an endocrine function, the secretion of the female and male sex hormones respectively.

SEX DETERMINATION AND DIFFERENTIATION.   The sex of the fetus is genetically determined. Of the 46 chromosomes normally present in each cell nucleus two are sex chromosomes. If two sex chromosomes of the fetus include both an X and a Y, the primordial gonad develops as a testis, while if the chromosomal constitution is XX, the gonad will develop as an ovary. In general, the Y chromosome is the male determiner, and the presence of a Y will result in a testis, while the absence of a Y (rather than the presence of one or more X chromosomes) favors development of the ovary. By conventional definition, a male is a person whose gonad is a testis, a female is an individual whose gonad is an ovary.

While sex is genetically determined, the differentiation during fetal life of the internal accessory reproductive organs and the external genitalia is not genetically determined, but seems to depend on whether a fetal testis is present or absent. The presence of a functioning fetal testis at a critical stage of fetal development leads to the development in utero of a prostate, ejaculatory ducts, penis, and scrotum, while the absence of a testis results in development of the fallopian tubes, uterus, and vagina. Recent embryological studies have shown that it is not the presence of the fetal ovary but the absence of the fetal testis which results in differentiation along female lines. The fetal testis, then, presumably by a hormonal mechanism, is of importance during fetal life for the appropriate differentiation of the male accessory reproductive organs; disturbances in utero of this function may lead to feminization of the male, while exposure of the female fetus to androgens in utero may lead to masculinization.

THE GONADS AND SEXUAL MATURATION.   During childhood, the endocrine function of the gonads is negligible. At adolescence, however, secretion of the gonadal hormones begins, and sexual maturation and the development of male or female secondary sex characteristics occur.

Adolescence is triggered by the secretion of the pituitary gonadotropins, which stimulate ovarian estrogen and testicular androgen production. Both estrogens and androgens are steroidal substances. The major ovarian hormones are estradiol and progesterone; the major testicular hormone is testosterone. In girls, the ovarian secretion of adolescence results in a spurt of linear growth, as well as growth and development of breasts and nipples, uterus and vagina, sexual hair (axillary and pubic), mature female body contour and habitus, and the onset of menstrual periods. The adolescent changes induced by testicular androgens in boys include a marked growth spurt, growth of penis and testes, development of sexual hair, deepening of the voice and the male pattern of muscular development, facial hair, and body contour. Some androgen is normally produced by the ovary, hence acne (the activity of sebaceous glands is enhanced by androgens) and body hair growth occur in female as well as male adolescents. The sex hormones not only accelerate bone growth at this time but also eventually lead to closure of the epiphyses of the long bones, so that further increase in height cannot occur. If the sex hormones are deficient during the growth period, bone growth is slower but the epiphyses remain open, so that a greater than average height may be achieved, largely because of long lower extremities.

In the mature male, the function of the testis normally persists to some degree throughout life without cyclic activity. Menstruation in girls and women is a cyclic process in which ovarian estrogens and progesterone lead to specific changes in the uterine lining, which is periodically shed at the time of menstruation. A delicate interplay of FSH and LH, with the ovarian follicular secretions of estradiol and progesterone, is necessary for a regular menstrual cycle. The time of ovulation is generally 14 days before the next menstrual period. Ovulation is detectable by the rise in body temperature that occurs at that time and persists through the latter half of the menstrual cycle. The secretion of estrogens and progesterone may be assessed by biopsy of the endometrium (uterine lining), by the microscopic examination of the cells obtained in vaginal smears, and by measurement of urinary pregnanediol (the excretion product of progesterone). Quantitative measurement of testicular androgen production in the male is more difficult and generally requires tedious bioassay of urine.

From what has been said about the changes induced by estrogens and androgens at adolescence, one may predict the consequence of gonadal endocrine deficit. If gonadal endocrine function is absent or inadequate at the usual age of puberty, there will be no development of secondary sex characteristics, no growth spurt, and sexual immaturity will persist; linear growth will continue, resulting in skeletal proportions in which the extremities are disporportionately long in comparison with the trunk—the so-called eunuchoid proportions (eunuchoid being the term describing the appearance, especially the skeletal proportions, characteristic of the adult male who has been castrated prepuberally). Once the secondary sex characteristics have been established, continued gonadal endocrine function is essential for their complete maintenance; however, acquired lack of sex hormones in the adult, sexually mature individual does not result in regression of skeletal proportions, pitch of the voice, bodily habitus, and other irreversible changes, although amenorrhea (absence of menstruation) and decrease in sexual hair, libido, and size of internal and external genitalia are observed.

THE PANCREAS

The pancreas is an abdominal organ which functions as both an endocrine and a digestive exocrine gland. The bulk of the pancreas is composed of exocrine glands which furnish to the intestine enzymes important in the digestion of dietary proteins, fat, and carbohydrates (sugars, starch, and chemically related substances). The endocrine portion of the pancreas is made up of the islets of Langerhans, which are microscopic areas containing the cells that produce insulin and glucagon. It has been known for 75 years that surgical removal of the pancreas of experimental animals leads to diabetes, and for 40 years that diabetes in human subjects responds to the injection of pancreatic extracts containing insulin. Insulin is a peptide hormone secreted into the blood stream whose primary effect is to facilitate the entry of glucose (sugar) from the body fluids into the cells. As a result of the improved cellular utilization of glucose, a host of metabolic consequences occur, such as synthesis of glycogen and fat from glucose, decrease in the body's utilization of fat as a fuel, and improvement in the synthesis of proteins. The secretion of insulin is chiefly regulated by the blood sugar level—when the value is high (as after a carbohydrate meal), the islet cells secrete more insulin and by promoting the utilization of glucose restore the normal blood sugar value; when the blood glucose falls below normal, insulin secretion diminishes and the decreased utilization of glucose aids in the restoration of the blood sugar level to normal. Although insulin is of prime importance as a regulator of the blood glucose concentration, other hormonal mechanisms are important; epinephrine, cortisol, and growth hormone all tend to increase the blood sugar. Although only a small fraction of the body's fuel requirements is normally supplied by glucose, it is of major importance because (a) brain metabolism is wholly dependent upon adequate supplies of glucose, and (b) the metabolism of fat is impaired when glucose utilization is impaired, an idea expressed in an old clinical aphorism that "the fats burn in the flame of the carbohydrates."

When the metabolism of glucose is impaired as a result of impaired cellular penetration, as in insulin deficiency, the blood sugar level rises. The rise in blood sugar level to a certain extent improves the cellular utilization of sugar, but at high blood sugar levels considerable glucose is excreted in the urine—much water is lost in the urine with the urinary sugar, and dehydration may occur, despite the compensatory water ingestion as a result of the dehydration-induced thirst. The impaired utilization of sugar necessitates an increased use of fat to supply bodily energy requirements. However, certain products of the oxidation of fat (ketone acids) are then produced more rapidly than they can be metabolically disposed of, and ketosis (an excess of ketones in the body fluids) results, which may progress to coma. Accumulation of ketone acids disturbs the acid-base balance of the body, the excess acid produced depletes the alkali reserves, and diabetic acidosis results. This clinical situation may be reversed by insulin administration.

When the blood sugar level falls to abnormally low levels, as from excessive doses of insulin, the major manifestations are related to impaired cerebral function (confusion, convulsions, coma), since glucose is the obligatory substrate for cerebral metabolism.

Glucagon is a second hormone produced by the pancreatic islets, by cells other than those producing insulin, and it seems to be of much less physiological importance. The primary effect of glucagon is the production of glucose in the liver from its storage form, glycogen, and the entry of glucose into the circulation; glucagon therefore tends to cause hyperglycemia (increased blood glucose level) and aids in maintaining the blood glucose level if hypoglycemia occurs.

DISEASE OF THE ENDOCRINE GLANDS

DISORDERS OF THE PITUITARY AND HYPOTHALAMUS

Because of the important endocrine regulatory functions of the anterior pituitary and hypothalamus, disease of these structures may result in profound disturbances of other endocrine functions. In addition, the anatomical closeness of the pituitary to major visual pathways explains certain disturbances of vision that may be associated with pituitary disease, especially tumors.

HYPOPITUITARY STATES. Deficiency of anterior lobe secretion may result from a variety of causes which may affect the anterior lobe, including tumors, chronic inflammatory states and infections (especially tuberculosis), degenerative lesions, injuries (both accidental and neurosurgical), circulatory disorders, and nutritional disturbances. The clinical manifestations of anterior lobe inadequacy vary, depending upon the severity and the age of onset. Of the adenohypophysial tropic functions, the gonadotropic is most easily disturbed, while loss of thyrotropic and adrenocorticotropic function occurs only when most of the anterior lobe is destroyed. In most instances of anterior lobe disorders, amenorrhea or testicular atrophy, loss of libido, and diminution in the quantity of axillary and pubic hair are observed, while in many cases, symptoms of TSH deficit (hypothyroidism) or ACTH deficit (hypoadrenocorticalism) may be in evidence. However, the symptoms of such secondary hypothyroidism are seldom as pronounced as they are in primary thyroid gland failure, and the manifestations of adrenal insufficiency secondary to pituitary disease differ in two important respects from primary deficiency of the adrenal cortex: (1) electrolyte disturbances in the body fluids are relatively mild in hypopituitarism, because adrenal aldosterone secretion, unlike cortisol secretion, is not under control of ACTH; and (2) patients with panhypopituitarism tend to be less pigmented than normal and to have a white, waxy appearance (due to MSH deficit), while patients with primary adrenal failure tend to be deeply pigmented (see below). When hypopituitarism occurs in childhood, the growth hormone deficit leads to dwarfism, in addition to the signs of thyroid and adrenal deficit. When hypopituitarism occurs during pregnancy of postpartum, absence of lactation is characteristic (prolactin deficit). The adult panhypopituitary patient tends to be a weak, lethargic individual with a waxy look to the cool, dry skin; the manifestations of hypogonadism (mentioned above) and of hypothyroidism and hypoadrenocorticalism (to be described below) are present, resulting in intolerance to cold, constipation, rather dull cerebration, and inability to withstand such stresses as infections, injuries, and starvation.

One of the important and striking situation in which hypophysial insufficiency occurs in women is called *Sheehan's syndrome* (syndrome = a constellation of symptoms and signs). This is due to postpartum necrosis (cell death) of the pituitary resulting from obstetrical hemorrhage at the time of childbirth; the pituitary toward the end of pregnancy is richly supplied with blood, so that the reduction in the blood supply to the pituitary resulting from hemorrhage elsewhere may lead to insufficient circulation to the pituitary, and the structure may degenerate. Should this occur, menstruation does not resume as it normally should, lactation does not occur, and decreased appetite, fatigue, irritability, intolerance to cold weather, dizziness, and loss of pubic and axillary hair occur. This clinical picture may be mistaken for a psychiatric disorder (such as postpartum depression); this is a tragic error, since endocrine replacement therapy for panhypopituitarism is excellent and may result in a remarkable transformation to vigorous good health.

Surgical hypophysectomy (removal of the pituitary) and transection of the pituitary stalk are sometimes done in the treatment of tumors or severe ocular complications of diabetes and as palliative treatment of various malignant tumors. In such cases, endocrine replacement therapy (described below) is mandatory, if life postoperatively is to be preserved.

Occasionally, monotropic pituitary deficits occur, instead of the more common panhypopituitarism. Although isolated deficits of ACTH and TSH have been described, the most common monotropic defect is that of gonadotropins. This occurs as a familial disorder affecting males, who suffer from "hypogonadotropic eunuchoidism." As a result of gonadotropic deficit, testicular atrophy results and secondary male sex characteristics do not develop.

The diagnosis of panhypopituitarism depends upon the detection of target organ deficiencies—that is, gonadal, thyroid, and adrenocortical failure—together with the demonstration that the administration of exogenous TSH and ACTH will restore thyroidal and adrenocortical secretion. The absence of gonadotropic hormones in the urine is also an important diagnostic finding.

The treatment of panhypopituitarism consists of replacing the deficient hormones of the target glands. Of these, the adrenocortical steroid deficit is most important, and cortisol is therefore given; the thyroid deficiency is treated by giving thyroid or thyroxine tablets, and androgens or estrogens are given for the gonadal failure. Cortisol, thyroxine, androgen or estrogen are given because orally ingested tablets of these hormonal preparations are effective, while replacement of the deficient tropic hormones (ACTH, TSH, gonadotropins) would require daily injections, since the tropic hormones are peptides which are not effective orally, presumably because of digestion in the intestine. The panhypopituitary patient who is continuously treated with cortisol, thyroid, and the sex hormones may lead a full vigorous life. Reproductive capacity is probably not restorable, but possibly newer preparations of human pituitary gonadotropin may eventually be helpful in this respect. In pituitary dwarfism, resulting from hypopituitarism acquired in childhood, treatment with injections of growth hormone made from human pituitary glands has stimulated growth, while growth hormone preparations made from beef or pork pituitaries are ineffective.

TUMORS OF THE PITUITARY. Tumors of the anterior pituitary are almost invariably benign. Three types are described, corresponding to the three major types of cell present in the adenohypophysis—the chromophil, the basophil, and the eosinophil cell, a classification based on their histological staining properties. The chromophobe adenoma is the most common tumor; it produces either no deficit or, by impinging upon the remaining normal pituitary, may cause varying degrees of panhypopituitarism. The basophilic adenoma is generally very small, sometimes microscopic; it occurs not infrequently in normal persons, but may be associated with adrenal cortical overactivity and *Cushing's disease* (discussed below). The eosinophilic adenoma is associated with the overproduction of growth hormone. If an eosinophilic tumor begins in childhood or adolescence, while linear growth is still possible, growth is greatly accelerated and gigantism may result. A giant, by definition, is an individual more than seven feet tall, and giants eight to nine feet tall have been described. If the hypersecretion of growth hormone begins at an age after the epiphyses of the long bones have fused (hence linear growth is no longer possible), then the condition called *acromegaly* (enlargement of the distal parts) results. This is characterized by broadening and thickening of bones, thickening of soft tissues, especially over bony prominences (the finger and jaw), and proportionate, general enlargement of the viscera. It is often associated with diabetes and thyroid glandular enlargement and overactivity. The acromegalic has a characteristic appearance—a protruding jaw (prognathism), with overgrowth of the bony prominence of the eyebrows, and massively widened hands and feet. In the early stages of the disease, the patient may be unusually strong because of increase in muscle mass. As the disease progresses, however, hypopituitarism generally supervenes and weakness together with signs of gonadal, adrenal, and thyroid deficiency are observed.

The pituitary, situated in the *sella turcica* in the base of the skull, lies just beneath the optic chiasm (the point of intersection on the floor of the skull of the nerve fibers constituting the visual pathways from the eyes to the brain). As a pituitary tumor enlarges, it widens and expands the bony sella turcica, producing a characteristic appearance in x-ray films of the skull, and may impinge upon the optic chiasm. Consequently, both headaches and disturbances in vision, commonly complicate pituitary tumors. The typical visual impairment is *bitemporal hemianopsia*, which is a restriction in the outer part of the field of vision of each eye, so that affected persons can see well straight ahead, but objects to either side may not be visible to them, and they are consequently subject to accidents.

Neurological disturbances, especially visual impairment, together with endocrine symptoms (generally endocrine deficit) are characteristic of pituitary tumors. The diagnosis of such tumors is aided by x-rays of the skull and by tests of thyroid, gonadal, and adrenal function. In cases where endocrine deficit of the target organs is minimal or lacking, much information can be obtained by recently devised tests of pituitary reserve, whereby the ability of the anterior pituitary to increase production of a tropic hormone (generally ACTH) is tested.

The treatment of pituitary tumors is either surgical or by irradiation. Removal of the pituitary (hypophysectomy) is a formidable neurosurgical procedure, which may be necessary if radiation therapy fails or if vision deteriorates rapidly. Irradiation of the pituitary has been accomplished by high-voltage x-ray therapy or by the implantation of a needle containing a radioactive substance (generally yttrium[90]) in the pituitary. Such therapy often not only halts the progressive visual impairment induced by pituitary tumors but also improves vision, but it seldom improves endocrine deficits. For the latter, replacement therapy with cortisol, thyroid, and the appropriate sex hormones is required.

Diseases of the Neurohypophysis and Hypothalamus. The posterior lobe of the pituitary, the pituitary stalk, and the adjacent hypothalamic centers, which are intimately concerned with the elaboration of vasopressin and oxytocin, are subject to a variety of disturbances that may lead to loss of function and deficit of vasopressin. Injuries, chronic infections (tuberculosis and fungal infections), primary tumors of the base of the brain, and metastatic tumors from cancer primary outside of the cranium may all lead to *diabetes insipidus* (the name indicates that urine so abundantly produced in the disease is tasteless, in contrast to the sweetness of the sugar-rich urine in diabetes mellitus). The major clinical manifestations are due to vasopressin, or antidiuretic hormone (ADH), deficiency. As a result of ADH lack, the kidneys produce a very dilute urine, water conservation is impaired, and dehydration may occur. In many cases, 6 to 12 liters of urine may be excreted daily; naturally, this depletes the body of water and results in continual thirst, satisfied only by drinking large quantities of water. Hence, polyuria (passing of excessive urine) and polydipsia (excessive drinking) are characteristic of diabetes insipidus. The patient is miserable because of the need to urinate every hour or so and the need to have large supplies of water available, night and day. The diagnosis most often confused with diabetes insipidus is "nervous water drinking"; in the latter, for psychological reasons, the patient consumes unusually large amounts of water and consequently passes large quantities of dilute urine. The distinction between diabetes insipidus and nervous water drinking is easily made by observing the response to water deprivation for 12 hours. The person who suffers from nervous water drinking will, under these conditions, generally pass a decreased volume of concentrated urine, which is an appropriate response to water deprivation mediated by increased ADH secretion. However, the patient with diabetes insipidus and ADH deficiency deprived of water, although he suffers greatly from dehydration and thirst, continues to excrete large volumes of dilute urine.

Treatment of diabetes insipidus is by the administration of Pitressin by injection, generally once daily, or by the nasal insufflation of crude posterior pituitary powder (taken like snuff) several times a day. Treatment is satisfactory, and the polyuria and polydipsia are eliminated.

A hereditary form of impaired ability to concentrate the urine which presents the clinical picture of diabetes insipidus is called *nephrogenic diabetes insipidus;* this is not due to neurohypophysial disease but to an inability of the kidney to respond to vasopressin. The condition consequently does not respond to therapy with posterior pituitary preparations, and other methods of managing this disorder must be used, such as dietary salt restriction.

Hypothalamic disorders of endocrine significance other than diabetes insipidus are rare but startling in the clinical disorders produced. Tumors of the hypothalamus may lead to stimulation of gonadotropic function of the anterior lobe of the pituitary; when this occurs in childhood, precocious puberty results, with sexual maturation occurring prematurely. In other cases, the tumor may impinge upon hypothalamic centers concerned with appetite regulation, and hyperphagia (excessive eating) with consequent obesity may result.

THYROID DISORDERS

The clinical thyroid disorders include goiter, hyperthyroidism, hypothyroidism, thyroiditis, and thyroid tumors.

GOITER.   An enlarged thyroid, *goiter,* is the most common abnormality of the thyroid. The synthesis of adequate quantities of thyroid hormone is the major function of the thyroid gland, and this the thyroid accomplishes by extracting iodide from the circulation and iodinating thyroglobulin, the protein in which the thyroid hormone, thyroxin, is stored in the gland. If the ability of the gland to make thyroxin were impaired to a significant degree, the plasma concentration of thyroxin would tend to fall, and by the operation of the negative feedback mechanism described previously, more TSH would be released from the pituitary. Thus the increased stimulation of the thyroid gland would result in enlargement of the gland as well as increased activity, which might compensate for the difficulty in hormone production under which the gland was laboring. Goiter is usually an indication of excessive thyrotropic stimulation of the gland; when the goiter is associated with neither overproduction nor deficiency of thyroid hormone, it is called *nontoxic goiter*. The causes of nontoxic goiter are many and include *dietary iodine deficiency* (particularly in regions where goiter is endemic, such as mountainous regions and other areas distant from the iodine-rich sea); *ingestion of certain drugs* that have an antithyroid effect (for example, thiocyanates); *ingestion of large quantities of certain raw vegetables* (rutabaga, cabbage, turnip), which contain naturally occurring goitrogenic substances; *hereditary defects in thyroidal enzymes* concerned with the iodination mechanism in the gland; and *chronic inflammatory processes* in the gland (chronic thyroiditis), which by destroying much of the thyroid glandular tissue lead to compensa-

tory enlargement of the remaining tissue. Goiter, like all thyroid dis- ✓
orders, is much more common among females than males.

The symptoms of simple goiter are only those associated with enlargement of the gland, which may become easily visible and may
attain such a large size as to constitute a cosmetic problem. Rarely does
simple goiter produce symptoms of tracheal compression or respiratory
embarrassment; hoarseness may occasionally be present. Malignant tumors of the thyroid are more likely to cause hoarseness, pain, and
difficulty in swallowing. Nontoxic goiter may be diffuse (the gland
as a whole is enlarged) or nodular (palpable, irregular masses), and
the latter is more likely to be neoplastic, particularly when only a single
nodule is present.

The functional status of the thyroid gland may be assessed in several
ways. (1) The serum protein-bound iodine (PBI) level is a measure of
the circulating thyroid hormone, and is normally 4 to 8 micrograms
per 100 ml. (2) The basal metabolic rate (BMR) reflects gross alterations in thyroid function; many other factors influence the metabolic rate, and the nonspecificity of the test as well as the wide range
of normal (plus 15 to minus 15 per cent of normal) diminishes the
usefulness of the BMR as an index of thyroid gland activity. (3) For
radioactive iodine (RaI) studies, of which the thyroidal RaI uptake is
the most widely used, a small quantity of an isotope of iodine that
emits gamma rays (generally I^{131}) is given to the patient, and 24 hours
later the RaI accumulated in the thyroid is determined by using a
geiger or scintillation detecting device positioned in front of the neck.
Normally 10 to 50 per cent of the administered dose is present in the
neck, higher and lower values being associated respectively with hyperthyroidism and hypothyroidism. (4) Devices that can map the distribution of RaI in the neck (scintillation scanners) are often used to
study nodular goiters; these provide information regarding the functional activity of various parts of the gland. In general, "cold" nodules—
those which accumulate less RaI than the surrounding thyroid tissue
and hence are less active than normal tissue—are viewed with more
concern (with regard to possible malignancy) than nodules which are
"warm"—that is, their level of activity is the same as that of the non-
nodular thyroid tissue. However, even most "cold" nodules are not
malignant, and, indeed, carcinoma of the thyroid is one of the least
frequently encountered cancers.

Since in most cases nontoxic goiter is a consequence of increased
thyrotropic stimulation, rational treatment would be to decrease the
pituitary release of TSH. This can be done by giving desiccated thyroid
gland preparations or thyroxin, by mouth, in dosage equivalent to the
normal daily secretion rate of thyroxin. The decrease in thyrotropic
stimulation of the gland that is achieved may result in substantial

decrease in goiter size. At the same time, goitrogenic influences (such as dietary iodine deficiency or antithyroid drug ingestion) should be eliminated. Since goiter is usually a compensatory phenomenon, not only is surgical removal of the thyroid generally unnecessary, but it may also be deleterious, since hypothyroidism may result.

HYPERTHYROIDISM (GRAVES' DISEASE, EXOPHTHALMIC GOITER). When the thyroid glandular secretion of thyroid hormone is excessive, the clinical condition of *hyperthyroidism,* or *Graves' disease,* results. The disorder is familial, occurs five times as frequently in women as in men, and is characterized by enlargement of the thyroid, nervousness, restlessness, irritability, weight loss despite an increased appetite, weakness, heat intolerance, sweating, a tremor of the hands and body, palpitation, and a rapid, often irregular heart rate. In addition to the signs of hypermetabolism, ocular manifestations of Graves' disease are striking; in the milder forms, there is retraction of the lids, so that more of the white of the eye (the sclera) is visible than normal, and the patient has an appearance of perpetual surprise or terror. In the more severe forms of ocular disturbances, there are exophthalmos (the eyeball is pushed outward from its bony socket, the orbit) and often paralysis of the ocular muscles, so that eye movements are limited and double vision may result. The exophthalmos sometimes becomes progressive and extreme to the point where vision may be threatened; such cases are examples of so-called malignant exophthalmos. Curiously, although hyperthyroidism is much more common among women, malignant exophthalmos tends to occur more frequently in men.

Certain variants of the typical clinical picture of Graves' disease occur. In some cases, the weight loss and wasting may suggest malignancy. Sometimes profound muscular wasting and weakness may be confused with a neurological disorder. Some cases have predominantly cardiac symptoms, and if the cardiac reserve is unable to keep pace with the hypermetabolism, congestive heart failure may occur that does not respond to cardiac therapeutic measures. In rare cases, hyperthyroidism may induce psychotic behavior. Recognition of hyperthyroidism is important because with proper treatment, recovery from most of the disability associated with the disease is the rule, while failure to make the diagnosis may lead to disability or death, particularly from cardiac causes.

The diagnosis can generally be documented by the elevated serum PBI, the greatly increased BMR, and the high glandular radioactive iodine uptake. Therapy of hyperthyroidism includes drugs, surgery, and radioactive iodine. (1) Drugs, such as propylthiouracil and potassium perchlorate, which interfere with the synthesis of thyroxin, can control the disease indefinitely; after starting such drugs, improvement is gradual and within two months most patients are euthyroid (normal thyroxin secretion rate). If treatment is continued for 9 to 12 months, 60 per cent of cases will thereafter remain well, while in 40 per cent hyperthyroidism will recur and further treatment will be necessary, either drugs or some destructive form of treatment. (2) Surgery: Removal of approximately 90 per cent of the thyroid in hyperthyroidism may achieve the euthyroid state. The operation should be undertaken only if the patient has been rendered euthyroid by a six- to eight-week course of antithyroid drug prior to operation, since unprepared hyperthyroid patients tolerate surgery (and other stresses) very poorly, and may develop, after operation, a dangerous and possibly fatal syndrome of high fever, coma, and shock ("thyroid storm"). The complications of subtotal thyroidectomy include hypothyroidism, hypoparathyroidism (from removal of too much thyroid or parathyroid tissue), and loss or impairment of the voice (from inadvertent injury to the laryngeal nerves). Recurrence of hyperthyroidism after operation is not unusual. (3) Radioactive iodine in recent years has been used increasingly in the treatment of hyperthyroidism. A single dose of RaI given orally is generally effective. The irradiation of the gland by the RaI accumulated in the gland produces a destructive effect which may cure the disease. The great advantage of RaI therapy is that recurrence of hyperthyroidism is very unusual. The chief drawback to this form of therapy is that 10 to 15 per cent of the patients develop hypothroidism. There is no evidence of a deleterious radiation effect of therapeutic doses of RaI to organs other than the thyroid. Nevertheless, the idea of giving RaI therapeutically to young hyperthyroid people is objectionable to many physicians, who consequently reserve this form of treatment for patients over age 40.

The further progession of exophthalmos in Graves' disease is generally halted by successful treatment of the hyperthyroidism, though appreciable decrease in the degree of ocular protrusion may not occur. In cases in which the exophthalmos continues to become worse after euthyroidism has been established, neurosurgical procedures (decompression of the bony orbit, hypophysial stalk section) or x-ray therapy (of the pituitary region) is sometimes required to preserve vision.

HYPOTHYROIDISM (MYXEDEMA). In hypothyroidism, glandular production of thyroid hormone is inadequate for bodily needs, and the clinical picture is in some ways the opposite of hyperthyroidism. Hypothyroidism may occur with or without goiter. (1) *Hypothyroidism without goiter* includes (a) idiopathic primary hypothyroidism in which, from unknown causes, the thyroid gland becomes atrophic and ceases to function; (b) hypothyroidism secondary to pituitary disease and TSH deficit as described above; (c) hypothyroidism secondary to loss of thyroid substance as a consequence of thyroid surgery or RaI therapy for hyperthyroidism or a nontoxic goiter. (2) *Hypothyroidism* with *goiter* may result from any of the various causes of nontoxic goiter listed above, the only difference being that in the latter the thyroid enlargement and functional activity are adequate to compensate for the difficulty in hormonogenesis, while in goitrous hypothyroidism compensation is inadequate. An additional cause of goitrous hypothyroidism is *Hashimoto's disease,* a form of chronic thyroiditis characterized by the occurrence in the blood of antibodies to human thyroglobulin; this has led to the idea that it is an *autoimmune disease*—that is, the body has somehow become sensitized to one of the thyroid gland proteins, and antibodies are formed which in reacting with the antigen (thyroglobulin) may lead to glandular damage.

The clinical manifestations of hypothyroidism in the adult are similar, regardless of cause, and reflect the decreased metabolic rate and the deposition of mucin in the skin and other organs. The patient presents a picture of lethargy, pallor, decreased appetite, decreased hearing, and constipation. The patient feels cold even in hot weather and rarely sweats. The face is puffy, and extremities are pale and present a dough-like consistency. There is a loss of scalp and body hair, the voice is hoarse and deep, the tongue is large. Contrary to a widely held notion, hypothyroid patients are seldom obese—although metabolic rate is reduced, appetite is generally commensurately decreased. The puffiness is caused by the widespread deposition of a peculiar gelatinous mucin which gives the disease its name (myxedema = mucinous edema).

In typical cases, diagnosis can be suspected merely by observing the patient, or even by hearing the gravel-like voice on the telephone. The diagnosis can be documented by the low serum PBI, low BMR, and low thyroidal RaI uptake.

Complications of Hypothyroidism. Myxedema coma is a rare but almost invariably fatal disorder. It occurs in untreated hypothyroid patients for no apparent cause, and is characterized by hypothermia (a subnormal body temperature), low blood pressure, and unconsciousness. Psychosis, picturesquely termed "myxedema madness," may accompany hypothyroidism, and often improves greatly with thyroid therapy.

Treatment. Therapy of myxedema with oral thyroid gland extract or thyroxin results in disappearance of most of the clinical manifestations, and in all of medical practice there is no more gratifying response to therapy. Within a few weeks, the patient is mentally and physically alert, vigorous, warmer, and the voice, skin, and hair changes begin to improve. Therapy with thyroid must be lifelong; unless emphasis is placed by the physician upon the need for continued daily thyroid replacement therapy, patients tend to discontinue thyroid medication after they have been restored to the euthyroid state, and may gradually slip back into hypothyroidism once again.

Cretinism. A form of myxedema that deserves special comment, cretinism is hypothyroidism which is present at birth; it may or may not be associated with goiter. The thyroid hormone is essential for the normal growth and maturation of the skeletal system and the brain; the cretin consequently suffers from physical and mental retardation. Unless cretinism is promptly recognized and treated (within the first few months after birth), a grotesque, dwarfed, mentally deficient child will result. Unfortunately, although most of the physical manifestations of myxedema are reversed by thyroid treatment, the mental damage that occurs during the development of the untreated cretin's brain is not reversible, so that early recognition and treatment of the slow, cold, potbellied, constipated, puffy, cretinous child is of critical importance, if severe mental changes are to be avoided.

THYROIDITIS. Two important inflammatory disorders of the thyroid deserve comment. (1) *Subacute thyroiditis* is caused by a viral infection of the thyroid that produces a painful, tender enlargement of the thyroid, often with hoarseness, fever, weight loss, and profound weakness. The disease may be protracted, with relapses for a period of months, but is generally self-limited, and complete recovery of glandular function is the rule. The severe inflammation in the gland may permit entry into the circulation of excessive quantities of thyroid hormone, with resultant manifestation of hyperthyroidism, but this is generally transient. (2) *Chronic thyroiditis* includes a number of diverse conditions; the most important is *chronic lymphocytic thyroiditis* or *Hashimoto's disease*. The disease tends to be familial and affects chiefly middle-aged women; for many years the only manifestation may be a slowly enlarging goiter. In many cases, hypothyroidism eventually supervenes. As previously mentioned, in most cases of Hashimoto's disease the serum titer of antithyroglobulin antibodies is very high, and it is possible that the disease is a form of autoimmunity, thyroglobulin being the sensitizing agent. The diagnosis is suspected from a high serum antibody and from the presence of abnormal iodoproteins in the circulation. It may be confirmed by biopsy of the thyroid, which presents a rather characteristic histological picture. Both the goiter and the hypothyroidism respond well to the administration of thyroid or thyroxin. Surgical removal of the goiter is unnecessary and may induce myxedema.

THYROID CANCER. Cancer of the thyroid is rarely of endocrine importance. Most thyroid neoplasms are nonfunctional although rarely a well-differentiated carcinoma of the thyroid and its metastases may produce excessive quantities of thyroid hormone and the clinical signs of hyperthyroidism. In such cases, radioactive iodine is useful in detecting the tumor and its metastases, since the functioning tissue accumulates RaI, and by scanning techniques the primary and metastatic lesions can be located and defined; RaI therapy of such tumors may eradicate the malignancy. Unfortunately, most thyroid carcinomas accumulate little iodine, and hence RaI is of limited value in therapy. However, many thyroid malignancies are often quite dependent upon TSH for their growth and invasiveness, and suppression of TSH release, by administered thyroid hormone, may slow the rate of growth of both the primary tumor and the metastases. Surgical removal of as much of the tumor as possible, followed by suppression of TSH by giving thyroid, is the usual method of treatment.

PARATHYROID DISORDERS

HYPERPARATHYROIDISM. An uncommon disease with disastrous effects if untreated but one that responds effectively to appropriate therapy, hyperparathyroidism is a disorder important to recognize. The clinical picture of excessive parathyroid hormone secretion is understandable in terms of the major effect of parathormone (PTH), which is demineralization and resorption of bone; most of the manifestations of hyperparathyroidism are secondary to the demineralization of bone and to the harmful effects of the excessive quantities of calcium thereby liberated into the body fluids. Hyperparathyroidism is generally caused by a tumor of one (occasionally more than one) of the parathyroid glands; these tumors are generally benign, quite small and neither visible nor palpable in the neck. The symptoms and signs include bone pain, fractures occurring after mild injury, lethargy, decreased appetite, abdominal discomfort (many cases have peptic ulcer), constipation, and recurrent kidney stones and signs of impaired kidney function, including a diabetes insipidus-like picture of nephrogenic type. Kidney stones and calcification of the kidney itself (nephrocalcinosis) are due to the excessive quantity of calcium liberated from bone which taxes the excretory capacity of the kidney; renal function may be further embarrassed by infections of the kidney to which persons with urinary tract stones are susceptible. Abnormal calcification may occur in soft tissues, especially around joints, in the stomach, and in the cornea of the eye. The diagnosis may be made by finding an elevated serum calcium level, a low serum phosphorus, and often increased serum levels of alkaline phosphatase; the latter is an enzyme that splits off phosphate from many phosphate esters, and it is increased when there is increased activity of bone-forming cells (osteoblasts). The condition must be differentiated from other diseases in which serum calcium is elevated, particularly excessive milk drinking, multiple myeloma and other tumors destructive of bone, and vitamin D poisoning; in most of these conditions, the serum phosphorus tends to be high as well as the calcium. Although bone disease secondary to hyperparathyroidism is classically described, it occurs most frequently in those regions where the dietary calcium is low. In the United States, where the per capita consumption of milk is high, demineralization of bone is masked by the calcium intake and the kidney complications predominate, while hyperparathyroid bone disease is less commonly seen.

The treatment of hyperparathyroidism is surgical removal of the parathyroid tumor; this effectively halts the disease and restores normal calcium levels. In rare cases, parathyroid tumors tend to be part of a "multiglandular syndrome" in which functioning adenomas (benign tumors) occur not only in the parathyroid but also in the anterior pituitary and the pancreatic islet cells.

HYPOPARATHYROIDISM. This is generally caused by the removal of too much parathyroid tissue at the time of surgical thyroidectomy, but a few cases are of unknown cause and characterized by atrophy of the glands. The major manifestations are those of increased neuromuscular irritability, particularly *tetany;* the latter takes the form of painful muscle spasm or cramps, especially in the hands and feet. In addition, generalized convulsive seizures occur, simulating epilepsy. In some cases, calcification in the brain occurs, as well as in soft tissues, intracranial pressure may be increased (producing headaches), and ocular cataracts are common. The combination of seizures and increased intracranial pressure may lead to an erroneous diagnosis of brain tumor. The diagnosis of hypoparathyroidism is confirmed by the coexistence of a low serum calcium level (the normal range is 9 to 11 mg/100 ml serum) and a high serum phosphate level.

Treatment of hypoparathyroidism is quite satisfactory. Since the availability of parathormone is limited and the material must be given by frequent injection, PTH is not used in therapy, but instead large doses of vitamin D are used; this can be given orally and has many of the effects of parathormone. The primary effect of vitamin D is to increase the absorption of calcium from the intestinal tract; this restores the serum calcium to normal and depresses the serum phosphorus as well. In addition to vitamin D, a high calcium, low phosphorus diet is prescribed. Therapy must generally be lifelong, and patients under treatment must be checked periodically to ensure that the serum calcium level is indeed normal; perhaps more dangerous than untreated hypocalcemia is hypercalcemia, resulting from overdosage of vitamin D used in treatment of hypoparathyroidism. Vitamin D intoxication may produce a clinical picture like hyperparathyroidism, with ultimate irreversible damage to the kidneys. Patients under treatment are therefore advised to check their urine for excessive calcium content from time to time, using a simple semiquantitative test (Sulkowich test), just as diabetic patients check their urine for sugar.

DISORDERS OF THE ADRENALS

THE ADRENAL CORTEX. Disorders of the adrenal cortex include states of overproduction and deficiency; the clinical pictures produced constitute a complex and interesting group. Since the three major products of the adrenal cortex are the catabolic hormone cortisol, the sodium-retaining hormone aldosterone, and several androgens, clinical manifestations of overproduction reflect the effects of excess of one or more of these secretory products.

Cushing's Syndrome. This term is applied to the disease state characterized chiefly by overproduction of cortisol. A clinical picture mimicking many features of this disorder may occur in patients with arthritis, asthma, and other diseases which are treated with large doses of corticosteroids. The characteristic features include high blood pressure; diabetes; wasting of muscle mass with resulting very thin extremities; a peculiar ruddy roundness of the face due to abnormal fat deposition; obesity of the trunk; psychiatric disturbances; amenorrhea; easy bruisability (so that minor injuries lead to subcutaneous bleeding or "black and blue" spots); thinning of the bones (osteoporosis) especially of the spine, so that fractures of the vertebral column are common; and dermal _striae_, which are striking, parallel, purple broad atrophic bands of skin, especially in the abdomen and thighs. There is often some evidence of mild androgen excess (amenorrhea, acne, and hirsutism or increased growth of body hair). Many of the clinical features are due to the catabolic effect of excess cortisol (especially the muscle wasting, osteoporosis, thin skin and fragile blood vessels, and the diabetes). The disease often runs a rapidly progressive course, with death or disability from the cardiac or renal complications of hypertension, or from psychosis, diabetes, or infections, to which such patients are very prone. The diagnosis is established by finding increased quantities of corticosteroid products in the urine or plasma (especially the 17-hydroxycorticosteroids) or by demonstrating an increase above normal in adrenal secretory rate of cortisol, using newer methods involving injection of a trace quantity of radioactive cortisol.

In about two-thirds of the cases, hypercortisolism of Cushing's disease results from _hyperplasia_ (increase in the number of cells and in the functional activity) of the adrenal cortex of both glands. Until recently it was believed that the hyperfunction of the adrenal cortex was due to a primary disorder of the adrenal glands, but it is now thought that it is secondary to a disorder of the pituitary and hypothalamus, which renders the latter less responsive than usual to normal plasma cortisol levels, with resultant hypersecretion of pituitary ACTH and overstimulation of the adrenal cortex. In one-third of the cases, an adrenal tumor is responsible for the excessive secretion; these tumors may be benign or malignant.

Treatment of Cushing's disease is generally surgical. If the disease is caused by an adrenal tumor (this can generally be diagnosed by study of the urinary steroids) removal of the tumor may be curative.

If the disease is caused by adrenal hyperplasia, total removal of both glands is performed; this means that the patient must be treated for the remainder of his life for adrenal insufficiency (see below). A complication that sometimes develops after bilateral adrenalectomy for Cushing's disease is pituitary tumor, with visual disturbances and intense pigmentation, the latter probably due to excessive ACTH secretion. Cushing's disease and adrenal hyperplasia may occur in association with certain malignant tumors of organs other than the adrenal, especially lung, kidney, and thymus; these tumors produce a substance that has an ACTH-like action in stimulating the adrenal and thus produce hypercortisolism. In such cases, removal of the primary tumor may ameliorate the Cushing's picture.

Adrenogenital Syndrome. This term includes several disorders, which have in common the adrenal production of excessive androgen, leading to virilization of the female or precocious sexual development in the male. Normally the production of androgenic substances by the adrenal cortex is of little clinical or physiological importance, but in certain disease states adrenal androgens may be produced in quantity.

Congenital adrenal hyperplasia is a familial disorder of recessive inheritance, in which adrenal cortical overproduction of androgens occurs because of inherited defects in the enzymes concerned with the synthesis of cortisol. The defect in cortisol synthesis is an impaired ability to introduce a hydroxyl group at one of several points of the steroid nucleus; this leads to compensatory stimulation of the adrenal cortex by pituitary ACTH in an effort to maintain adequate adrenal secretion of cortisol, but the enhanced stimulation of the defective adrenal cortex causes the over production of androgenic steroids. If the fetal adrenal produces excess androgen, virilization of the female fetus occurs *in utero,* so that at birth, the newborn's clitoris may be enlarged. The vaginal libia may be fused and resemble a scrotum, and the general appearance of the genitalia may be so ambiguous as to render difficult the correct assignment of gender. This is an example of female *pseudohermaphroditism.* (A pseudohermaphrodite is an individual of one sex whose genital development presents features of the other sex; thus a female pseudohermaphrodite is a subject with ovaries whose genitalia are masculine in appearance; a male pseudohermaphrodite is a person with testes whose genitalia have some female features.) If the overproduction of adrenal androgen persists during infancy and early childhood, somatic growth is accelerated, but because early closure of epiphyses occurs, the eventual height achieved is subnormal; in addition, virilization occurs (enhanced muscle bulk, deep voice, phallic enlargement), and normal development of female secondary sex characteristics will not occur at the expected age of puberty.

In males, congenital adrenal hyperplasia is difficult to diagnose at birth, because the genitalia appear normal, but within one to two years, evidence of unusually rapid growth and sexual precocity (large penis, sexual hair, mature male appearance) calls attention to the disorder, which in males descriptively is termed *macrogenitosomia praecox*. In many cases of virilizing adrenal hyperplasia there is a tendency for body sodium depletion to occur due to excessive urinary sodium loss, and dehydration and death may occur unless the true nature of the disorder is recognized and appropriate therapy instituted; the diagnosis is especially difficult in young boys, in whom the sexual precocity is much less apparent than is virilization in girls. The diagnosis of congenital adrenal hyperplasia is confirmed by the increased urinary excretion of 17-ketosteroids (these correlate roughly with adrenal androgen production) and of pregnanetriol.

Treatment of virilizing hyperplasia is very effective; cortisone or a synthetic corticosteroid analogue is given in modest doses just large enough to suppress pituitary ACTH secretion; by this means, stimulation of the adrenal gland is diminished and the abnormal secretion of androgen halted. With successful therapy the manifestations of virilization in the female slowly regress (although plastic reconstruction of the vagina and clitoris may be necessary) and normal growth and development in childhood with normal adolescent maturation and reproductive life is possible. Adrenal suppressive therapy must be lifelong, since the enzymatic defects leading to androgen excess are not cured by the corticosteroid therapy; because of the dangers of Cushing's syndrome from cortisone overdosage, careful regulation of dosage is essential, especially in childhood and adolescence. A variant form of congenital adrenal hyperplasia is associated with severe hypertension, and this also responds well to cortisone therapy.

In children and adults certain tumors of the adrenal cortex may produce an acquired form of the *adrenogenital syndrome*. In adult females the virilization is expressed in such clinical features as deepening of the voice, male pattern baldness and body hair distribution, hirsutism (increased body hair), and amenorrhea. In adult males, instead of the "superman" one might expect, the clinical signs are often those of feminization (testicular atrophy, enlargement of the breasts, and so on) presumably because these tumors secrete estrogens as well as androgens. The treatment of such functioning tumors of the adrenal is surgical removal; the tumors are seldom under ACTH control, hence cortisone therapy is not effective.

Aldosteronism. In recent years, a number of cases have been reported in which hypertension was secondary to the increased adrenocortical secretion of aldosterone, the salt-retaining steroid of the adrenal cortex. An adrenocortical tumor, usually benign, which secretes aldosterone is found in such cases, and the disorder is therefore called *primary aldosteronism.* These tumors occur chiefly in young adults, the hypertension may be severe and progressive, and usually there is found a high serum sodium and low serum potassium level and an alkaline urine, reflecting the effects of aldosterone on the renal excretion of sodium and potassium. Although primary aldosteronism is an unusual disease, it is important that it be recognized, since prompt surgical removal of the tumor may cure both the hypertension and the electrolyte abnormalities. The diagnosis is confirmed by finding increased quantities of aldosterone metabolites in the urine.

Adrenocortical Deficiency. Deficiency of adrenocortical secretion results in *Addison's disease,* in which the adrenal glands undergo atrophy of unknown cause, are destroyed by disease (tuberculosis, infiltration with metastatic tumor, amyloid or other materials), or are surgically removed, as in the treatment of Cushing's disease. The predominant symptoms and signs are due to lack of cortisol and of aldosterone. Thus, the typical clinical features include weakness, decreased blood pressure, hypoglycemia, a variety of gastrointestinal symptoms, and a brownish pigmentation of the skin (especially prominent on the exposed parts of face, neck, hands, and on pressure points such as elbows) and in the mouth; dehydration and salt depletion secondary to large losses of sodium in the urine may lead to collapse. In addition, there is a remarkable inability to withstand stress, so that death may result from a mild respiratory infection or a minor surgical procedure. The increased pigmentation is often extreme and probably is due to increased secretion of pituitary ACTH elicited by the primary cortisol deficiency; ACTH has an intrinsic melanocyte-stimulating effect.

The diagnosis of Addison's disease is supported by finding very low levels of 17-hydroxycorticosteroids in the urine and by the failure of urine steroids to rise after ACTH injections are given. Although the disease carries a high mortality and morbidity if untreated, replacement therapy of the cortisol and aldosterone deficits results in remarkable improvement. Within a very short time, often a few hours after starting therapy, the patient has more strength, a sense of well-being, and the blood pressure rises. After prolonged therapy, the pigmentation tends to decrease. Therapy must continue for the remainder of the patient's life; usually cortisone and a synthetic salt-retaining steroid are used. In hot weather, when sodium losses may be excessive, extra salt is provided in the diet, and in times of illness, surgery, or other stress, the dose of cortisone must be increased. In successful therapy the cortisone dosage is just sufficient to replace the cortisol deficit without producing signs of cortisolism.

THE ADRENAL MEDULLA. *Pheochromocytoma* is a tumor of the adrenal medulla, generally benign, sometimes multiple, which is a rare but remediable cause of hypertension. The hypertension may be sustained or intermittent and paroxysmal. The symptoms and signs are caused by the excessive production of epinephrine and norepinephrine by the tumor, and the manifestations include rapid heart rate, hypertension, hyperglycemia, hypermetabolism with consequently increased sweating. The clinical picture (except for the hypertension) is somewhat like hyperthyroidism. Sometimes massage of the abdomen, intentional or accidental, over the tumor may produce a violent rise in blood pressure, a very rapid pulse, profuse sweating, tremor, and convulsions. The tumor is rarely large enough to be felt on abdominal examinations, but its presence may be suggested by x-ray study of the abdomen. A characteristic diagnostic laboratory finding is a high urinary excretion of catecholamines or of one of their main degradation products, especially vanillinmandelic acid (VMA), a metabolite of epinephrine and norepinephrine. Therapy consists of prompt surgical removal of the tumor; if the hypertension has persisted for a long time before the operation, irreversible cardiac and renal complications of hypertension may have occurred.

ENDOCRINE DISORDER OF THE GONADS

THE OVARIES. Alterations in the ovarian production of estrogen and progesterone may result either from primary disorders of the ovary or from abnormalities of the gonadotropic functions of the hypothalamic pituitary system. The latter have been mentioned in the section on the hypophysis. It may be added that minor degrees of hypophysial disturbance, such as may be secondary to nutritional, emotional, constitutional, and other factors, may interfere with gonadotropin release sufficiently to result in such conditions as delayed puberty, menstrual disturbances such as amenorrhea and excessive menstrual bleeding, failure of ovulation and infertility. Of the primary disorders of the ovary, the following are of the major clinical importance.

Ovarian Agenesis (Turner's Syndrome). Although the clinical picture of this congenital disorder has been recognized for some years, the profound genetic abnormality responsible for it has only recently been defined. The typical history in a case of Turner's syndrome is that of a phenotypic female (that is, the appearance is female) child who may have been born with some congenital physical defects of varying severity, who is generally shorter than average throughout childhood, and who fails to undergo the normal female sexual maturation at the time of puberty, so that breasts, vagina, uterus, remained undeveloped. The congenital malformation may include a rather striking skin fold on either side of the neck (termed webbed neck), asymmetry of the face, widespread eyes, a broad shieldlike chest, and narrowing of the aorta, the great artery emerging from the heart. The final height achieved by these patients is usually about four and a half feet. These patients have no ovarian tissue, and the primary ovarian defect is reflected in the high urinary titer of pituitary gonadotropin.

Studies of the chromosomes in these patients have shown that their cell nuclei contain not the normal human chromosome number of 46 but only 45; this is made up of the 22 pairs of somatic chromosomes, together with a single sex chromosome—which is an X chromosome— rather than two X chromosomes as in the normal female. It is now believed that because of the lack of a sex chromosome, the fetal gonad does not undergo differentiation and does not develop, and in the absence of a fetal testis the differentiation of the embryonic sexual duct system is along female lines, so that fallopian tubes, uterus, and vagina are normally formed. The lack of ovarian tissue precludes development of the pubertal secondary sex characteristics. Since the missing sex chromosome could be a Y as well as an X, and the absent gonad a testis as well as an ovary, the disorder is now called *gonadal dysgenesis* rather than ovarian agenesis.

The chromosomal abnormality in Turner's syndrome probably stems from a faulty cell division in the process leading to production either of the ovum or of the sperm whose fusion formed the zygote (the fertilized ovum) from which the patient developed. In both oogenesis and spermatogenesis, cells with 46 chromosomes give rise to ova and sperm with 23; this reduction division results in ova which have 22 somatic chromosomes plus an X chromosome $(22 + X)$, and sperm which have either $22 + X$, or $22 + Y$. A zygote would then have $44 + XX$ (normal female genotype) or $44 + XY$ (normal male genotype). If nondisjunction occurs, an ovum or sperm may have genotypes $22 + O$, $22 + XY$, $22 + XX$. Fertilization of a $22 + X$ ovum by an abnormal $22 + O$ sperm could result in the $44 + XO$ genotype of the Turner's syndrome patient. Nondisjunction may occur in either parent, but in Turner's disease, genetic studies suggest the defective cell division is in the father, a normal egg being fertilized by a defective sperm.

The diagnosis of Turner's syndrome is made from the clinical picture, the high urinary gonadotropin value, and a simple procedure called nuclear sexing. When cells, generally scraped from the inside of the cheek, of normal female individuals are suitably stained, a small dark nuclear chromatin mass is visible under the microscope; such cells are called chromatin positive. Stained cells of normal males do not show this chromatic mass and are therefore chromatin negative. It is believed the XX pair is necessary for chromatin positivity. Cells from Turner's syndrome patients, being XO, are chromatin negative. A phenotypic female who is chromatin negative may be presumed to have gonadal dysgenesis, and the diagnosis may be made at birth, long before the endocrine deficit becomes evident.

The patient with gonadal dysgenesis should be treated with estrogens at the usual age of puberty, so that normal female maturation will occur and appropriate cyclic courses of estrogens given with progestational steroids will result in cyclic menstrual bleeding. Such patients often marry, have normal sexual activity, and lead normal feminine lives, although reproductive activity is impossible. Because of the potentially disastrous psychological effect that awareness of her abnormal genotype could produce, the patient should not be told of this, but only that her ovarian function is limited and that fertility is remote.

Stein-Leventhal Syndrome (Polycystic Ovary Syndrome). The clinical picture presented by this disorder of adult females is very varied but may include menstrual irregularities; hirsutism (increased growth of body hair, especially in male pattern) without other signs of masculinization; obesity; infertility due to lack of ovulation and large, pale ovaries, with many cysts. Most patients consult physicians because of menstrual irregularity. The cause of the disorder is not agreed upon. Some feel it is due to ovarian production of excessive androgen, others that it is a disease in which the adrenal cortex produces a mild excess of androgen which secondarily affects ovulation. The condition sometimes responds to corticosteroid therapy which suppresses the adrenal gland (as in virilizing adrenal hyperplasia) and sometimes responds to surgical removal of a portion of the ovary (especially the hilar portion believed to contain androgen-secreting cells). In successfully treated cases, ovulation, fertility, and menstrual disturbances improve, but hirsutism usually is little affected.

The Menopause. The reproductive life of women ends in middle life, usually in the fifth decade. Associated with the failure of ovulation is a sharp decline in ovarian estrogen production. Although these changes are physiological, the estrogen deficit may give rise to such phenomena as atrophy of the skin; demineralization of bone (osteoporosis) especially of the vertebral column, with back pain; "hot flashes," which are sudden sensations of warmth, often with sweating and a red flush of the skin; and psychological depression. The hot flashes generally last one to two years. Many menopausal symptoms are not reflective of estrogen deficit but are of emotional origin, especially the depression associated with the end of reproductive life and the feeling of having outlived one's usefulness, and psychotherapy may be useful in some cases. Estrogen therapy may improve the psychological picture and modify or prevent the annoying hot flashes, and a few months of treatment may be useful in tiding the patient over this transition period in ovarian function. Longer-term estrogen therapy for menopausal osteoporosis has been beneficial in some cases. There is some suspicion that prolonged estrogen therapy may increase the incidence of cancer of the uterus and breast; although this may be true in experimental animals, the evidence for a potential danger of prolonged estrogen treatment in women is incomplete.

Functioning Ovarian Tumors. Of the many neoplasms that may involve the ovary, relatively few secrete estrogen or androgen; when such tumors do occur, however, the clinical picture is so striking, that some mention of them may be desirable.

Feminizing tumors include theca cell and granulosa cell tumors which secrete large quantities of estrogens. Since the manifestations of estrogen excess would be masked in females of the reproductive age, these tumors are particularly apparent in childhood and in the postmenopausal period. In female children, in the first decade, these tumors produce precocious puberty, with development of the female secondary sex characteristics and vaginal bleeding. The condition may be differentiated from constitutional or hypothalamic causes of premature puberty by the fact that in estrogen-producing tumors, gonadotropin is suppressed and none is present in the urine, while in precocious puberty of hypothalamic origin, gonadotropin is present in the urine. Such tumors in menopausal females are manifested chiefly by resumption of vaginal bleeding, generally on an irregular basis.

Virilizing tumors of the ovary, of which the arrhenoblastoma is best known, are rare. They produce symptoms of androgen excess, similar to those of virilizing adrenal tumors in adult females, with resulting hirsutism, clitoral enlargement, and amenorrhea. The diagnosis is suspected from the clinical picture of androgen excess, the presence of an ovarian mass, and the relatively normal or only slightly increased urinary 17-ketosteroids, the latter being much higher in adrenal virilizing tumors.

THE TESTES. As in the case of the ovary, endocrine disorders of the testis may be secondary to pituitary disease, or may be primary in the testes. Disorders of the pituitary generally result in both spermatogenic and endocrine testicular deficit, while primary testicular disorders may affect one or both testicular functions. Many of the primary testicular disorders affect mainly spermatogenesis while androgenic function is preserved. Thus, the testicular damage resulting from mumps and other forms of *orchitis (inflammation of the testes)*, injuries, infections, and irradiation of the testes generally results in spermatogenic deficit alone, and patients present with sterility problems rather than diminished libido or absence of male secondary sex characteristics. These disorders are generally characterized by small testes (since the bulk of the testis is composed of spermatogenic elements), and the diagnosis can be made by studies of sperm number and motility in semen specimens and by testicular biopsy.

Among the primary testicular disturbances that are endocrinologically important are *Klinefelter's syndrome* and the *testicular feminization syndrome*.

Klinefelter's Syndrome (Seminiferous Tubule Dysgenesis). This is a condition characterized by very small testes, varying degrees of development of the male secondary sex characteristics (ranging from eunuchoidism to relatively mild deficit), gynecomastia (enlargement of the breasts), increased urine gonadotropic titer, and a characteristic pathology of hyalinization of the seminiferous tubules, so that there is virtually no sperm formation with variable degrees of sparing of the Leydig cells. *Klinefelter's syndrome* is one of the more common causes of male infertility. It is often associated with mental retardation. A characteristic finding in most cases is chromatin-positive smears studied by nuclear sexing techniques, in contrast to the normal male chromatin-negative pattern. Chromosome analysis has shown that in most cases of this disease, there are 47 chromosomes per nucleus, occasionally 48, and even 49; the chromosome pattern is 44 somatic chromosomes + XXY (the two X's account for the chromatin positivity). The disorder is believed to result, like *Turner's syndrome*, from a faulty cell division leading to nondisjunction in the cell divisions which produce the ovum— that is, a 22 + XX ovum is fertilized by a 22 + Y sperm, to yield a 44 + XXY zygote. Chromosome study techniques now permit the establishment of the diagnosis in infancy, before the possible androgen deficit is apparent. Treatment consists of inducing appropriate male maturation at the time of puberty and maintaining the secondary sex characteristics thereafter by testosterone or other androgenic compounds. Fertility is highly improbable.

Testicular Feminization. This is an unusual familial disorder of apparent sex reversal and is an extreme form of male pseudohermaphroditism. The patients at birth are phenotypic females, with fairly normal female external genitalia, although uterus and tubes may be absent. At the normal time of puberty, apparently appropriate female secondary sex characteristics develop but no menstrual periods. Examination may reveal masses in the groin which if exposed turn out to be normal-looking testes, and no ovarian tissue is present. Nuclear sexing shows a negative chromatin pattern and chromosome analysis reveals the normal male pattern (44 autosomes + XXY). The cause of the female appearance and of the pubertal female development may be a faulty testis that secretes estrogens rather than androgens. The patients with this disorder, although genetic males, have almost invariably been raised as females; in order to avoid the emotional upheaval consequent to assignment of a male gender after a previous life with a female orientation, it is customary to remove the testes, reconstruct the external genitalia if necessary, and provide estrogenic hormones to maintain the female sex characteristics. Such patients are feminine in their outlook, and cases of this disorder demonstrate that in areas where the attitudes of men and women differ, it is not the type of gonad that is responsible for the differences.

Testicular Tumors. Most testicular tumors are nonfunctional from an endocrine viewpoint; they arise from germinal cells rather than from

Leydig cells. The rare Leydig cell tumors may be either masculinizing or feminizing. The masculinizing variety produces notable changes only in childhood, were precocious male pubertal changes may occur. The feminizing variety tend to occur in adult males, where the excessive estrogen produced may lead to decreased libido, impotence, decrease in body hair, and some enlargement of the breasts. Another tumor of the testis is the malignant choriocarcinoma, composed of chorionic cells similar to those present in the normal placenta. Choriocarcinomas exert an endocrine effect by virtue of the fact that the tumor may secrete large quantities of gonadotropins which stimulate the Leydig cells to produce androgens and estrogens; enlargement of the breasts may result. Therapy is surgical removal followed by x-ray therapy.

DISORDERS OF THE PANCREAS

DIABETES MELLITUS. One of the commonest endocrine disorders is diabetes mellitus. It is estimated that there are nearly two million diabetics in the United States. There is a strong familial tendency, and the disease appears to be inherited as a Mendelian recessive. Diabetes may be a manifestation of other primary diseases. Thus, it is seen frequently with acromegaly, Cushing's disease, pheochromocytoma, hemochromatosis, and chronic pancreatic inflammatory diseases.

Diabetes is caused by a relative or absolute deficiency of the pancreatic islet cell hormone insulin; as a consequence of the insulin deficiency, carbohydrate utilization is inefficient, and there is a wasting both of glucose of dietary origin and of that produced via metabolism of protein and lipids. The major manifestations of diabetes include the so-called diabetic triad of *polyphagia* (increased food consumption), *polydipsia* (increased thirst and drinking), and *polyuria* (increased urine volume); in addition, loss of weight, weakness, fatigability, and itching frequently occur. The polyuria results from the obligatory renal excretion of much water imposed by the large quantity of glucose excreted, and the polydipsia is compensatory for the dehydration.

Two general clinical types of diabetes are described, the maturity-onset type and the juvenile-onset type. The maturity-onset type of diabetes generally begins rather gradually in middle life, tends to occur in obese persons, the glycosuria tends to respond to dietary restriction, there is little tendency for development of ketoacidosis, and the patients are relatively resistant to the effects of administered insulin. Plasma insulin levels tend to be normal or even high. In these cases, insulin antagonists may be responsible for the relative insulin deficiency. Diabetes of the juvenile-onset type is characterized by a more rapid onset of diabetic symptoms in the first or second decades of life, there is a strong tendency to develop acidosis, and the patients are very sensitive to the effects of administered insulin. Plasma insulin values tend to be low, implying an absolute insulin deficiency.

Diagnosis of Diabetes. In most diabetics, the blood sugar after an overnight fast exceeds the normal range of 60 to 100 mg/100 ml, and there is glycosuria, especially after a meal. In borderline or early cases, the fasting blood sugar may be normal, but if the patient's efficiency in utilizing glucose is tested by having him consume a standard dose of glucose or a meal rich in sugar (glucose tolerance test), the blood sugar reaches abnormally high values (more than 140 mg/100 ml two hours after the meal), and glycosuria may occur. An elevated fasting blood sugar, persistent glycosuria with hyperglycemia, or persistently impaired glucose tolerance establish the diagnosis of diabetes. It should be pointed out that glycosuria *per se* need not mean that diabetes is present—there are many persons who have glycosuria but with normal blood sugar values; this is primarily caused by a renal defect in glucose conservation and is called renal glycosuria.

Treatment of Diabetes. Treatment aims at improving carbohydrate utilization and diminishing the diabetic symptoms. The most important aspects of treatment are concerned with diet, insulin, and hypoglycemic agents.

1. Diet. Caloric restriction and reduction of body weight to normal are often helpful in obese diabetics of the maturity-onset type; glycosuria may disappear on such a regimen alone. Regular exercise, which improves the utilization of glucose, is a helpful adjunct in treatment.

2. Insulin. Insulin by injection is essential for the control of diabetic symptoms in most diabetics of the juvenile type and in many maturity-onset diabetics. Patients are taught to self-administer the insulin. Many insulin preparations are available; they range from relatively short-acting insulins such as crystalline, or "regular" insulin, with a duration of action of four to eight hours, to long-acting insulin, such as protamine-zinc insulin (duration of action 24 to 36 hours). Most patients require a single daily morning injection of a moderately long-acting preparation (NPH insulin is most widely used) for effective control of hyperglycemia and glycosuria, but some labile diabetics may require additional injections of regular insulin once or twice more during the day.

3. Oral Hypoglycemic Agents. Several substances chemically related to sulfonylurea lower the blood sugar after oral ingestion. These agents, of which tolbutamide and chlorpropamide are best known, lower the blood sugar chiefly by stimulating the release of insulin from the pancreas. They are very useful in treatment of maturity-onset diabetes, in conjunction with dietary regulation. Perhaps 80 per cent of such cases can be maintained without insulin. They are of little effectiveness in juvenile-onset type diabetes, in which pancreatic insulin reserves are presumably exhausted. An orally effective adjunct in the treat-

ment of diabetics of both types (usually in association with insulin or sufonylurea drug) is phenylethyl-guanide, which promotes partial degradation of glucose.

4. Education. In addition to diet, drugs, and insulin, education of the diabetic patient is an essential part of the therapeutic program. Patients must be taught to give themselves insulin, to understand the principles of diet therapy, and to test their urine for sugar. They must know how to modify insulin dosage appropriately in the face of varying degrees of glycosuria; they must be particularly wary of infections and injuries, which may lead to disastrous results in poorly controlled diabetics; and they must be alert to the symptoms and management of hypoglycemic reactions.

Complications of Diabetes. Complications of the disease may be categorized as *acute* or as *chronic*.

1. Acute Complications. The major complication is diabetes acidosis, which may be precipitated by infections, injuries, or negligence in insulin dosage. The mechanism of diabetic acidosis has been discussed in the section on pancreatic physiology; it is essentially a flooding of the body with ketone acids as a consequence of impaired glucose utilization. The clinical signs of diabetic acidosis may develop very rapidly and include dehydration, circulatory collapse, very rapid deep breathing, dulling of the sensorium, and coma. The fruity odor of acetone is usually perceptible on the breath, and the urine contains not only sugar but acetone. Diabetic acidosis and coma are major medical emergencies with a high mortality if treatment is delayed. Hospitalization is usually advisable, and the injection of insulin, often in large quantities, together with appropriate restoration of losses of water and electrolytes incurred during the development of acidosis, is mandatory. In addition, discovery and treatment of the infection and other situations that provoked the acidosis are essential.

Hypoglycemia may occur in diabetics as a result of overdosage with insulin or oral hypoglycemic agents. The symptoms, referable to non-availability of glucose to the brain, range from relatively mild reactions such as pallor, tremulousness, and numbness of the lips and hands, to more profound disturbances such as confusion, instability of gait, convulsions, and loss of consciousness. Since diabetics taking insulin are subject to both hypoglycemic coma and diabetic coma, these two disorders must be carefully differentiated; this can be done by noting absence of sugar and acetone from the urine of the hypoglycemic patient. Hypoglycemia usually responds dramatically to the administration of glucose or sugar-rich foods.

2. Chronic Complications. Diabetes tends to be associated with a number of degenerative and other sequelae. It is these chronic degenerative complications, especially those involving blood vessels, which

constitute the major causes of morbidity and mortality from diabetes. The acute complications of diabetes, such as acidosis, are now readily controlled by insulin therapy; and the control of infections, to which diabetics are particularly vulnerable, has been improved by antibiotics. Consequently, diabetics rarely succumb to these acute problems; they are more subject to the chronic complications of the disease.

(a) Coexisting diseases. The incidence of pulmonary tuberculosis and of hypertension is higher among diabetics than among nondiabetics. For this reason, periodic general health examinations and chest x-rays are advisable for diabetic patients so that these diseases may be recognized early and appropriate therapy begun.

(b) Ocular complications. Diabetics are subject to *cataract formation* in the lens of the eye and to *diabetic retinopathy*, which is a result of small hemorrhages from the retinal vessels. Cataracts tend to occur when diabetes is poorly controlled; thus careful diabetic regulation may reduce the frequency of cataract. Retinopathy, however, results from disease of the retinal blood vessels which may be modified relatively little by careful diabetic control. The incidence of retinal changes increases with the duration of diabetes, and is disappointingly unrelated to the meticulousness with which glycosuria has been controlled. Indeed, there is some suggestion that the retinal vascular changes may even precede the onset of frank diabetes, since these changes have been noted in some relatives of diabetic persons whose carbohydrate tolerance has been normal. Diabetic retinopathy leads to impaired vision and sometimes blindness.

(c) Atherosclerosis. The accumulation of cholesterol and other materials in the wall of arteries, and the subsequent narrowing of such vessels, occur frequently among diabetics and are responsible for the impaired circulation which is an important factor in many of the complications. Diminution in blood flow to essential organs, such as the brain, may give rise to "strokes" with partial or complete paralysis of extremities, to sensory deficit, and to disturbances of speech and comprehension. Arteriosclerosis of the coronary arteries supplying the heart muscle may lead to angina pectoris, congestive heart failure, and infarction of the myocardium. Involvement of the kidneys by the arterial occlusive disease leads to nephrosclerosis and impaired renal function. When the vessels of the legs are affected by severe arteriosclerosis, such circulatory disturbances as pain or exercise (intermittent claudication) and ischemic gangrene (death of tissue due to insufficiency of blood supply) of the toes and feet may occur. The poor circulation in the lower extremities leads to impaired wound healing and impaired resistance to infections.

(d) Renal disease. Kidney disorders are frequently encountered among diabetics. Chronic urinary tract infections are especially common (pyelonephritis), and acute renal infections sometimes are complicated by necrotizing papillitis of the kidney, in which necrosis of kidney occurs, a condition that may run a rapidly progressive course with complete cessation of urine formation, shock, and death within a few days of onset. A form of chronic renal disease characteristic of diabetes is *intercapillary glomerulosclerosis (Kimmelstiel-Wilson disease)*, which tends to occur in patients who have had diabetes for a number of years. It has a characteristic pathological picture associated with much albumin in the urine, generalized edema, hypertension, and anemia. The disorder tends to occur in patients who have extensive diabetic retinopathy, and, indeed, similar pathological changes are seen in the small blood vessels in both the kidney and the retina. Renal function may become so limited as to produce uremia.

(e) Diabetic neuropathy. This is a complication of diabetes that may produce a variety of clinical manifestations, such as pain in the extremities, muscular weakness and atrophy, sensory changes such as numbness, disturbances in the function of the urinary bladder, paralysis of the eye muscles, and difficulties in gait. The neuritic changes are at least in part a reflection of lesions in small blood vessels which interfere with adequate nutrition of the nerves.

Although many of the chronic sequelae of diabetes seem to occur even in well-regulated diabetics, the aim of therapy in this disease is to restore efficient utilization of glucose and to treat the complications as they occur.

HYPERINSULINISM. *Insulinomas* are pancreatic tumors of islet tissue, generally benign but occasionally malignant, which secrete excessive quantities of insulin and consequently produce hypoglycemic symptoms. The clinical picture, which may include sudden episodes of bizarre or psychotic behavior, unsteady gait or convulsions, as well as milder manifestations of hypoglycemia, is often confusing; and patients suffering from such tumors have been erroneously considered to be epileptics, psychotics, or alcoholics. The hyperglycemic episodes tend to be most marked after fasting and are promptly relieved by the administration of glucose. Patients sometimes become obese because of the large sugar intake needed to prevent hypoglycemia. The diagnosis may be made by reproducing the hypoglycemic blood level and symptoms on depriving the patient of food (24 to 72 hours). Such patients are extremely sensitive to tolbutamide, which produces an exaggerated fall in blood sugar; this is a helpful diagnostic test for insulinoma. Therapy consists of surgical removal of the tumor, which generally relieves the hyperinsulinism.

VIII

THE CENTRAL NERVOUS SYSTEM: DISORDERS OF THE BRAIN

The central nervous system consists of the brain, located in the cranium (skull); the spinal cord, enclosed by the vertebral column; 12 paired cranial nerves; and 31 paired spinal nerves. Although they are integral parts of the same system, the brain and spinal cord are discussed in separate chapters.

ANATOMY OF THE BRAIN

The brain is the most highly developed and uppermost portion of the central nervous system. It is encased and protected by the bony skull. The skull articulates with the first cervical vertebra, known as the atlas, which in turn articulates with the second cervical vertebra, the axis. The lowest portion of the brain emerges through the foramen magnum, an opening at the base of the skull, and continues as the spinal cord down into the spinal canal. There are other bilateral paired openings or foramina in the skull through which the 12 paired cranial nerves emerge to innervate the various structures of the head and neck. The spinal cord terminates at the level between the first and second lumbar vertebral bodies; the remaining lumbar, sacral, and coccygeal nerves continue as the cauda equina. The spinal cord is a continuation of the brainstem consisting of 31 spinal cord segments or neurotomes.

EMBRYOLOGY

The embryo is made up of individual units known as somites or metameres. Each of these includes a unit of nervous tissue (neurotome), a unit of cutaneous tissue (dermatome), and a unit of muscle tissue

By EDWARD J. LORENZE, M.D., Medical Director, The Burke Foundation, White Plains, New York.

(myotome). Each segment of the spinal cord sends out motor fibers arising from the anterior horn cells, which pass out combining as peripheral nerves to innervate corresponding muscle segments of the same somite. The same segment of the spinal cord will receive posterior root fibers carrying sensory impulses arising from the corresponding cutaneous segment or dermatome. Thus, all three of these body structures are closely related with one another.

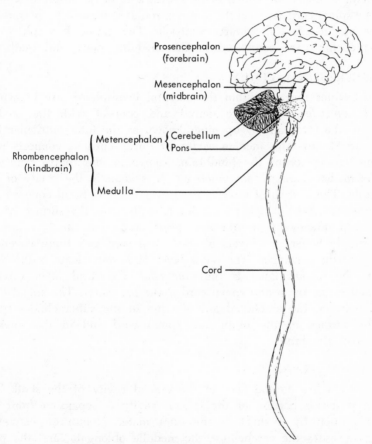

Figure 8. Diagram illustrating gross divisions of the central nervous system. (Courtesy of Diana Clifford Kimber, Carolyn E. Gray, Caroline E. Stackpole, and Lutie C. Leavell, *Anatomy and Physiology*, 14th ed., New York: The Macmillan Company, 1961.)

Embryologically the nervous system develops by an infolding along the midline of the embryo which becomes the neural tube. The uppermost part of this tube develops three swellings which ultimately form the brain, while the lower portion of the neural tube becomes the spinal cord. The three swellings from top downward are known as the *prosencephalon* (forebrain), *mesencephalon* (midbrain), and *rhomben-cephalon* (hindbrain). The forebrain develops two paired optic cups which extend out by stalks. These cups ultimately become the retinas of the eyes; the stalks become the optic nerve. The forebrain forms the masses of the cerebral hemispheres which include the cerebral cortex, internal capsule, thalamus, and basal ganglia. The midbrain forms the stalk that connects the forebrain and hindbrain.

The rhombencephalon, or hindbrain, forms the cerebellum, pons, and the medulla oblongata, which is the lowest area of the brain, extending into the spinal cord. The cerebellum is a rounded mass lying posteriorly to the medulla and the fourth ventricle. The paired hemispheres of the cerebellum are connected to the medulla, pons, and midbrain.

CEREBROSPINAL FLUID

The cavities formed within the cerebral hemispheres are known as *lateral ventricles*. These are paired and connect with the median cavity of the forebrain by openings known as the interventricular foramina of Monro. This median cavity, or third ventricle, connects with the median cavity of the hindbrain, known as the fourth ventricle, by the median cerebral aqueduct, which is actually the cavity of the midbrain. This system of internal cavities within the brain contains the *cerebrospinal fluid,* which passes out laterally over the surface of the brain and downward around the spinal cord. This fluid is located between the inner two layers of the spinal cord and brain coverings known as the *meninges.* The outer layer of fibrous tissue is the *dura mater,* the second layer is the *arachnoid,* the third layer directly attached to the brain and spinal cord is the *pia mater.* The spinal fluid flows between the arachnoid and the pia in the subarachnoid space on the surface of the brain and spinal cord and in the internal cavities of the brain.

SURFACE ANATOMY

The brain lies on the floor of the cranial cavity of the skull. The lowest posterior portion of the cranial cavity is separated from the upper portion by a sheet of the dura mater (tentorium cerebelli) which separates the cerebellum, the medulla oblongata, and the pons from the cerebral hemispheres above. This cavity of the skull, known as the posterior fossa, contains those areas of the brain that have developed from the hindbrain. The midbrain extends through the tentorium cerebelli connecting the hindbrain with the forebrain. The latter occupies the anterior and middle cranial fossae. The cerebral hemispheres make up the main portions of the prosencephalon and cover the rest of the brain.

CEREBRAL HEMISPHERES. The right and left cerebral hemispheres are separated from each other by the longitudinal fissure. When viewing the lateral surface of either hemisphere, we note that it is divided by fissures into four areas or lobes. The lateral cerebral fissure (fissure of Sylvius) runs anteroposteriorly, separating the temporal lobe below from the frontal lobe and parietal lobes above. These latter two lobes are separated by the central sulcus (fissure of Rolando), which runs down across the lateral surface of the hemisphere toward the lateral fissure. The occipital lobe posteriorly is separated from the parietal lobe above and the temporal lobe below by the parieto-occipital fissure. The basal surfaces of the hemisphere consist of the ventral (front) surfaces of the temporal lobes posteriorly and the orbital surfaces of the frontal lobes. The former lie upon the tentorium cerebelli in the middle cranial fossa, while the latter lie on the floor of the anterior cranial fossa.

The cerebral hemispheres cover the other parts of the brain over the entire dorsal (back) or convex surface. The layer of gray matter on the surface of these hemispheres is the *cerebral cortex,* which contains the motor and sensory cell bodies. The thalamus and basal ganglia lie deep in each cerebral hemisphere.

The base of the brain resting on the floor of the cranial cavity as seen from below consists of the medulla oblongata, the pons, the hypothalamus, optic chiasm, optic nerves (vision), and olfactory tracts, (smell); emerging on the lateral and ventral surfaces are the paired cranial nerves. The cerebellum lies posterior to the medulla and pons extending laterally.

INTERNAL STRUCTURE

Basal Ganglia. These are bilateral masses of gray matter located deep in the substance of the cerebral hemisphere. They are paired structures occurring in each hemisphere, consisting of the caudate nucleus, which lies adjacent to the lateral ventricle, and the lenticular nucleus, which is lateral to the caudate nucleus. The internal capsule, containing the motor and sensory pathway from the cerebral cortex, separates them. The lenticular nucleus is divided into a lateral putamen and a medial globus pallidus. The caudate and lenticular nuclei form a mass with the fibers of the internal capsule that separate them, known as the corpus striatum.

Disease in this region gives rise to involuntary movements such as Parkinson's syndrome, athetosis, chorea, rigidity of muscle tone and slowness of voluntary movements.

Internal Capsule. The internal capsule lies between the caudate nucleus and thalamus medially and the lenticular nucleus laterally. A bilateral structure, it contains the thalamic radiation of sensory pathways from the thalamus to the cerebral cortex; the descending pathways from the cerebral cortex to the cranial nerve nuclei in the midbrain, pons, and medulla; and the corticospinal tract, which arises from motor cells in the cerebral cortex and descends through the cerebral peduncles of the midbrain and, as the pyramidal tracts, through the brainstem and spinal cord. Through these motor pathways impulses for movements of the structures innervated by the cranial nerves are carried as well as motor impulses to the anterior horn cells of the spinal cord for movement of the muscles of the trunk and extremities. The pyramidal tracts *decussate,* or cross over, to the opposite half of the central nervous system for the most part at the lower level of the

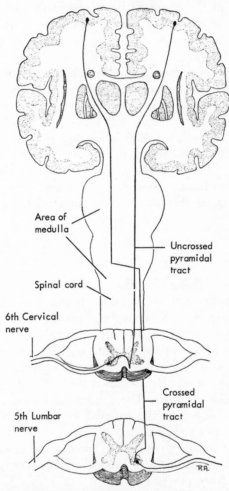

Area of medulla

Uncrossed pyramidal tract

Spinal cord

6th Cervical nerve

Crossed pyramidal tract

5th Lumbar nerve

Figure 9. Descending tracts (two shown): the lateral corticospinal tract (crossed pyramidal) and the ventral corticospinal tract (direct pyramidal). These tracts contain motor fibers to skeletal muscles. (Courtesy of Diana Clifford Kimber, Carolyn E. Gray, Caroline E. Stackpole, and Lutie C. Leavell, *Anatomy and Physiology,* 14th ed., New York: The Macmillan Company, 1961.)

medulla, thus giving rise to the cross-representation of the motor system. A few of the corticospinal fibers continue down without crossing until they terminate. It is for this reason that injury to one cerebral cortex or internal capsule causes paralysis or loss of sensation on the opposite side of the body.

EXTRAPYRAMIDAL SYSTEM. In addition to the main motor pathway or pyramidal tracts, there are several secondary motor tracts known as extrapyramidal tracts, which in large part take origin from cells in the premotor area of the cerebral cortex. They descend and connect with the red nucleus, the tegmental cells in the midbrain, and Deiters' nucleus. They then continue down the spinal cord as the rubrospinal, tegmentospinal, and vestibulospinal tracts. This system helps in producing smooth coordination of motion through the regulation of antagonistic muscle groups. This smooth control of movements is further aided by integrating impulses from the cerebellum, visual impulses from the optic apparatus, impulses arising from the extraocular muscles, and impulses from the labyrinth (inner ear).

THALAMUS. The right and left thalamus lie on either side of the third ventricle at the upper end of the midbrain. They lie under the floor of the lateral ventricle with the medial surface of each thalamus constituting the lateral wall of the third ventricle. The lateral surface of the thalamus is adjacent to the internal capsule, which is formed by the long tracts that connect the cerebral cortex with the levels below. Sensory pathways enter the internal capsule from the thalamus as the thalamic radiation and course to the sensory cortex of the cerebral hemispheres.

The lateral and medial geniculate bodies lie lateral to the structures above and may be considered specialized thalamic nuclei. The lateral geniculate body receives sensory fibers from the optic tract, which pass from there to the cortex of the occipital lobe, the visual area. Visual impulses from the eye follow this pathway to consciousness. The medial geniculate body receives fibers via the lateral lemniscus from the cochlear nuclei of the opposite side, and from the medial geniculate body fibers pass to the auditory area of the cerebral cortex. This is the pathway for hearing. The other thalamic nuclei receive the sensory pathways from the spinal cord which pass up through the brainstem and midbrain.

MIDBRAIN. This, the downward extension of the forebrain, connects with the pons, which in turn connects with the medulla. In the center of the midbrain is the cerebral aqueduct connecting the third and fourth ventricles. The anterior portion of the midbrain is made up of the cerebral peduncles. The cerebral peduncles of the midbrain contain motor pathways from the cerebral cortex that have descended from the internal capsule and then continue through the brainstem. The midportion is formed by the corticospinal tract, and continues as the pyramidal tracts of the medulla oblongata and the spinal cord. The pyramidal system also includes the corticobulbar tracts which carry conscious motor impulses to the cranial nerves. Note that these efferent motor pathways cross at the levels of the cranial nerve nuclei and at the lower level of the medulla to innervate contralateral muscles. This is the crossed cerebral representation.

The medial longitudinal fasciculus is located close to the midline, descending through the midbrain to the spinal cord. The nucleus of the ocular motor (third cranial) nerve is adjacent to this structure in the midbrain, as is the nucleus of the abducens (sixth cranial) nerve and the nucleus of the trochlear (fourth cranial) nerve in the pons. This medial longitudinal fasciculus mediates reflex eye and head movements, and serves as a connecting pathway between the nuclei of eye movements and the vestibular nucleus (balance) in the pons.

The medial lemniscus, made up of sensory fibers that crossed from the opposite side of the medulla, constitutes the sensory pathway for touch and position sense which ascended in the posterior columns of the spinal cord. The medial lemniscus ascends through the pons and midbrain to end in the thalamus. The spinothalamic tracts of crossed pain, temperature, and touch sensations merge with it.

PONS. The motor pathways continue down as corticospinal and corticobulbar fibers. At the level between the pons and the medulla lie the dorsal and ventral cochlear nuclei of the cochlear nerve (hearing) and the nuclei of the vestibular nerve (balance). These two nerves form the acoustic (eighth cranial) nerve. In the medial longitudinal fasciculus is a bundle of fibers extending from the upper spinal cord to the floor of the third ventricle in the midbrain. It receives fibers from the vestibular nuclei which connect with the nuclei of the abducens nerve, trochlear nerve, and ocular motor nerve. Some of the fibers cross the midline to enter the nuclei on the opposite side. Others descend to the nucleus of the spinal accessory (eleventh cranial) nerve. In this way, there is reflex control of the movements of head, neck, and eyes arising from stimuli from the semicircular canal of the ears. Also located in the pons are the nucleus of the facial (seventh cranial) nerve, the nucleus of the abducens (sixth cranial) nerve, and the motor and sensory nuclei of the trigeminal (fifth cranial) nerve.

MEDULLA OBLONGATA. At the lower level of the medulla the pyramidal tracts in most part cross over to the opposite side of the brainstem to continue in the spinal cord as the lateral corticospinal tracts. These tracts finally terminate in the anterior horn cells at the various levels of the spinal cord. A small portion of the motor pathway which continues into the spinal cord as the ventral corticospinal tract decussates just before ending in the gray matter of anterior horn cells.

The posterior columns of the spinal cord terminate in the medulla. These sensory fibers decussate and ascend to the thalamus as the medial lemniscus. In the medulla are located the nucleus of the hypoglossal (twelfth cranial) nerve; the nucleus ambiguous, from which motor fibers innervate the musculature of the pharynx and larynx; and the dorsal motor nucleus of the vagus (tenth cranial) nerve, which innervates the smooth muscle of the stomach and intestines. In the medulla is located a vasomotor center that is necessary for the maintenance of blood pressure and a respiratory center that controls breathing.

CEREBELLUM. The central portion of the cerebellum is the white matter with a thin outside layer of gray matter, the cerebellar cortex. There is a median portion called the vermis and two lateral masses, the right and left cerebellar hemispheres. The dentate nucleus is one of several located in each cerebellar hemisphere. Fibers run from the dentate nucleus across the midline of the midbrain to the red nucleus and to the lateral ventral nucleus of the thalamus.

Each cerebellar hemisphere is connected by the three cerebellar peduncles to the rest of the brain.

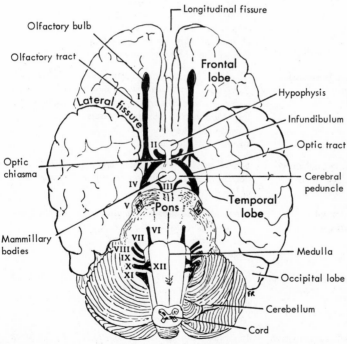

Figure 10. Undersurface of the brain showing cerebrum, cerebellum, the pons, and medulla. The numerals indicate the cranial nerves. (Courtesy of Diana Clifford Kimber, Carolyn E. Gray, Caroline E. Stackpole, and Lutie C. Leavell, *Anatomy and Physiology,* 14th ed., New York: The Macmillan Company, 1961.)

Dysfunction of the cerebellum gives rise to disturbances of equilibrium, unsteadiness on the feet, incoordination of movement. Thus there may be ataxia of gait, impaired finger-nose testing, and difficulty with rapid rhythmic movements of the hands (dysdiadochokinesia).

CRANIAL NERVES AND THEIR NUCLEI

Name	Function	Location of Nucleus
First cranial nerve (olfactory nerve)	Sense of smell	
Second cranial nerve (optic nerve)	Sense of vision	
Third cranial nerve (oculomotor nerve)	Supplies motor innervation to the muscles of the eye, except for the lateral rectus and superior oblique muscles, and to the levator palpebrae muscle, which lifts the eyelid. It also carries fibers to the ciliary ganglion causing constriction of the pupil. The nuclei are innervated by the cortical motor fibers arising in the contralateral cerebral cortex. Paralysis causes lid droop (ptosis), dilatation of pupil, and abduction of the eye due to unopposed action of the abducens nerve.	Close to the cerebral aqueduct in the midbrain
Edinger-Westphal nucleus	Gives rise to parasympathetic fibers that pass with the oculomotor nerve to the ciliary ganglion for the innervation of the intrinsic muscles of the eye—that is, constriction of the pupil.	Rostral to the nucleus of the oculomotor nerve in the midbrain
Fourth cranial nerve (trochlear nerve)	Fibers arising from this nucleus decussate and supply the superior oblique muscle of the eye.	Below the oculomotor nucleus in midbrain
Fifth cranial nerve (trigeminal nerve)	Innervates the muscles of chewing and carries sensation from the face and mucous membranes of the mouth.	In the pons
Sixth cranial nerve (abducens nerve)	Gives rise to fibers that innervate the lateral rectus muscle of the eye causing abduction of the eye (movement outward).	In the pons
Seventh cranial nerve (facial nerve)	Innervates the muscles of the face including closing of the eyes.	In the pons
Eighth cranial nerve (acoustic nerve)	The cochlear nerve carries impulses of sound from the cochlea	Cochlear nucleus and vestibular nucleus at

Name	Function	Location of Nucleus
	of the ear, and the vestibular nerve carries impulses from the semicircular canal giving information concerning movement and posture of the head. Fibers carrying sound decussate and ascend to the midbrain terminating in the inferior colliculus and the medial geniculate body. From the latter they pass to the cerebral cortex. Fibers from the vestibular nuclei, including Deiters' nucleus, pass to the cerebellum. Other fibers run in the medial longitudinal fasciculus and reach the motor nuclei of the ocular muscles. Still others pass down into the spinal cord as the vestibulospinal tract, bringing the motor neurons of the spinal cord under reflex control of the vestibular apparatus.	lateral upper portion of the medulla
Ninth cranial nerve (glossopharyngeal nerve)	Primarily sensory for the upper respiratory tract, middle and inner ear, and taste for the posterior third of tongue.	
Tenth cranial nerve	Innervates the heart, gastro intestinal tract, and the muscles of swallowing and vocal cords. Receives sensory fibers from the same structures.	Medulla
Eleventh cranial nerve (accessory nerve)	Innervates the upper trapezius muscle and the sternocleidomastoid muscle of the neck, which shrug the shoulder and rotate the neck.	Medulla
Twelfth cranial nerve (hypoglossal nucleus)	Produces movements of the tongue.	Medulla

Long Sensory Tracts. Sensory impulses arising in the periphery are of different types and are picked up by different sensory nerve endings in the skin and other tissues. They pass along the mixed peripheral nerve, terminate in individual cell bodies in the posterior sensory ganglia, and then pass through the posterior root into the spinal cord. Depending on the type of sensibility the fibers carry they will ascend in the spinal cord in different long tracts. These ascending sensory pathways are located in specific areas of the spinal cord. Superficial sensibility includes touch, temperature, and pain sensations.

Diminished tactile sensibility is known as tactile *hypesthesia* or, if complete, *anesthesia*. Increased sensitivity is known as tactile *hyperesthesia*. Diminished pain sensation is *hypalgesia*, and its absence *analgesia*.

Touch fibers pass up the ipsilateral posterior column to the lowest portion of the brain, the medulla oblongata, where they then decussate and ascend to the thalamus in the medial lemniscus tract. Other touch fibers cross to the opposite side of the spinal cord at their level of entrance, ascend in the contralateral anterior spinothalamic tract, join the medial lemniscus in the brainstem, and terminate in the thalamus. Pain and temperature fibers end about posterior horn cells; then neurons cross the midline, ascend in the lateral spinothalamic tract, and end in the thalamus.

Deep sensibility (proprioception) refers to impulses arising from muscles, tendons, periosteum, and joints that enter consciousness in terms of position sense. Vibration also is in this group, as is pressure pain. These fibers ascend the ipsilateral posterior column to the medulla; then cross the midline and ascend in the medial lemniscus to the thalamus.

The sensory nerve fibers of the mixed spinal nerve carry conscious and subconscious impulses. The latter, originating in deep structures such as muscles, tendons, and joints, give rise to information that constitutes the afferent intake that makes possible the maintenance of equilibrium, ease of locomotion, and synergistic (smooth) movements. These fibers ascend in the ipsilateral spinocerebellar tracts and enter the cerebellum.

MOTOR APPARATUS. Motor impulses that are under conscious control originate in cells in the motor areas of the cerebral cortex. The motor fibers pass from the cerebral cortex to the anterior horn cells located in the contralateral anterior horn (central gray matter) of the spinal cord at the various segmental levels. This is known as the main motor pathway and the *upper motor neuron*. The anterior horn cell in the spinal cord and the peripheral motor nerve fiber that pass from it to the individual muscle fibers are known as the *lower motor neuron*. The motor nerve fibers thus pass from the cerebral cortex as the corticospinal or pyramidal tracts, decussate at the lower level of the medulla oblongata, and then continue down in the spinal cord as the lateral corticospinal tract, ending in the anterior horn cells. There are also pathways for conscious movement of muscles innervated by cranial nerves. These pathways, called the corticobulbar tracts, terminate in the appropriate cranial nerve nuclei decussating at the appropriate level in the brain.

AUTONOMIC NERVOUS SYSTEM. The sympathetic pathways are part of the autonomic nervous system, which is under reflex rather than voluntary control. They originate from the lateral horn cells of the gray matter of the spinal cord from the first thoracic segment through the second lumbar segment. These fibers pass out through the anterior spinal root and enter the respective sympathetic ganglion. From the ganglion, fibers pass to constrict blood vessels and stimulate sweat glands and the erector muscles of the hair. This portion of the autonomic nervous system is called the *sympathetic nervous system*. Sympathetic fibers innervate certain structures of the head in connection with cranial nerves. These fibers arise from the first and second thoracic segments, enter the respective sympathetic ganglia, then pass through the sympathetic chain, ascending to the stellate ganglion at the first thoracic segment, then the middle cervical sympathetic ganglion, and finally the superior cervical sympathetic ganglion, where they terminate. Post-ganglionic fibers arising here are located on the outer surface of the internal carotid and ophthalmic arteries, and thus enter the skull, where they innervate the dilator muscle of the pupil, the smooth muscle of the upper eyelid, and the smooth muscle in the back of the orbit. When these sympathetic structures are interrupted anywhere in the chain, Horner's syndrome occurs with drooping of the eyelid (ptosis), constriction of the pupil, loss of sweating on the forehead, and enophthalmos, or sinking of the eyeball into the orbit. The other portion of the autonomic nervous system which is not under conscious control is called the *parasympathetic nervous system*. Parasympathetic nerves cause constriction of the pupil, tearing of the eye, salivation, and emptying of the bladder.

PATHOGENESIS

Pathogenesis refers to the method of causation or development of a disease process. Disease or damage to the brain may be due to a variety of causative factors.

The pathological lesions (abnormal changes in the tissue) may be acquired before birth or at any time during life. For example, cerebral palsy is present at birth, dystonia musculorum deformans develops later in childhood, and Huntington's chorea in later adulthood. They may result from anoxia, trauma, infection, insufficient blood supply, degeneration of brain tissue of unknown cause, benign and malignant tumors. They may be due to hereditary defects and disorders genetically transferred from one generation to another. It would appear that many of the so-called hereditary diseases are due to inborn errors of metabolism that are genetically determined. In infectious cases we may be able to diagnose the specific causative agent such as the tuberculosis bacillus or the spirochete of syphilis. In many cases, the exact cause is unknown, although much may be known about the disease, including its clinical manifestations, course, and outcome. The condition may be static as in cerebral palsy or progressive as in multiple sclerosis.

The clinical signs on neurological examination will depend upon the localization of the pathological lesion in the brain. Thus the manifestations will depend upon the part of the brain that is injured and not on a specific etiological factor. The exact nature of the pathological lesion may be determined by such factors as the age at onset, sudden or gradual onset, whether the course is static or progressive, relapsing or spontaneously improving, whether single or multiple areas of the brain are involved, and the particular areas damaged.

These characteristics, in addition to the neurological signs, will determine diagnosis of the condition. The ultimate prognosis and course will be determined by the diagnosis even if the etiological factor is not known. Thus we may diagnose a brain tumor or multiple sclerosis, the specific causes of which are unknown.

LOCALIZING SYMPTOMATOLOGY

CORTICOSPINAL LESIONS. A lesion anywhere in the motor pathways of the cerebral cortex, internal capsule, corticospinal and pyramidal tracts will give rise to spastic paralysis of the muscles affected. This upper motor neuron type of paralysis is characterized by increased stretch reflexes and resistance to passive stretch, hyperactive deep tendon reflexes, clonus, and pathological reflexes such as the Babinski sign. If localized, it may affect only the hand, but if more extensive, it may involve the entire half of the body. If the lesion involves the motor pathway above the point of origin of corticobulbar fibers to the cranial nerves, these may also be involved. If the lesion occurs below the outflow level of a particular cranial nerve, that function will not be affected. Because of the crossed pathways, a lesion on the right side of the brain will cause paralysis of the structures of the left side of the body and vice versa. Thus the typical unilateral supranuclear lesion will give rise to hemiplegia with contralateral paresis of the lower face, the tongue, the arm, and the leg. The other cranial nerve functions are usually not significantly involved in unilateral supranuclear lesions because they receive a bilateral cortical innervation, and the fibers coming from the opposite cerebral cortex can take over the function. This is not true to a significant degree for the arm and the leg. Thus eye movements, swallowing, and upper face are not usually significantly involved. If there are, however, bilateral supranuclear lesions, the patient will have a double hemiplegia or quadriplegia involving all four extremities and difficulty with eye movements, swallowing, movements of the tongue; upper and lower facial weakness will be noted. If there were a complete bilateral interruption of these motor pathways, the patient would die due to involvement of the vagus nerve, with its effect on the heart, and interference with the muscles of respiration.

When the lesion of the motor tracts is not supranuclear but occurs in the midbrain or below, the exact localization will be identified by specific cranial nerve involvement and may give rise to the various syndromes of hemiplegia alterna, which will be described under the vascular disorders.

SENSORY LESIONS. Lesions in the cerebral cortex, internal capsule, and brainstem may in addition involve not only the motor pathways but the sensory pathways, giving rise to a hemisensory defect on the contralateral side of the body with various impairments of pain, touch, position, and temperature sensation. Thus the awareness of a pin prick may be diminished or completely absent.

EXTRAPYRAMIDAL LESIONS. The basal ganglia described above give rise to muscular rigidity without the characteristic findings of the cortical spinal or pyramidal lesions such as hyperreflexia, clonus, and Babinski sign. Difficulty in initiating voluntary movement, tendency for the extremities to assume fixed positions, loss of automatic movements such as the swinging movements of the arms when walking, cog-wheel rigidity, and tremor of head and hands are characteristic. The involuntary movements of chorea, athetosis, dystonic torsions, and hemiballismus involving the spontaneous violent movements of the extremities on one side of the body arise from lesions located in various portions of the basal ganglia or the associated connecting structures of the thalamus, red nucleus, and corpus luysi. Thus, a variety of different clinical types of involuntary movements arise from lesions in these areas. The clinical conditions include Parkinson's syndrome, Huntington's chorea, dystonia musculorum deformans, Sydenham's chorea associated with rheumatic fever, athetoid form of cerebral palsy, Wilson's disease.

CEREBELLAR LESIONS. The cerebellum serves to influence synergistic movements of muscle groups and the strength of their contraction so that balance of the body and equilibrium are maintained. The cerebellum receives afferent impulses from the muscles and joints of the body via the spinocerebellar tracts and impulses from the semicircular canals (vestibular nerve) in regard to the spatial position of the head and body. Impulses from the eye muscles also pass to the cerebellum and affect orientation in space.

The efferent pathways from the cerebellum to the anterior horn cell and thence to the peripheral muscles affect the same side of the body as the cerebellar hemisphere via the vestibulospinal tract. Note that Deiters' nucleus receives impulses from the vestibular nuclei and transmits them to the cerebellum and also serves as the origin of the vestibular spinal tract to the anterior horn cells. From Deiters' nucleus some fibers pass through the medial longitudinal fasciculus to the nuclei of the cranial nerves to the eye muscles. Others cross to the opposite red nucleus and thalamus through the superior cerebellar peduncle and then to the motor areas of the cortex. It is felt that in this way the cerebellum affects the muscles of the extremities, trunk, and the eyes so that equilibrium is maintained.

The signs that occur with cerebellar lesions include impaired coordination of rapid rhythmic movements of dysdiadochokinesis, cerebellar ataxia or incoordination particularly of lower extremity movements, cerebellar hypermetria noted in exaggerated opening of the hand or increase in the size of the handwriting, hypotonia, and pendular or absent knee jerks as a result of hypotonia. The signs are located on the same side of the body as the cerebellar lesion. Nystagmus or rhythmic movements of the eyes may occur in any direction. Nystagmus occurs in other conditions as a result of stimulation of the semicircular canals, Deiters' nucleus, or the medial longitudinal bundle. It is thus felt that nystagmus in the presence of a cerebellar lesion is due to direct or indirect involvement of distant structures.

LESIONS OF THE BRAINSTEM. The brainstem refers to the medulla oblongata, the pons, and the midbrain. All of the nuclei of the cranial nerves except those of the olfactory and optic nerves are located in the brainstem. Lesions in this area, regardless of cause, will give rise to symptoms of spastic paralysis if corticospinal or pyramidal tracts are involved, contralateral sensory disturbance if the spinothalamic tracts and the lemniscus are involved, and specific cranial nerve palsies depending upon the nuclei involved. These lesions will be discussed under vascular lesions. Once again, the specific etiological factors will give rise to the same signs if the lesion is in the same area.

DIAGNOSTIC PROCEDURES

The *spinal tap,* in which a needle is inserted into the subarachnoid space, measures changes in intracranial pressure, indicates interference with the normal flow of the cerebrospinal fluid, and may reveal infectious organisms and increases in protein and white cells, denoting infection, or red blood cells, signifying hemorrhage. Spinal fluid is removed for microscopic examination and for culture of infecting bacteria.

Electroencephalography (EEG), the recording of electrical activity of the various surface areas of the brain, may reveal the location of areas of local damage in the cerebral cortex, such as a tumor. It also is of diagnostic aid in the various types of epilepsy.

Pneumoencephalography is a procedure in which spinal fluid is removed and the ventricular system of the brain is filled with air so that contrast studies of the brain tissue and the ventricular system can be made by x-ray. This may reveal distortions in the normal architecture of the brain. In this way masses, such as tumors that extend into the ventricles, can be identified as well as loss of brain substance.

Cerebral arteriography, in which radiopaque substances are injected into the arteries of the neck, reveals on x-ray displacement of these arteries by tumors or other enlarging lesions of the brain that force them out of their normal position. It also may reveal congenital malformation such as a hemangioma, which is a tumor of dilated blood vessels, or an aneurysm, which is a localized dilatation and weakness of the arterial wall.

The *deep tendon reflexes* include the biceps, triceps (of the arm), and the knee and ankle jerks. The tendons of these muscles are tapped with a rubber hammer which stretches the tendon and results in a stretch reflex of contraction of the muscle. Increased response may indicate upper motor neuron disease, and diminished or absent reflexes indicate lower motor neuron disease.

DISEASES OF UNKNOWN CAUSE

HUNTINGTON'S CHOREA

This is a degeneration of the basal ganglia and cerebral cortex of unknown cause that develops usually in the third decade, after a normal development.

It begins with mental symptoms of poor concentration or memory loss. This is followed by involuntary movements of the extremities, which become progressively stronger and involve more areas of the body. Initially, these may be only small movements of the hands or face, but subsequently they involve rotation of the head. Eventually this disturbs ambulation and gait. Associated with this is progressive mental deterioration. The course of complete disability and loss of mental function may progress over 10 to 15 years.

There is no specific treatment for this progressive condition. Little in the way of rehabilitation from a physical point of view can be achieved, as difficulty in walking is primarily related to the incoordination and violent movements of the extremities. Weakness and deformity are not a major part of the disability until late, and at that point weakness is not amenable to improvement with therapeutic exercise. The associated mental defects also preclude satisfactory rehabilitation. In the earlier phases when disability is not too great, appropriate vocational placement which would take into consideration the incoordination and involuntary movements in upper extremity function and in ambulation should be considered. As in all progressive conditions there may be stages in the early phases when some type of productive activity is still possible, but intensive vocational training is limited, as progressive disability will develop.

PARKINSON'S SYNDROME

This syndrome, originally described by James Parkinson in 1817, is a slowly progressive condition that usually develops in the later period of life and involves the extrapyramidal system; it in general excludes the pyramidal tracts. It is characterized by a rhythmic resting tremor (so-called pill-rolling tremor), rigidity of muscle tone, and slowness and difficulty in initiating voluntary movements. As originally described by Parkinson, its cause was unknown. Pathologically, there are abnormalities in various areas of the brain, including the substantia nigra and basal ganglia. In younger people this has been known to develop following encephalitis (postencephalitic Parkinson syndrome). It may also be caused by arteriosclerosis involving this general region of the brain.

The tremor, noted at rest, affects primarily the hands, although the tongue and other muscles may become involved. First one extremity is involved and then one side; eventually bilateral involvement may occur. This causes slowness in walking; difficulty with writing, fine movements, and feeding; pseudobulbar palsy characterized by slurred speech; and difficulty in chewing and swallowing. There is a tendency for drooling of saliva. The facial muscles do not contract much so that there is little facial expression; the patient has the so-called mask-like facies. Ambulation is characterized by small steps, walking backward or retropulsion, and short running steps forward (festination or propulsive gait).

The diagnosis is based on the history and physical findings. There is no specific cure, but muscle rigidity and tremor are at times helped by a variety of drugs. The operation of chemothalamectomy has been developed in which a lesion placed in one thalamus causes a disappearance of the contralateral tremor and rigidity without causing paralysis. In a high proportion of properly selected cases, the results have been very good, particularly for unilateral involvement. The procedure can, however, be performed bilaterally under suitable conditions.

Physical rehabilitation in the form of physical therapy and therapeutic exercise to decrease rigidity and maintain functional range of motion and functional use of the extremities is very desirable. Many of these patients, if the rigidity is left unaltered, will develop contractures and deformities which will preclude ambulation and self-care. A sustained program of physical therapy to prevent contractures and atrophy of disuse is extremely useful.

If the patient has been allowed to deteriorate, an intensive program of physical rehabilitation may be indicated to regain the lost functional status in ambulation, self-care, and upper extremity function that has come through disuse and that may be more extensive than is actually warranted by the degree of disease present. As in other conditions, the patient may have latent functional capacity that has been allowed to deteriorate and that can be brought back through practice and training. Likewise, the patient's psychological outlook may be improved through an activity program and a concerned staff of therapists who can help the patient to improve and maintain his functional level.

In the Parkinson's syndrome associated with atherosclerosis there may be progressive loss of intellectual function and minimal extension into the pyramidal tracts. In advanced Parkinson's disease there can be progressive deterioration physically and mentally, leading to total incapacity.

Since this syndrome tends to come on in the later part of life, vocational rehabilitation is frequently not a consideration. However, its course is generally slow, so that an onset during the working years would raise questions as to whether surgical therapy or drug treatment was in order.

MYASTHENIA GRAVIS

This disease is included in disorders of the brain since various cranial nerve functions are impaired. However, skeletal muscles of the extremities and trunk are also involved. It is a chronic disorder involving muscles of the eye, of the face, and of swallowing, as well as the muscles of the extremities. It is characterized by easy fatigability of the muscle after a few contractions. Onset is in the third decade and later. There is a failure of neuromuscular conduction from the nerve ending to the muscle, perhaps due to a defect in the acetylcholine and cholinesterase mechanisms. Because of this chemical failure there is interference with transmission of the nerve impulse to the muscle, resulting in weakness of the muscles. The condition can be improved to a major degree by the drug neostigmine, an anticholinesterase compound. While it does not cure the condition, it markedly improves the functional ability. The drug must be taken on a regular daily basis, just as insulin is used in diabetes.

Ptosis (drooping) of the eyelids and diplopia (double vision) due to involvement of the eye muscle are frequent symptoms. Bilateral facial weakness results in a blank facial expression. Nasality of speech may develop due to involvement of the soft palate. The arms and legs may become weak and easily fatigued, so that walking and function of the upper extremities are impaired. The course may be slow or rapid, but there are frequently fluctuations in the severity of the symptoms from day to day. The condition may also become static for long periods of time. Except in severe fulminating cases, one can estimate perhaps 10 to 20 or more years of activity if the patient is under adequate treatment. A therapeutic trial by an injection of neostigmine gives marked improvement in the muscle strength within ten minutes and is a diagnostic test.

The onset usually comes in women in the third decade and in men from that age onward. Therefore, these are patients who may have problems in the vocational area. Proper guidance in regard to following the drug regimen and in training or placement in a vocation that will not put severe physical demands on the patient are in order. There are no intellectual defects in this disease, and any emotional disorder would be a reaction to the illness, so that proper placement on a job or as a homemaker is quite feasible. This disease actually has a more effective method of treatment than most of the neurological conditions. For the woman who is functioning as a homemaker, the training in a rehabilitation kitchen in terms of time-energy studies and work simplification are very much in order. These patients tend to fatigue easily with therapeutic exercise, but since they do not have abnormalities of muscle tone or true paralysis, they rarely develop deformities.

HEREDITARY ATAXIAS

MARIE'S HEREDITARY CEREBELLAR ATAXIA. This condition involves a degeneration in the cerebellum, the pyramidal tracts, and the optic nerve. It is characterized by progressive deterioration in balance, cerebellar function, and vision. The onset is in the fourth to sixth decade.

FRIEDREICH'S ATAXIA. This is the most common form of hereditary ataxia—a degeneration of the cerebellum and posterior spinal cord. Several children in the same family may be affected. The ataxia develops between the ages of 7 and 15 years. As in all ataxias, the gait is staggering and broad-based, simulating the gait of an intoxicated person. The other manifestations of cerebellar disease as described above subsequently develop. The feet show a high arch (pes cavus) and later may show a marked footdrop and inversion (pes equinovarus). Nystagmus, choreiform movements, optic atrophy with impairment of vision, and double vision may develop. The course is slowly progressive over 20 to 30 years.

The ataxias resembling both Friedreich's and Marie's type that may also occur in middle life are also slowly progressive. There is no specific treatment for any of these conditions.

From a treatment point of view, physical rehabilitation offers prevention of deformity or correction of deformity if it has developed. In addition, it attempts to maintain muscle power and coordination through exercise and training. Since the disease is progressive, results will vary, depending on whether the gains of the training program are being exceeded by the degenerative process. Vocational objectives in the younger person would have to be selected carefully in the light of slow progression over several decades, particularly impairment of balance, ambulation, and fine finger-hand coordination.

AMYOTROPHIC LATERAL SCLEROSIS

This is a fairly rapidly progressive disease of unknown cause with death occurring within five years in the majority of instances. However, as in many of these conditions, there are cases where patients live for many years. The degeneration occurs in the anterior horn cells, the pyramidal tracts, and the cranial nerve nuclei of the brainstem.

The condition occurs in the fourth or fifth decade. It is considered by many to be a composite of three conditions: (1) progressive muscular atrophy (a degenerative disease of the anterior horn cells) causing a progressive flaccid paralysis of the extremities with a rather prolonged course over several decades; (2) primary lateral sclerosis, an isolated degeneration of the pyramidal tracts giving rise to spastic paralysis of the lower extremities with a slowly progressive course; and (3) progressive bulbar palsy, a degeneration of the motor nuclei of the brainstem resulting in difficulty in swallowing, hoarseness, articulation, facial weakness. These three conditions when present in one individual constitute amyotrophic lateral sclerosis with its more rapid course. It may start in one form and progress to include the others.

No specific therapy is available for any of these conditions. The rehabilitation procedures will depend upon the physical disability found. Basically, spastic or flaccid paresis of the lower extremities would be managed like any other paraplegia—by a trial of therapeutic exercise to correct or prevent deformities and improve strength within the patient's capacity, use of braces for the lower extremities if indicated, and crutch walking if the upper extremities retain sufficient strength to use them. If the patient is unable to walk because of a combination of lower and upper extremity weakness, training for independence in the wheel chair may be feasible.

These conditions are slowly progressive, but since their course extends over a long period of time, the possibility of help and improved function cannot be dismissed. Objectives should be within the individual's ability, taking into account the probability of progressive loss of ambulatory function as well as possible impairment of strength and coordination in the upper extremities. Bulbar palsy when present, is a dangerous disease, with impairment of swallowing a serious problem. Speech therapy is usually not of help in these progressive dysarthrias.

MULTIPLE SCLEROSIS

This is a demyelinating disease involving a loss of the myelin sheath about the tracts of the white matter of the central nervous system. It is characterized by remissions and exacerbations but by a gradually progressive course. Episodes may be acute and terminate fatally, or the disease may be arrested for many years. After each recurrence, although the patient may improve, he usually does not achieve the level of function that he had previously. The disease may progress over several decades. There may be remissions with marked recovery of function throughout its course. There usually are manifestations of involvement of multiple areas of the central nervous system rather than one location or system. The onset is usually in early or middle adult life. There are associated generalized weakness and fatigability.

Common findings include spastic paraplegia, transient optic atrophy with impairment of vision, numbness, and paresthesias, and urinary incontinence or urgency. Cerebellar signs with incoordination, scanning or slurring of speech, ataxia and intention tremor of the upper and lower extremities, and nystagmus are frequent. Diplopia (double vision) due to involvement of the nerves to the muscles of the eyes may develop. Emotional symptoms and later intellectual deficits may occur. In the acute progressive stages, the patient has generalized weakness, often severe mental impairment, and progressive deterioration with decubiti (bed sores) and urinary incontinence.

There is no specific treatment of this condition. Management is based on the handling of the individual's disorders as they develop. Urinary infections are treated by catheter drainage and appropriate antibiotics. General hygienic measures for the maintenance of good skin condition and prevention of decubiti are important. If neurogenic (reflex) bladder develops, as in any type of paraplegia, periodic urological check-up with cystoscopy, intravenous pyelograms, and retrograde pyelograms may be necessary, particularly for the detection of renal or bladder stones.

Rehabilitation treatment likewise is aimed at the disability. If the primary manifestation is a spastic paraplegia and there is not significant ataxia or involvement of the upper extremities, the patient will be managed as in any other type of paraplegia. This involves training in personal activities of daily living using braces, crutches, or wheel chair. Incoordination and intention tremor cannot be corrected but practice, repetition, adaptive devices, and techniques of retraining will improve functional capacity.

Since this may be a slowly progressive disease there are for individual cases possibilities of training in a vocation if the disease occurs in early adult life. Particularly if the manifestations involve only one system, such as a spastic paraplegia, the opportunities for physical rehabilitation and for continuing in a vocation are good. The primary obstacle is the fact that the disease may, and eventually does, involve many systems so that there are, in addition to the spastic paraplegia, the complications of ataxia and incoordination in the use of the upper extremities. To this may be added a visual disturbance due to optic atrophy or to double vision. Thus, the rehabilitation possibilities must be weighed against the multisystem involvement of the central nervous system, which makes this one of the most difficult disabilities to deal with. There are not only weakness and spastic paralysis but also incoordination and special sense involvement. Nevertheless, some patients can perform successfully for many years. They should not be arbitrarily dismissed from rehabilitation consideration because the disease is progressive.

INFECTIOUS DISEASES OF THE BRAIN

MENINGITIS

Inflammation or infection of the meninges, or covering of the brain and spinal cord, by specific bacteria, viruses, parasites, or fungi is called meningitis. Common agents are the tuberculosis bacillus, meningococcus, streptococcus, and staphylococcus. Formerly, it frequently occurred as an extension of middle ear or mastoid process infection.

Signs and symptoms include alteration in state of consciousness such as stupor or coma, convulsions, elevated temperature, and signs of meningeal irritation—spasm with pain in the neck, back muscles, and hamstring muscles.

Diagnosis is made by the history, the clinical findings, spinal tap with examination of the spinal fluid that shows increase in the cell count and protein, Gram-stained smears, and culture of spinal fluid for identification of the bacteria.

Identification of the bacteria permits the use of an antimicrobial agent specific for the particular bacteria. Depending upon the bacteria and the specificity of the drug used, the patient may completely recover or may be left with focal neurological signs if there has been extension of the infection into the brain tissue causing encephalitis or brain abscess. The residua would depend upon the area affected. If specific treatment is not carried out, the patient may die from the infection.

BRAIN ABSCESS

Bacterial infection of the brain may give rise to focal signs as a result of localized accumulation of purulent material. As this expands, it encroaches on important brain structure giving rise to neurological focal signs such as hemiplegia, fever, and signs of meningeal irritation.

Identification of bacteria and the use of the appropriate antimicrobial agent or surgical drainage of the abscess are the treatment. If suitable treatment is instituted there may be full recovery, residual hemiplegia, or other neurological signs, depending on the areas involved.

ASEPTIC NONBACTERIAL MENINGITIS

This may occur secondary to viral infection such as in infectious mononucleosis, infectious atypical pneumonia, mumps, and measles. These usually carry a good prognosis for recovery without disability unless there is extension into the brain tissue itself. These cases do not show bacteria on examination or culture of the spinal fluid, and usually the cell counts do not show as much of an increase of the white cells as in bacterial meningitis.

ENCEPHALITIS

This is an infection of the brain itself that may be localized or diffuse throughout the brain. It may extend or be associated with meningitis and also with myelitis (infection of the spinal cord). Some forms are due to specific viral infection. During the acute stages these forms are difficult to differentiate, but this may be done by study of the spinal fluid using various complement-fixation tests.

Signs and symptoms include fever, convulsions, alteration in state of consciousness, lethargy, and sometimes focal paralysis. Specific types include poliomyelitis; St. Louis encephalitis; postinfection encephalitis following such viral diseases as measles, German measles, chickenpox, mumps, or influenza. It may occur also during the course of, or after, vaccination against smallpox and rabies. This would not appear to be a direct invasion of the brain by the virus, but possibly it is a toxic allergic reaction. The postinfection encephalitis is more likely to give rise to various forms of paralysis, ataxia, and incoordination. Treatment requires the appropriate drug if due to a specific organism sensitive to a chemotherapeutic agent. Viruses are not usually affected by chemotherapy.

The patients, if they recover, may have neurological, intellectual, or emotional deficits as a result of organic brain damage. The complications of meningoencephalitis may include transient paralyses; permanent monoplegias, hemiplegias, quadriplegias, paraplegias; intellectual and emotional changes; convulsive disorders; cranial nerve involvements; blindness; aphasia; deafness; and hydrocephalus.

Rehabilitation is dependent entirely upon residual neurological defects, the management of which will be covered in other sections. Intellectual and emotional disturbances secondary to encephalitis with organic brain syndrome may occur.

ACUTE IDIOPATHIC POLIOMYELITIS

This has also been called Landry's ascending paralysis and Guillain-Barré syndrome. It is included here under diseases of the brain although it also involves the spinal cord. It is an infectious disorder, probably of viral origin.

The signs and symptoms consist of a symmetrical ascending motor paralysis starting with the legs and later involving the arms. This is a flaccid type of paralysis with loss of the deep tendon reflexes and usually paresthesias or minimal sensory losses. The sensory changes tend to differentiate it from poliomyelitis. This condition is due to involvement of the spinal roots, thus giving rise to the term *radiculitis*. The condition may ascend into the brain resulting in dysarthria, dysphonia, dysphasia due to paresis of the muscles of the tongue, pharynx, or larynx. Less frequently there may be paresis of the eye muscles and of the face. Respiratory failure may develop because of paralysis of the respiratory muscles.

There is no specific treatment, although corticosteroid therapy has been considered helpful, and respirators are essential if respiratory muscles fail. Most patients spontaneously recover if they do not die of respiratory failure during the acute phase. During the period of recuperation, a program of therapeutic exercises in physical and occupational therapy will aid in the recovery of strength, and progressive ambulation training using such aids as parallel bars, crutches, and walkers will improve walking.

In those cases in which residual paralysis occurs, management would depend upon the particular disability as covered under hemiplegia, monoplegia, paraplegia, and quadriplegia. In brief, this would consist of the use of supportive bracing, crutches, or canes, as indicated. No intellectual deficits would be expected; emotional problems would be those reactive to the residual disability. This condition carries a more favorable prognosis for recovery over weeks and months than does poliomyelitis.

ACUTE CHOREA

This is also known as St. Vitus' dance and Sydenham's chorea. It occurs most commonly between 5 and 15 years of age and is not usually seen in infants where the more common congenital form or those secondary to degenerative types of encephalitis are observed. More common in females, it also may develop or recur during pregnancy. In pregnant women there is usually a history of rheumatic fever and rheumatic heart disease.

It may develop as a complication of acute infections with toxic effects on the central nervous system. These would include scarlet fever, pneumonia, measles, and most commonly rheumatic fever. It is frequently considered a form of rheumatic fever in childhood due to toxins of hemolytic streptococcus. Examination of the brain in these cases reveals vascular disease such as thrombosis and hemorrhage as well as cellular degeneration in the cortex, basal ganglia, and cerebellum. It is thought that the symptoms are due to involvement of the basal ganglia and their connections.

The signs and symptoms include spontaneous involuntary movements that are rapid and purposeless, involving the face, tongue, head, fingers, and then the limbs and trunk. There may be irritability and restlessness. In severe cases the involuntary movements may interfere with ambulation and functional self-care.

There is no specific treatment, and the symptoms may run from several weeks to many months but gradually disappear. It is rarely fatal and usually leaves no significant neurological residual, although personality changes may continue.

There are no specific physical disabilities. However, since many cases are associated with rheumatic fever, there may be disabilities due to rheumatic heart disease.

Cerebral Palsy

The broad term "cerebral palsy" refers to some form of congenital brain damage resulting in a motor disability. It occurs during intrauterine life, during delivery, or in the immediate postnatal period. The various causes include anoxia, hemorrhage, trauma, prematurity, infection, toxemia of pregnancy, Rh factor incompatibility, and developmental anomalies.

The course is usually static and nonprogressive, although some brain-injured children later have progressive deterioration and seizures. Certain clinical types occur with predominant neurological findings of spasticity, athetosis, ataxia, and rigidity. These disturbances may involve one limb (monoplegia), one side (hemiplegia), both lower extremities (paraplegia), three extremities (triplegia), or all four extremities (quadriplegia). The degree may vary from mild, with no functional incapacity or obvious disability, to severe with little or no functional ability. The spastic patient may show increased muscle tone and weakness of the involved muscles. The athetoid patient manifests involuntary movements of the extremities which may be hardly noticeable or severe constant thrashing movements of the head, trunk, and extremities that prevent head control and sitting balance. This is due to primary damage in the basal ganglia. The ataxic patient has primary damage in the cerebellar system of the brain manifested by ataxia with poor balance. This too may delay or prevent walking and fine coordination in the upper extremities. In addition to the motor problem, there may be any of the other concomitants of brain damage: personality or intellectual defects, delayed language development, hearing losses, sensory defects, and epileptic seizures.

Little in the way of specific curative treatment can be carried out, since the damage is already done. The condition may be observed at birth, or it may not be noticed until months or even years later when the child does not develop in a normal fashion. Rehabilitation treatment or management in the early years centers about therapeutic exercises to prevent deformity and develop muscle strength and coordination. Training in the progressive developmental activities of head control, sitting control, standing control, and walking is carried out.

When necessary, footdrop braces, long leg braces and double long leg braces with pelvic bands may be used to prevent deformity due to muscle tightness. Braces are used to support the body weight in the standing position if the muscles are too weak. Such bracing is also used to prevent excessive strain in the joints, such as hyperextension of the knee (genu recurvatum), which may occur when the leg muscles are weak and stretch the capsule and ligaments of the knee joint. Standing and walking training is usually performed beginning with parallel bars; then the patient progresses to crutches and eventually to a cane. Initially, if a paraplegia is present, double-bar long leg braces and pelvic bands may be necessary. Under these circumstances, the child will usually have to walk with crutches with either a four-point or "drag-to" type of gait. As the child grows and develops, the braces may be cut down, starting from the top, and may eventually be done away with.

Occupational therapy is used in evaluating the activities of daily living and training the child to do upper extremity activities such as feeding, dressing, bathing, and writing. The child may have delayed development of skills due to the neurological involvement, lack of opportunity, or mild intellectual deficit, all of which may respond to intensive training. At other times, the disability may prevent the child from developing normal performance so that special techniques for dressing may be necessary. Adaptive clothing is sometimes of value. Many methods of exercise have been developed such as the Bobath techniques, but none have been shown to have specific value over the others. The basic fundamentals of therapeutic exercise remain the same.

Throughout the growth period there is constant danger of deformity, since the bones tend to lengthen faster than the muscles, and the deforming forces become greater. Various types of orthopedic surgery are frequently of value if braces fail to prevent deformity or if the braces can be suitably removed as the result of a surgical procedure. These include bone fusions, usually in the foot to provide lateral stability, heel cord lengthening, lengthening of the hamstring muscles to prevent knee flexion contractures, adductor muscle tenotomies, and obturator neurectomies in which the muscle itself is cut as well as the nerve to reduce the tendency of adduction of the thighs—a common deformity.

The most common speech problem in these children is delayed language development and defective articulation (dysarthria). Speech evaluation is important to determine if the language delay is due to intellectual deficit, severe involvement of the articulators, deafness, auditory perceptual deficits, or aphasic language disturbances. Based on these findings, speech therapy is useful in stimulating language development and improving vocabulary and articulation. Where deafness is a problem, the use of a hearing aid and special techniques for the hard of hearing are of value.

As the child develops, psychological evaluation is important to assess the actual intellectual capacity of the child so that function that is beyond the child's intellectual level is not attempted. This is of importance in the guidance of the parents and also for the planning of future education. Psychological counseling with the parents and the child may prevent or correct situations leading to emotional disturbance.

Little can be done to control the involuntary movements of the athetoid, but with training, functional development can occur. Ataxic cerebral palsy involves primary balance disturbance that can be improved with training and often aided with crutches.

One must determine whether the adult cerebral palsied individual has received maximum results from physical rehabilitation. Through procedures of physical medicine, orthopedic surgery, drug control of seizures, and/or psychotherapy for the improvement of emotional reactions, a previously neglected patient may be brought to a higher level of function. Correction of deformities, bracing, training in the activities of daily living including wheel chair independence, and training in ambulation all help to improve the individual's functional capacity.

Assuming that the individual has achieved the maximum functional level, it is helpful to determine vocational potentials through prevocational exploration, vocational workshop activities that actually test functional capacity, and intellectual and aptitude testing. For many, depending upon the particular disability and residual capacity, employment in industry is possible; for others further education is desirable; for still others with severe disability sheltered workshop or homebound programs may be the only answer. There are also those who, because of the severity of their disabilities, will be essentially homebound or only able to participate in activity programs aimed at maintaining them in a good psychological and physical state without any consideration of productive employment. Such a determination, however, must come after careful evaluation of the patient and his residual problems. Many mildly disabled individuals are handicapped by immature attitudes and dependency reactions which interfere with work performance well within their physical and intellectual capacity. Others are handicapped by perceptual disturbances and poor eye-hand coordination.

HYDROCEPHALUS

Hydrocephalus occurs as a result of accumulation of fluid in the ventricles of the brain which causes increased pressure. Enlargement of the head in children, often with atrophy of brain tissue, occurs. The latter frequently results in impairment of intellectual function and may give rise to cerebral palsy in the form of varying degrees of spastic paralysis of the extremities.

The condition may be spontaneously arrested so that the patient shows only a large head without evidence of brain damage. In this case prognosis for life function is good. Such a condition is not progressive. Internal hydrocephalus is caused by obstruction of the aqueduct of Sylvius, and cerebrospinal fluid produced by the choroid plexuses of the lateral and third ventricles accumulates. This may be due to a congenital constriction or later in life to a tumor. Since the fluid cannot pass to the subarachnoid space where it is normally absorbed, there are constant pressure and atrophy of brain tissue. This in turn will lead to progressive deterioration and eventual death.

If congenital hydrocephalus is spontaneously arrested, the individual may function at a generally satisfactory level. If it is progressive, there are several operative procedures that may be performed in children. When the block or obstruction is in the aqueduct of Sylvius, a Torkildsen procedure may be performed. A catheter is placed connecting the lateral ventricle with the cisterna magna so that the fluid may be removed from the lateral ventricle and pass beneath the scalp to empty into an area from which it may be absorbed. As long as this bypass functions, the patient will develop satisfactorily. This technique is also used when hydrocephalus is due to an unremovable tumor blocking the aqueduct of Sylvius.

BRAIN TUMORS

Tumors are an abnormal overgrowth of cells in the different tissues of the body. The cells continue to multiply excessively. They are independent of the normal rate of growth for such tissues and have no normal physiological function. Primary tumors develop from brain cells. Secondary tumors are metastatic and spread from a tumor in another area of the body. They may be benign and circumscribed, correctable by surgical excision, or they may be malignant with extreme invasiveness and a tendency to spread, thus not easily or completely removed.

Primary brain tumors do not usually spread outside of the skull or spinal canal. The brain tumors are named according to the type of cell from which they arise. They include gliomas, menigiomas (arising from the coverings of the brain), pituitary adenomas (arising from the pituitary gland), and acoustic neurinomas (arising from the acoustic nerve). One-fifth of all brain tumors are metastatic. The original tumor in these cases is most commonly in the lung but may also come from the gastrointestinal tract and other systems.

Tumors may occur in various areas of the brain; depending upon the area involved, related functions will be impaired. Acoustic neurinomas arising from the acoustic nerve will cause tinnitus (ringing in the ears), deafness, and ataxia of the arm and leg on the involved side. Cerebellar tumors will give rise to cerebellar signs including hypotonia, ataxia, and nystagmus.

Tumors of the pons, while benign, may cause death because they cannot be surgically removed, owing to their location. They cause palsies of the eye muscles, trigeminal nerve, facial nerve, and the muscles of swallowing and phonation. Cerebellar signs may also develop because of interference with the connecting pathways. Hemiplegia is common due to involvement of the pyramidal tracts.

Tumors of the cerebral hemispheres give rise to progressive hemiplegia, starting with focal weakness and increasing to involve the entire side of the body. If located in the frontal lobes, personality changes characterized by apathy or facetiousness are frequent. Various forms of aphasia will develop from tumors in the dominant temporal lobe.

The course is usually one of gradual onset and progression as the lesion expands. The patient with a brain tumor shows progressive signs and symptoms as the tumor enlarges and encroaches on vital areas of the brain or increases intracranial pressure. These include progressive paralysis, impairment of consciousness progressing to coma, double vision, and impaired vision. Impaired vision is due to pressure on the optic nerve by the tumor. Double vision is due to increased intracranial pressure. When intracranial pressure increases, the patient will manifest headache, vomiting, papilledema, elevation of blood pressure, and slowing of respiratory and heart rates.

X-rays of the skull, electroencephalography, and angiography may help to locate the tumor. Pneumoencephalography, by revealing displacement of the ventricles, also helps in localization. Radioactive isotopes concentrate in tumors, and detectors may be used to find the area of concentration.

The treatment of tumors is surgical removal. In many instances this can be complete, with partial or complete recovery. In other cases, because of the invasiveness of the tumor or its location, it may be only partially removable, so that there will be progression of the disease. Meningiomas, acoustic neurinomas and cerebellar astrocytomas are frequently completely removable. Some tumors if partially removed may be further limited in their development by x-ray therapy. When internal hydrocephalus occurs the use of the Torkildsen procedure may reduce the pressure and relieve the symptoms.

In those cases where the tumor is nonmalignant and can be removed, the patient may have a complete recovery without residua. If, on the other hand, the tumor cannot be completely removed and is malignant or continues to expand, ultimately the patient may become completely disabled and die.

In those cases where the tumor is removed or arrested but the patient has residual neuromuscular deficits, the usual physical rehabilitation approach to the problem is used. Thus, in paralysis, the type of management that is given to the hemiplegic, paraplegic, or the quadriplegic patient would be in order.

Bilateral interruption of the motor tracts in the brain gives rise to double hemiplegia or quadriplegia. Bilateral cerebral cortical lesions involving the leg areas will give rise to paraplegia. The physical rehabilitation management of these disabilities is essentially the same as paraplegia or quadriplegia due to spinal cord disease and is discussed elsewhere.

Following removal of the brain tumor, there usually will be a period of spontaneous recovery of neurological function. This can be increased and extended by proper physical rehabilitation procedures. If there is an aphasic disturbance or a dysarthria in which there is partial paresis of the articulators, speech therapy may be indicated. Training in the techniques of the activities of daily living appropriate to each type of disability would be in order. The prognosis for functional recovery would depend upon the actual damage to the central nervous system in terms of paralysis or balance disturbance (ataxia) and to the intellectual function of the patient. If not enough motor function can be recovered or balance regained, the specific upper extremity activities of daily living and the lower extremity activities of ambulation may be precluded. Bracing and adaptive devices suitable to the particular disability and condition are used. In addition to the intellectual disturbances and speech disturbances, patients frequently may have disturbances in the form of loss of vision due to optic atrophy and various types of visual field defects. Many patients, however, following successful brain tumor removal may have completely normal function and be able to return to work.

APHASIA AND RELATED DISORDERS

Aphasia is not a disease but an impairment of language or symbolization resulting from neurological damage to the areas of the brain associated with language function. It is important to recognize that it is not due to impairment of the sensory organs nor to paralysis of the articulators or muscles of speech but rather to dysfunction of the higher levels of the brain. In effect, the aphasic is a person who has lost fully or partially the ability to deal with the symbols of the language he once knew.

Aphasia may result from cerebral vascular accidents, brain tumors, or traumatic injuries to the dominant hemisphere—the hemisphere in which the language centers have developed. The dominant hemisphere is usually the left one; thus, aphasia and its associated disorders usually occur with a right hemiplegia caused by a lesion in the left cerebral cortex or subcortical pathways. Partial loss is indicated by the prefix "dys," total loss by the prefix "a." For example, dysphasia refers to the partial loss of the ability to understand or express language, whereas aphasia indicates total loss.

Aphasia is the inability to transmit or receive ideas through any form of language communication, such as speaking, writing, reading, or listening. *Receptive* or *sensory aphasia* is the inability to understand language. It includes such categories as auditory aphasia, the inability to comprehend speech, and visual aphasia, the inability to read (*alexia*). *Expressive* or *motor aphasia* refers to the inability to express oneself. Forms of expressive aphasia include *anomia,* the inability to initiate meaningful words (that is, to name objects); *amnestic (amnesic) aphasia,* difficulty in word finding; and *agraphia,* the inability to write. *Mixed aphasia* refers to a combination of expressive and receptive aphasia, in which one form may predominate. *Global aphasia* denotes severe impairment in both forms.

Related disorders include agnosia and apraxia. *Agnosia* is the total or partial loss of recognition through perception. For example, tactile agnosia is loss of recognition through the sense of touch; visual agnosia is the inability to recognize objects through sight; and auditory agnosia is the inability to recognize sounds—for example, the jingling of keys. Visual agnosia dealing with reading, and auditory agnosia for words are forms of receptive aphasia. *Apraxia* is the inability to perform purposeful movements although, again, no paralysis is involved. Verbal apraxia refers to the organs of speech; for example, the patient will be unable to move his tongue at will or on command, although reflex swallowing and chewing may be unimpaired. An examiner would test for this by asking the patient to repeat words and phrases. Other forms of voluntary movement may be affected in apraxia, including movements of the upper and lower extremities. Tests for these forms of apraxia would require the patient to follow simple instructions, such as handing the examiner a pencil or putting the uninvolved foot in a certain spot. Apraxia in its pure form would presume that the patient's inability to follow instructions is not based upon a receptive aphasia. In actual practice, combinations of aphasia, agnosia, and apraxia are most common; it is sometimes difficult to delineate all forms of these disorders. This is particularly true in view of the fact that generalized impairment of intellectual functioning is frequently a concomitant of brain injury.

Speech therapy may be of considerable value to aphasic patients. The degree of improvement that may be expected is difficult to predict in advance. In general, the less severe the aphasic disturbance and the greater the patient's overall comprehension and motivation, the better the results will be. Treatment is based upon a good interpersonal relationship between patient and therapist, one which will permit the patient to better tolerate the frustrations of language and retraining. In this framework, treatment is primarily one of language reeducation directed toward helping the patient regain the skills he has lost. Automatic speech—that is, speech involving serial repetition (for example, days of the week)—is the last form of speech to be impaired. Verbal expressions of strong emotions—for example, profanity—also are usually well retained so that aphasic patients are frequently able to swear fluently. However, propositional speech—that is, speech expressing the complicated interactions of thought and language to convey ideas—is easily impaired and presents the greatest problem in speech retraining.

Impairment of the ability to communicate constitutes for most patients a severely depressing and frustrating experience. This is particularly true for the individual who was highly verbal before he became aphasic. In turn, the depression and frustration of the patient are communicated to the family. For this reason, counseling with members of the family, as well as orienting and educating them to the nature of the disability and the needs of the patient, will help in achieving the overall rehabilitation goals. The value of continuing speech therapy is determined largely by the progress of the patient over a period of time. While it is difficult to determine to what extent progress is a result of speech therapy and to what extent it reflects spontaneous recovery, there appears to be little question that the patient makes greater progress when he receives language reeducation beginning soon after the acute phase of the illness subsides.

Vascular Disease of the Brain

CEREBRAL VASCULAR ACCIDENTS

Cerebral vascular accidents are caused by a failure of arterial circulation to areas of the brain causing damage or death of brain cells. This results most commonly in hemiplegia. Cerebral vascular accidents, or "strokes," are due to hemorrhage if the blood vessel bursts, thrombosis when a blood clot forms locally in a cerebral artery, or embolism when a blood clot forms in the heart and travels to a cerebral artery causing a blockage or occlusion. In any situations the pathological process is the same; there is a cerebral infarct or failure of circulation to an area of the brain with resultant localized damage.

In hemorrhage, there is bleeding into the substance of the brain; this may form an expanding lesion of increasing size and increasing symptoms as it encroaches upon the brain tissue, in much the same way as a tumor would do. If such an expanding blood clot can be localized by electroencephalography and cerebral angiography, it may be removed surgically with remission of the patient's symptoms. If the hemorrhage extends into the ventricular system of the brain, as it frequently does, a bloody spinal fluid which is diagnostic will be obtained on spinal tap.

Some hemorrhages arise from congenital aneurysms (defects in the arterial wall) leading to rupture. This may occur in younger persons and if identified by cerebral angiography may be surgically repaired. Thrombosis and hemorrhage usually occur in arteriosclerotic cerebral vessels with or without hypertension.

Cerebral embolism occurs in cases of rheumatic heart disease and in cases of arteriosclerotic cardiovascular disease following myocardial infarction of atrial (auricular) fibrillation. The incidence of cerebral emboli from the heart in rheumatic heart disease with mitral stenosis may be diminished by surgical correction of the mitral stenosis and removal of clots in the auricular appendage. Cerebral arterial occlusion may also occur in systemic disease such as the collagen diseases (polyarteritis), leukemia, and polycythemia vera.

SUBDURAL HEMATOMA

This is the formation of a blood clot in the subdural space between the outer and middle layer of meninges. It is due to hemorrhage, occurring frequently as a result of head trauma. There is usually a clear period without symptoms following the initial injury, and then subsequently, days or weeks after the injury, the patient develops headache, alteration in state of consciousness, convulsive seizures, and hemiplegia. This syndrome is similar to that seen with other types of expanding lesions of the brain.

The presence of the lesion is determined by the clinical course and the findings of xanthochromic or yellowish spinal fluid as a result of extravasation of the blood into the spinal fluid. Electroencephalography, pneumoencephalography, and carotid angiograms may help localize the clot, as in the case of other expanding lesions. Treatment is the surgical removal of the blood clot through openings in the skull.

SUBARACHNOID HEMORRHAGE

This occurs as a result of hemorrhage into the subarachnoid space where the spinal fluid is located. It usually is caused by a rupture of an aneurysm of the circle of Willis. Symptoms include neck stiffness, alteration in the state of consciousness, and focal neurological paralysis. If the aneurysm can be identified by cerebral angiography, surgical correction may prevent recurrences.

CLINICAL SYNDROMES

Most cerebral vascular accidents involve the corticobulbar and corticospinal tracts, thus giving rise to hemiplegia. If they occur above the level of the brainstem there will be a contralateral paralysis of the arm and leg, contralateral lower facial paresis, and possibly contralateral hemisensory loss. If the lesion occurs on the left or dominant side of the brain, the patient may develop aphasia (described above), so that there may be various combinations of loss of speech, loss of comprehension, inability to read, inability to write, and so forth.

Certain well-defined clinical syndromes occur in association with occlusion of specific arteries of the cerebral circulation:

INTERNAL CAROTID ARTERY SYNDROME. This syndrome occurs frequently with several transient attacks of visual disturbance or contralateral hemiplegia, as described above. When complete occlusion occurs the hemiplegia remains. Blindness may occur on the side of the lesion when the ophthalmic artery, which arises from the internal carotid artery, is involved. Aphasia may or may not be present, depending upon whether or not the lesion is on the dominant or left side. On physical examination there may be a loss of pulsation in the internal carotid artery in the neck, and cerebral angiography may reveal an occlusion. If diagnosed early enough, surgical treatment may be beneficial with removal of the thrombosis or a bypass arterial graft.

ANTERIOR CEREBRAL ARTERY SYNDROME. This artery gives off perforating branches to the internal capsule and carries circulation to the leg area of the cerebral cortex; if the penetrating branches are involved, a typical hemiplegia will develop. If the occlusion, however, is distal to these penetrating branches, only the leg area of the cerebral cortex will be involved. The patient will have primarily a monoplegia involving the leg, while the arm will be spared. In most other syndromes, the arm and hand are more severely affected than the leg, and they are least likely to recover function.

MIDDLE CEREBRAL ARTERY SYNDROME. This artery is a direct continuation of the internal carotid artery, which supplies the lateral area of the cerebral cortex of the frontal, temporal, parietal, and occipital lobes. It also gives off penetrating branches to the internal capsule. Occlusion results in typical hemiplegia. There also may be a homonymous hemianopsia or loss of vision for the visual field on the side opposite the lesion. If the dominant side is involved, there may be aphasia. This artery is most commonly involved in strokes.

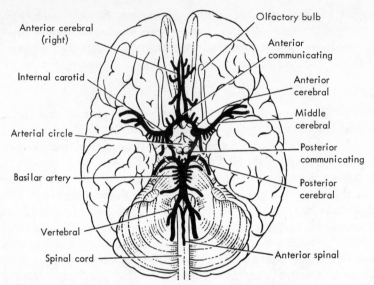

Figure 11. Diagram of the arterial circulation at the base of the brain, showing the arterial circle of Willis. From this circle the anterior, middle, and posterior cerebral arteries extend to each cerebral hemisphere. The anterior spinal artery supplies the cord. (Courtesy of Diana Clifford Kimber, Carolyn E. Gray, Caroline E. Stackpole, and Lutie C. Leavell, *Anatomy and Physiology*, 14th ed., New York: The Macmillan Company, 1961.)

POSTERIOR CEREBRAL ARTERY SYNDROME.   This artery arises from the basilar artery. On each side it is connected to the corresponding middle cerebral artery by the posterior communicating arteries. Similarly, the anterior cerebral arteries which arise from the internal carotid are connected by the anterior communicating artery. Thus, at the base of the brain there is a complete communication between the arterial system of the left side and the right side of the brain. Those arteries arising from the internal carotid artery and from the basilar artery are also connected. This is known as the circle of Willis; it serves to protect the brain by permitting the two arterial systems and the left and right arterial systems to communicate. Arterial blood may flow in either direction.

If the main posterior cerebral artery is occluded there will be a contralateral homonymous hemianopsia (loss of right or left field of vision in each eye) due to destruction of the ipsilateral occipital lobe. The thalamic syndrome occurs if there is impairment of the thalamus. The thalamic syndrome includes transient contralateral hemiparesis; contralateral impairment of sensation; contralateral intolerable pains; choreoathetoid involuntary movements, tremor, or ataxia due to involvement of the rubrothalamic tracts.

VASCULAR LESIONS OF THE BRAINSTEM.   The basilar artery, formed by the joining of the two vertebral arteries, lies on the anterior surface of the brainstem. Partial occlusion may permit recovery, but after several transient episodes major occlusion will lead to death. Various combinations of cranial nerve paralyses, hemiplegia, facial paralyses, quadriplegia, double vision (diplopia), and disturbance of swallowing may develop. This results from failure of the arteries that arise from the basilar artery to maintain the circulation to various areas of the brainstem.

Arising from the basilar artery are two arterial systems. One paramedian group supplies bilateral paired arteries to the midline structures of the medulla, the pons, and the midbrain. If this is obstructed, it gives rise to hemiplegia alternans, in which cranial nerves are paralyzed on one side and the extremities on the other. The second group of paired bilateral arteries maintains the circulation of the lateral aspect of the three levels of the brainstem and the cerebellum and gives rise to ataxia when occluded.

Weber's Syndrome. The highest midline artery arising from the basilar artery supplies the ocular motor nucleus (third nerve nucleus) in the midbrain giving rise, when occluded, to ipsilateral paralysis of the third nerve and contralateral hemiplegia. This will include drooping or ptosis of the eyelid due to paralysis of the levator palpebrae muscle, dilatation of the pupil due to paralysis of the parasympathetic constrictors of the pupil, and paralysis of eye movements except those controlled by the lateral rectus muscle, which is innervated by the sixth cranial nerve. Thus the eye will turn laterally. If the lesion involves the red nucleus, there will be contralateral involuntary movements (Benedikt syndrome).

Millard-Gubler Syndrome. The occlusion of the paramedian artery arising from the basilar artery at the level of the pons will involve the sixth and seventh cranial nerves, giving rise to ipsilateral paralysis of abduction of the eye, an upper and lower facial paralysis, and a contralateral hemiplegia.

Jackson's Syndrome. The occlusion of the midline artery at the level of the medulla will involve the twelfth cranial nerve, causing an ipsilateral paralysis of the tongue and contralateral hemiplegia.

Wallenberg's Syndrome. The most frequently involved of the arteries supplying the lateral aspect of the brainstem and cerebellum is the posterior inferior cerebellar artery, which supplies the lateral medulla. Occlusion causes Wallenberg's syndrome with difficulty in swallowing due to paralysis of the tenth cranial nerve, Horner's syndrome due to involvement of the sympathetic fibers, nystagmus due to involvement of the vestibular nuclei, ipsilateral hemiataxia, and contralateral sensory loss. Slightly higher lesions may cause ipsilateral facial paralysis, deafness, and ipsilateral involuntary movements.

Thus, we see again the specific manifestations of the pathological process will depend upon the particular anatomical area that is involved. These lesions, which involve the specific cranial nerve nuclei, cause impaired function of the cranial nerves because they interfere with the normal bilateral cortical innervation of these nuclei. Since the brainstem is a small area, frequently lesions will cause bilateral involvement resulting in even further impairment of functions such as swallowing, tongue movements, facial movements. When bulbar palsy occurs the nuclei are involved bilaterally. If the lesion occurs bilaterally involving the corticobulbar fibers on each side above the level of the nuclei, we have a condition called pseudobulbar palsy, with difficulty in swallowing, difficulty in articulation, and facial paralysis.

Epilepsy

Epilepsy is a chronic disorder of the brain characterized by recurrent attacks involving impairment of consciousness and/or convulsions. It is classified in two categories. Idiopathic epilepsy has no known cause and probably is an inborn hereditary tendency. Acquired or symptomatic epilepsy is due to specific organic disease or damage in the brain that causes the seizures.

There is an abnormality of discharge of the cells of the cerebral cortex, which can be recorded by the electroencephalograph. In addition to focal lesions such as tumors or scarring of the cortex due to injury, such generalized disturbances as syncope (fainting) or insulin shock may be associated with impairment of consciousness or convulsions. Seizure is a synonym for epilepsy.

The syndrome may consist of (a) involuntary tonic or clonic movements of the skeletal muscle (convulsion), (b) impairment of the state of consciousness, and (c) impairment of autonomic nervous function. Among patients having idiopathic epilepsy, there is a higher familial incidence of the disorder, particularly of abnormal electroencephalographic tracings. Onset of seizures is usually in childhood; the petit mal form tends to disappear after adolescence. Idiopathic epilepsy is frequently preceded by an aura in which the patient is aware of warning symptoms that may include dizziness or numbness of the extremities.

GRAND MAL TYPE

This is the most common type of convulsion. It is frequently preceded by an aura warning that the attack is coming on. The patient loses consciousness, the muscles become rigid (tonic convulsion), and there are rhythmic contractions of the muscles of the extremities (clonic convulsion). The seizure may last from a few minutes to several hours. Following the seizure, the patient may go into a deep sleep. Such attacks may be very infrequent, less than once a year, or may occur several times a day. *Status epilepticus* refers to the situation in which the seizures persist without regaining of consciousness. Such episodes require intensive treatment, whereas the isolated grand mal seizure may pass without any specific treatment whatsoever.

JACKSONIAN EPILEPSY

This is a form of acquired epilepsy of the grand mal type in which the convulsion starts in one portion of the body (for example, a twitching of the fingers) and gradually spreads out to involve the entire extremity. It may spread to involve the leg and then the entire body. This type of focal seizure indicates the localization of the lesion in the brain, as it is usually in the area of the cerebral cortex corresponding to the body area initially involved.

PETIT MAL EPILEPSY

This is manifested by a temporary loss or impairment of consciousness without significant convulsions. It may last only a few seconds, with the only external manifestations being rhythmic movements of the eyelids. The patient may lose posture control and fall (akinetic seizure). It is usually a form of idiopathic epilepsy that may recur frequently each day. Sudden muscular contractions that are not sustained may occur; these are called myoclonic jerks. There is a tendency for these seizures to disappear after adolescence, although grand mal or psychomotor epilepsy may develop. Petit mal has a characteristic type of electroencephalographic tracing called the spike wave pattern.

PSYCHOMOTOR EPILEPSY

This may include dream states, hallucinations, alterations in state of consciousness, amnesia, disturbance of muscular activity with rigidity or fits of running and other physical dysfunction. The condition is more common in adult males. Electroencephalography may reveal an abnormal focus, particularly in the temporal lobe.

Diagnosis is based on the history of the patient, family history, observation of the seizures, and particularly the electroencephalogram. This apparatus records the electrical potentials of the brain that result from the discharge of cortical cells in the brain. Abnormalities appear in terms of the rhythm, appearance, and excessive voltage. In idiopathic epilepsy there are usually no focal neurological findings and no observable organic abnormalities in the brain.

If neurological examination reveals focal neurological signs, further work-up in the form of pneumoencephalography or angiography and spinal tap may be necessary.

Brain injury may result in damage to an area of the cerebral cortex and serve as an irritating focus. This region can at times be removed successfully through surgery with cure of seizures. In some cases of cerebral palsy with uncontrolled seizures and hemiplegia, a hemispherectomy (removal of one-half of the cerebral hemisphere) can be performed with control of the seizures and improvement in associated behavior. Successful removal of a tumor would remove the cause of the seizures secondary to such a growth.

If the seizure cannot be managed by surgical correction of the cause, then various types of drugs are used, with a very high proportion of satisfactory control of the seizures. These drugs include Dilantin and phenobarbital. Tridione is used particularly for petit mal. Determining the proper medication, particularly the proper dosage, requires faithful visits on the part of the patient to his physician over a prolonged period of time.

The majority of cases of idiopathic epilepsy can be adequately controlled with drugs; with proper vocational placement the individual can do a very satisfactory job. If complete control is not possible, placement must take into consideration the possible danger to the individual or others if seizures occur at the place of work. Fortunately, most seizures of this type occur at night during sleep with the patient often unaware of them. The greatest obstacles to the vocational rehabilitation of patients with epilepsy are negative attitudes on the part of society, which in turn breed unfavorable attitudes on the part of the patient. This obviously makes suitable placement difficult. In a small number of cases there may be subsequent deterioration with further impairment of intellectual functioning and worsening of the seizure control.

Some patients with epilepsy may have varying degrees of mental retardation or reactive emotional problems. Particularly if the seizure is associated with organic brain damage and neurological findings, the possibility of intellectual deficit exists. At times psychotherapy and counseling may be of help in dealing with the associated emotional problems of epilepsy. Improved emotional adjustment may also raise the threshold at which seizures occur, thus providing an important contribution to management.

MANAGEMENT OF HEMIPLEGIA

Hemiplegia describes the paralysis of the muscles of one side of the body as a result of pathology involving the cerebral cortex or pyramidal tracts in the brain. Any pathological cause in these areas such as a stroke (apoplexy), tumor, trauma, or anoxia may give rise to hemiplegia.

This disorder has been described under cerebral vascular accidents in detail. It causes loss or impairment of the ability to walk and to use the upper extremity on the affected side. Thus, bimanual activities are limited. Aphasia, intellectual defects, perceptual defects, emotional lability, and visual disturbances are frequently associated.

Trauma and anoxia are causes of hemiplegia in cerebral palsy, while cerebral vascular accidents frequently cause hemiplegia in adults. Usually in these instances there is gradual improvement from the original condition involving complete paralysis (loss of all active movement on the involved side) or paresis (partial paralysis with varying degrees of functional use of the extremities). If the hemiplegia is caused by a tumor that has been completely removed there may be improvement, depending on the extent of the permanent brain damage.

These remarks about physical rehabilitation assume that any corrective procedures, such as surgery for tumor or aneurysm, have been performed. We are dealing with the residual motor defects that are either permanent, improving, or not deteriorating too rapidly to preclude at least temporary improvement in function.

PREVENTION OF CONTRACTURES

There is a tendency to flexion-adduction of the shoulder, pronation of forearm, flexion of the wrist and fingers, flexion contracture of the hip and knee, and equinovarus deformity of the foot (footdrop). If these develop, they will preclude function, even if motor power returns. For example, footdrop interferes with safe balance of weight borne on the inverted ankle. The swing phase of ambulation is impeded by the drop-foot dragging on the ground and not clearing properly when advanced. Contractures are prevented by proper bed positioning, therapeutic exercise, foot board, splinting for hand and wrist, and the use either of footdrop or long leg braces.

PAINFUL SHOULDER

The paralyzed shoulder frequently develops inflammatory periarthritis with limitation in range of motion. This interferes with functional use of the extremity, and the pain impedes the participation of the patient in the physical rehabilitation program. Treatment includes physical medicine modalities of heat and cold, as well as therapeutic exercise— active exercises in which the patient voluntarily moves the extremities, or passive exercises in which the therapist moves the extremity through the range of motion when the patient is unable to do so.

REGAINING VOLUNTARY FUNCTION

The recovery of active control of the involved extremities is the objective of physical rehabilitation. When the course is not progressive, gradual recovery can be expected. This is aided by therapeutic exercises which stimulate maximal strength and coordination. Muscle function improves with use, and exercises under a skilled therapist hasten the process in the early phases, when the patient can produce little active movement himself. Atrophy and weakness due to disuse are avoided, and strength in remaining or recovering neuromuscular units is developed. Perhaps with exercise and training, motor impulses find new pathways around the damaged area of the brain.

Special techniques of neuromuscular reeducation are used which incorporate gross mass movements, resistance, proprioceptive facilitation, and tonic neck reflexes. They are helpful when there is little independent active movement. The objective is to refine gross mass movements of the entire extremities into voluntary isolated purposeful movements.

AMBULATION

Ambulation training, starting in parallel bars for support, with or without temporary supporting braces at the knee and ankle, develops balance. Gait training is then started. As the patient improves in muscle strength, coordination, and balance he may progress outside the bars. Here he may ambulate with a cane or walkerette, with or without assistance. From this he progresses to ambulation without assistance and eventually to independent ambulation. At this time, training in stair climbing and ramp climbing is also included. Approximately 70 per cent of patients who do not die during the acute episode of a cerebral vascular accident will achieve independent ambulation with a cane and a footdrop brace.

ACTIVITIES OF DAILY LIVING

In occupational therapy, the patient is given tasks to stimulate the use of the affected extremity within its limitations, and also training in the personal activities of daily living such as feeding and dressing. This includes the use of adaptive clothing and training in substitute techniques that permit the individual to perform a function even though one of the extremities may be useless. The patient, without recovery of any function in the upper extremity, may still achieve complete independence in self-care with adaptive devices. This is usually achieved more frequently and more quickly in patients with right hemiplegia than in those with left hemiplegia.

PROGNOSIS

Prognosis for recovery of voluntary control is best when return is noted early and continues. Therapy is indicated as long as progress is being made. When recovery has stabilized and function has not returned, the physician should counsel the patient toward acceptance of the disability and not stress useless therapeutic efforts on the arm. Many psychological problems revolve around the patient's focus on complete functional recovery of the arm, which rarely occurs in middle cerebral artery involvement. Usually the upper extremity is a greater functional and psychological problem than the lower extremity. Even with return of motor power, sensory and coordination deficits interfere with completely normal feeling and function, so that at times the patient prefers to use the nonaffected member. Early in the course of training, the use of the nondominant hand is stressed in case of failure of recovery in the affected dominant hand. Functional independence in activities of daily living, regardless of the paralysis, is completely possible without any assistance from the dominant hand. Impaired balance, obesity, lack of motivation, intellectual deterioration, and specific perceptual dysfunctions are the factors that may preclude this.

IX

THE CENTRAL NERVOUS SYSTEM: DISORDERS OF THE SPINAL CORD

Man's spinal cord, a cylindrical mass of nervous tissue 17 to 18 inches long, is a continuation of the brain above and is subject to its control. The combination of the two constitutes the central nervous system. In the process of evolution, the precursor of the spinal cord was a flexible strut, which constituted the entire central nervous system in a primordial crawling insect. From this simple beginning, development through fish, amphibians, reptiles, and mammals has been a gradual aggregation of constant changes. The early nervous structures were utilized to new ends, and new structures were elaborated for new demands. Thus, there is the anticipation that man of the future will have a nervous system more highly developed and of superior function. In man, the highest level creature, the brain is the seat of decision or will. The cord relays, as one of its major functions, input from sensory reception to the brain and after organization of information by the brain it transmits impulses resulting in motor activity or series of activities.

STRUCTURE AND FUNCTION

VERTEBRAL COLUMN

The spinal cord lies within the canal of the vertebral or spinal column. The column is made up of a succession of bones designated as vertebrae. Each vertebra is separated from the next by fibrocartilage—

By Murray M. Freed, m.d., Assistant Professor of Rehabilitation Medicine, Boston University School of Medicine, and Chief, Rehabilitation and Physical Medicine, Massachusetts Memorial Hospitals, Boston University Medical Center; Physician-in-Chief for Physical Medicine and Rehabilitation, Boston City Hospital, Boston, Massachusetts.

intervertebral disc—which provides a cushioning effect. There are a total of 33 vertebrae consisting of 7 *cervical* in the neck, *12 thoracic* in the upper back, 5 *lumbar* in the lower back, 5 *sacral* within the pelvis, and 4 *coccygeal* which constitute the vestige of the tail. In the adult, the five sacral vertebrae are fused into a single bone to form the *sacrum*. The vertebral column serves to support the trunk and to protect the spinal cord (see Figure 4, p. 108).

The cord is located in the upper two-thirds of the canal, extending in the adult from the upper border of the first cervical vertebra to the junction between the first and second lumbar vertebrae. In the embryo, the cord extends to the base of the sacrum. During subsequent fetal development the vertebral column grows in length at a more rapid rate than the cord, so that at birth the cord ends at the level of the third lumbar vertebra, and ultimately one vertebra higher at the completion of growth and development. The cord tapers to a conical end, the *conus medullaris*. A fine thread, the *filum terminale*, extends from the conus and is attached to the end of the canal. The cord is separated from the bony walls of the canal and its ligaments, first by a layer of areolar tissue, and then by a set of enveloping membranes or covers called meninges.

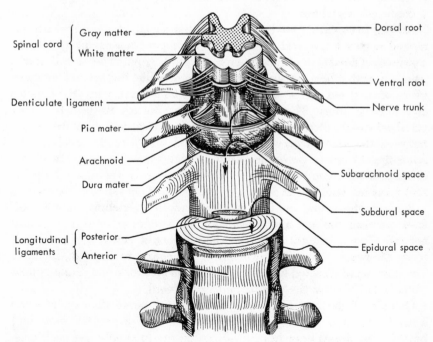

Figure 12. Spinal meninges and their spaces. (Courtesy of Ben Pansky and Earl Lawrence House, *Review of Gross Anatomy*, New York: The Macmillan Company, 1964.)

The outermost membrane, the *dura mater,* is a tubular sheath of strong connective tissue which is a continuation of a similar layer within the skull that extends downward to the level of the second sacral vertebra ending in a closed sac. Inside the dura, and separated only by the very thin subdural space containing fluid, is the *arachnoid.* The arachnoid is also a tubular sheath but much thinner than the dura. Separating the arachnoid from the innermost membrane, the pia mater, is the *subarachnoid* space, which is filled with cerebrospinal fluid. The *pia mater,* also a thin sheath, is firmly bound to the spinal cord. Bathed in the spinal fluid of the subarachnoid space, the cord with its attached pia mater is suspended by denticulate ligaments which project at intervals from each side of the cord along its entire length to penetrate the arachnoid and attach to the dura.

SPINAL CORD

As is the vertebral column, the cord is divided into divisions or segments. The segments are referred to as cervical (8), thoracic (12), lumbar (5), sacral (5), and coccygeal (1). The numbers within each region correspond to those of the vertebral column with the exception of the cervical, which has 8, one more than the number of cervical vertebrae, and the coccygeal, which has 1 segment as compared with 4 coccygeal vertebrae.

Arising from each spinal cord segment is a pair of symmetrically arranged nerves for a total of 31 pairs. Each pair consists of two roots, a sensory (dorsal) root and motor (ventral) root. The dorsal has a ganglion with fibers passing into the cord, while the ventral contains fibers coming out of the cord. Thus the spinal nerve consists of motor and sensory fibers. The first cervical nerve makes its exit from the vertebral canal between the skull and first cervical vertebra; the eighth between the seventh cervical vertebra and first thoracic. Each of the remaining 29 spinal nerves leaves the canal below the vertebra of the corresponding name and number. The nerves leave through intervertebral foramina with the exception of the first and second cervical nerves.

Because the spinal cord is shorter than the vertebral column and ends between the first and second lumbar vertebrae, only the cervical nerves follow a straight course to their points of egress. The more inferior the nerve, the more downward is the course to reach its foramen. The downward directed lumbar and sacral nerves form the *cauda equina* (horse's tail) below the termination of the cord.

Outside of the vertebral column the spinal nerve divides into two main branches, a dorsal (posterior) branch and a ventral (anterior) branch. The dorsal branches course posteriorly to supply the back muscles and continue to the skin of the back. The ventral branches continue to the side and then anteriorly to supply the muscles of the limbs, chest, and abdomen and the overlying skin.

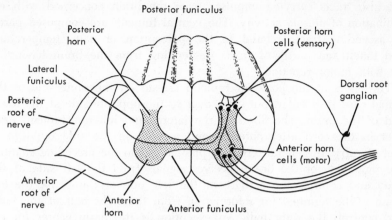

Figure 13. Cross section of the spinal cord.

In cross section the spinal cord, on inspection, is made up of an internal mass of gray substance, known as the gray matter, shaped in a distorted form of the letter "H." This portion is made up of symmetrical halves joined across the midline by a horizontal connection through which runs a very narrow central canal. Surrounding the gray matter is a glistening white area designated as the white matter.

FUNCTION

From the standpoint of function, the anterior gray column (anterior horn), which lies in front of the central canal, contains the motor or anterior horn cells, which give rise to the ventral roots. These serve to innervate voluntary muscle. The lateral gray column contains cells of the autonomic nervous system which controls function of smooth muscle, cardiac muscle, and some glands. The posterior gray column (dorsal horn) is concerned with relaying sensory impulses which enter the cord over the spinal nerves, either upward to the brain or to other cells within the spinal cord. The gray matter consists essentially of nerve cell bodies and of the fibers that leave the cell bodies or that enter the gray matter to terminate on the cell bodies. The white matter is made up of myriads of nerve fibers whose course may extend up or down the cord for varying distances, to the brain from the cord or from the brain to the spinal cord.

The white matter is divided into three bundles of fibers (funiculi). The posterior is made up of fibers concerned with muscle and joint perception and some involved in touch that are routed to the brain to areas of consciousness. The lateral contains tracts that convey impulses from musculoskeletal structures to centers for coordination. The lateral funiculi are also the location of descending tracts from the motor areas of the central cortex, which bring to the spinal cord impulses for voluntary muscle activity of the neck, trunk, and limbs. Finally, there are also tracts carrying impulses from the brain concerned with co-ordination of muscle activity. The ventral funiculi are composed partly of ascending tracts related to the perception of pain, temperature, and touch and partly of tracts descending from the brain having to do with motor function.

The fibers of the posterior funiculi ascend on the same side of the spinal cord they enter, but cross over to the opposite side at the lower end of the brain. The fibers of the lateral and anterior funiculi cross over in the cord after entering and ascend on the side opposite to that of entry. In general terms, as pointed out in the preceding chapter, the right side of the brain receives signals from the left side of the body and controls the activity of the left side of the body; the left brain is the terminal for information from the right half of the body and controls the right half. An exception is the brain center for co-ordination (cerebellum), the two halves of which contribute to controlling muscle activity on their corresponding sides (see Figure 9, p. 220).

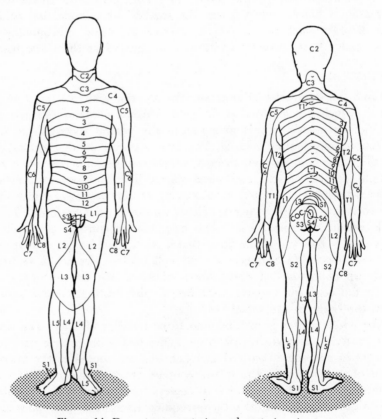

Figure 14. Dermatomes—anterior and posterior views.

For clearer understanding of the signs and symptoms of spinal cord disorders discussed later in this section, it would be germane to describe a general scheme of segmental distribution. The skin regions of the body supplied by the sensory roots of a spinal cord segment, through the spinal nerves, are called dermatomes. These have been determined by clinical means and have been charted (see Figure 14). The segmental innervation of voluntary muscles has also been recorded. Most muscles are innervated from two or more cord segments.

SEGMENTAL INNERVATION OF MUSCLES

Neck	Flexion ⎞ Extension ⎬ Rotation ⎠	C 1,2,3,4,
Shoulder	Flexion	C 5,6
	Abduction	C 5,6
	Adduction	C 5,6,7,8
	Extension	C 5,6,7,8
Elbow	Flexion	C 5,6
	Extension	C 7,8
Forearm	Pronation	C 6,7
	Supination	C 5,6,7
Wrist	Extension	C 6,7
	Flexion	C 6,7, T 1
Hand	Gross extension of fingers	C 6,7,8
	Gross flexion of fingers	C 7,8, T 1
	Fine digital motion	C 8, T 1
Back	Extension	C 4 to L 1
Chest muscles for breathing		T 2 to T 12
Diaphragm		C 2,3,4,
Abdominal muscles		T 6 to L 1
Hip	Flexion	L 2,3,4
	Abduction	L 4,5, S 1
	Adduction	L 2,3,4
	Extension	L 4,5, S 1
	Rotation	L 4,5, S 1,2
Knee	Extension	L 2,3,4
	Flexion	L 4,5, S 1
Ankle		L 4,5, S 1,2
Foot		L 5, S 1,2
Bladder		S 2,3,4
Bowel	Rectum and Anal Sphincter	S 2,3,4
Generative system		
ERECTION	Sacral Cord	S 2,3,4
EJACULATION	Lumbar Cord	L 1,3

In summary the nervous system consists of central and peripheral divisions, the former made up of the brain and spinal cord and the latter of the spinal nerves and autonomic nervous system. Both systems are interdependent for normal body function. The central nervous system depends on the peripheral for receipt of information from all parts of the body and exerts its effect by transmission of impulses through the peripheral system. Within the central nervous system there is also interdependence between the brain and spinal cord. Certain basic signals or impulses leaving the spinal cord must be modified by impulses from the brain in order that there may be smooth, co-ordinated and purposeful muscle activity.

ETIOLOGY AND PATHOLOGY

Those pathological changes that present the most commonly encountered problems will be discussed. The variety of spinal cord lesions will be presented on an etiological basis.

CONGENITAL DEFECTS

SPINA BIFIDA.   Failure of closure of the vertebral canal, spina bifida, is due to a defect in vertebral development. When only a bony defect occurs without protrusion of any elements of the cord or its meninges the condition is designated as *spina bifida occulta*. The error is as a rule located in the lumbar or sacral spine and is often noted as an incidental finding in an x-ray examination of this area. Spina bifida occulta as such is compatible with normal function. Spina bifida may be associated with additional defects.

MENINGOCELE.   In spina bifida with meningocele there exists in addition to the bony defect a protrusion of the meninges through the opening, resulting in a saclike tumor in the midline of the low back. The cord is unaffected.

MENINGOMYELOCELE.   A more severe form of developmental defect is meningomyelocele, wherein the spinal cord and nerve roots together with the covering meninges protrude through the bony defect. In meningomyelocele there is sensory and motor loss in the peripheral areas innervated by the involved spinal cord and nerve roots, including bowel and bladder incontinence and interference with sexual function. Surgical repair of the protruding sac along with closure of the defect is performed early in life. When the sac contains elements of the cord and roots, varying degrees of permanent impairment of function result.

SYRINGOMYELIA.   Cavitation of the cord or syringomyelia is associated with proliferation of cells that surround the central canal of the spinal cord. In the embryo, the precursor of the spinal cord, the neural tube, closes, and thereafter further growth involves the multiplication and development of cells in the vicinity of the central canal. Conditions are favorable in the location for areas of primitive tissue to remain. There exists the theory that the primitive tissue gives rise to proliferation of glial cells in the region about the central canal. These cells degenerate, producing a cystic cavity containing a thick yellow fluid, thus the name syringomyelia (syrinx = tube or cavity, myelia = related to the spinal cord).

The cell proliferation may extend out in fingerlike projections into the anterior and posterior gray matter and thence into the ventral, lateral, and dorsal white matter. The lower cervical segments of the cord are affected. However, there may be involvement of the lumbar segments of the cord and lower brain.

The signs and symptoms customarily become manifest during the second and third decades of life. There is usually rapid progression at the outset, then a slower course followed by a fairly stable period. The initial manifestations, loss of pain and temperature sense with preservation of touch and deep pressure, are usually obvious in the arms and upper chest. From a functional standpoint, because of loss of temperature and pain perception, the individual may burn himself without realizing it, or he is unable to appreciate the temperature of water.

The process may extend to, or develop in, the anterior gray matter of the cord, so that weakness and paralysis present themselves in the affected parts of the extremities. The cord pathology involves one side before crossing to the opposite side, so that motor function abnormality is initially present in one hand. The same process may involve the cord segments innervating the upper back muscles, so that one-sided weakness produces curvature of the spine. With possible further extension into the white matter there results interference with tracts communicating with the brain. There may thus occur development of generalized paralysis, spasticity, and incoordination in the body segments, including the bladder, which receive innervation from spinal cord segments below the area of damage.

When the lumbar and sacral portions of the cord are involved, the same findings are present in the legs and bladder. If the process is present in the lower brain (syringobulbia) there may be noted tongue weakness, loss of facial pain and temperature perception, interference with the peripheral speech mechanism, and eye-fixation abnormality.

Treatment of syringomyelia, which has included surgical evacuation of the cyst or deep x-ray therapy, has produced only temporary improvement. Furthermore, efficacy of treatment is difficult to assess due to the natural history of this ailment, which is characterized by slow progression and not infrequent stationary stages.

INFECTIOUS DISORDERS

Although it is protected by the vertebral column, access to the cord and its coverings may be gained by organisms or by their toxins through the blood stream in systemic infections or by direct extension along the spinal nerves from adjacent areas of infection.

BACTERIAL DISEASE.   Bacterial infection resulting in *meningitis* (inflammation of the covering membranes of the spinal cord) is most commonly due to the meningococcus, pneumococcus, streptococcus, or influenza bacillus. With the help of appropriate antibacterial therapy, the prognosis is relatively good for survival and function.

Epidural abscess, a rare occurrence, is a localized area of suppuration in the space between the dura mater and vertebral column which may develop from extension of local skin infection, from perforating wounds, or by seeding through the blood stream from a remote infection. Paralysis of the legs may develop, along with fever, local pain, and headache. The most common area of abscess formation is at the midthoracic spinal cord level. Treatment includes immediate surgical drainage and use of indicated antibacterial agents. In spite of the above measures, permanent damage to the cord may occur as a result of a myelitis or the plugging of infected vessels supplying the cord.

Tuberculous infection involving the spinal cord may arise as a result of epidural space involvement by direct extension from tuberculosis of adjacent vertebrae (Pott's disease). The process appears in children and results in collapse of the involved vertebrae or vertebra. Paralysis may result from sudden collapse and dislocation of an involved vertebra. More usually, the deformity develops very slowly and the cord is able to adapt itself to angulation. When paralysis does develop in the lower extremities, it results from compression of the cord by abscess or granulation tissue.

VIRAL DISEASE.   *Anterior Poliomyelitis.*   The most widely recognized viral infection of the cord is that of anterior poliomyelitis. The recently developed Salk and Sabin vaccines have been instrumental in decreasing dramatically the incidence of this infection. The site of the lesion is localized to the gray matter of the anterior horn cells, most frequently in the cervical and lumbar segments. There may also be involvement of the brainstem with production of circulatory and respiratory difficulty as well as weakness of facial movements, swallowing, and articulation function.

Permanent destruction of the anterior horn cells may result, or merely temporary dysfunction with ultimate recovery as the mild inflammatory changes recede. With comprehensive and conservative care, maximum recovery of muscle function is reached within one and one-half years after onset; about 75 per cent of the potential recovery occurs within the first nine months. Bladder dysfunction, characterized by urinary retention which may be present in the early stages of the illness, usually resolves itself. Bowel difficulty, manifested as constipation, is not due to an intrinsic defect but rather to the combination of curtailed mobility and depressed abdominal and diaphragmatic muscle function. Prolonged immobilization as well as neurogenic factors with resultant bone demineralization, coupled with urinary stasis, provides the background for urinary tract stone formation and infection.

In summary, anterior poliomyelitis is a viral infection that produces lesions in the anterior horn cells of the spinal cord and to a lesser degree in lower brain centers with varying degrees of residual involvement—from no residual paralysis to involvement of the trunk and all limbs. The paralysis is asymmetrical in that there is weakness of isolated muscles or individual limbs. Certain muscle groups—such as the abductor of the shoulder, thumb opponens, dorsiflexors of the ankles, and abductors of the hip—are more frequently involved than others. It is interesting to note that these are phylogenetically newer muscle groups in the evolutionary scale. Since the virus spares the posterior gray matter, there is no sensory involvement.

Ascending Polyneuritis. Guillain-Barré syndrome, or ascending polyneuritis, is considered to be a viral inflammation involving the peripheral nerves, the spinal nerve roots, and the spinal cord, either singly or in combination. The manifestations vary from mild temporary disturbances of muscle power and sensation to severe motor and sensory loss including respiratory paralysis. The course is characterized by progressive paralysis beginning in the lower extremities and ascending to involve the trunk, arms, and at times the facial muscles. The disease may last for weeks or months; if the patient survives the early acute stage, the outlook for survival is excellent and prognosis for recovery of motor and sensory function is favorable.

Viral Transverse Myelitis. Viral transverse myelitis of the cord is manifested by a sudden onset of complete paralysis of body segments innervated by the spinal cord segments at and below the level of infection, including loss of voluntary bowel and bladder function and disorder of the generative system. Complete loss of sensory function accompanies the motor loss. The onset may be preceded or accompanied by an upper respiratory infection. The site of spinal cord involvement is usually in the midthoracic region. The prognosis for recovery of sensorimotor function is poor.

NEOPLASTIC DISEASE

Tumors may affect function of the spinal cord by virtue of their location within the spinal canal. Classification is based on location—extradural growths are located outside of the dura mater and intradural are found within the dura. Intradural tumors are further subdivided into extramedullary (outside of the cord, but within the dura) and intramedullary (within the spinal cord substance).

The intradural extramedullary growths are most common, comprising about two-thirds to five-eighths of spinal tumors. As a group they are relatively benign in that symptoms result from pressure rather than direct invasion. These tumors arise from the meninges or sheaths of the nerve roots and are designated as *meningiomas* and *neurinomas* respectively. They carry the most favorable prognosis in that they are amenable to surgical removal.

Extradural tumors are chiefly *sarcomas*. The development of symptoms and disability is usually more rapid with extradural than with intradural tumors, and lead to eventual development of a total sensorimotor paraplegia. The extradural tumors may arise primarily in the spinal canal or metastasize from a remote source.

From a prognostic standpoint, the best outlook is in the presence of an intradural extramedullary growth because it lends itself to satisfactory management by surgical intervention. In intramedullary tumors some improvement results with surgical removal and radiation therapy.

DEGENERATIVE DISEASES

The central nervous system is subject to a variety of disorders, a significant number of unknown cause, which involve the anterior horn cells and tracts. Dissolution of nerve tissue occurs with replacement by patches of scarring.

MULTIPLE SCLEROSIS. One of the more frequent neurological diseases, multiple sclerosis, usually has its onset between the ages of 20 and 40 years. The cause of multiple sclerosis is unknown. Pathologically, there are irregular patches of degeneration throughout the brain and spinal cord, customarily found in the white matter, sparing the gray matter. In the early stages there is loss of myelin in the nerve bundle sheaths; later there may be disappearance of the nerve tissue with replacement by scar formation.

The clinical manifestations are exceedingly variable with regard to time and involved body segments, since multiple combinations of nervous system areas can be the site of pathological changes. Ordinarily the first symptoms are those of motor weakness, visual disturbances (double vision, blurred vision, or impaired color perception), intention tremor, or coordination difficulties. The natural history of the disease is characterized by remissions and exacerbations. Early in the disease, symptoms are fleeting and the remissions are almost complete. As the disease proceeds, the remissions are less striking, although relatively long quiescent periods are not unusual.

Spastic weakness of the lower extremities is one of the more common manifestations. Occasionally, this also occurs in the upper extremities. In the early stages, the weakness is minimal, with spasticity being a greater cause of impaired function. Tremor, which is more usual in the later stages, is of the intention or activity type in that it is absent at rest. However, when the individual attempts a volitional activity of an extremity the tremor develops and becomes more pronounced as the voluntary movement continues.

In some cases slow, slurred speech of a monotone character is present. Scanning speech is a more advanced type of disorder in which the speech sounds as though each word is spelled out. The lesion that is the basis for speech disorder is located in the brain and produces an incoordination of the vocal cords and respiratory mechanism.

Emotional symptoms may occur, the most common of which is euphoria. This is characterized by a feeling of well-being and optimism in spite of the physical impairment. In other instances, there may be mental deterioration or depression. Mild bladder dysfunction may be present to some degree. However, if the disease goes on to an advanced stage, urgency, frequency, and incontinence may develop.

The prognosis in multiple sclerosis is good for a considerable lifespan. In some patients, one or two attacks may be followed by no subsequent progression, or an onset early in life may be followed by many years of normal function and then an exacerbation late in life. The time element is not completely predictable. However, because of the progressive nature, partial disability usually results.

SPINAL MUSCULAR ATROPHY. Primary spinal muscular atrophy is a rare degenerative disorder of the anterior horn cells that generally occurs late in life and is manifested by a gradual increase of muscular weakness and wasting, starting usually in the small muscles of both hands. There is subsequently a slow proximal spread to involve the entire extremity. *Primary lateral sclerosis* is a disorder of the lateral spinal cord tracts that produces a spastic paraplegia.

Most authorities feel that primary spinal muscular atrophy and primary lateral sclerosis are both part of the degenerative disorder designated as *amyotrophic lateral sclerosis,* which is characterized by anterior horn cell degeneration as well as degeneration of the lateral tracts of the spinal cord. The onset may be manifested by one or the other; ultimately both become manifest, and the course is rapidly progressive without remission.

PERNICIOUS ANEMIA. Pernicious anemia may be characterized by a neurological complication designated as *subacute combined system disease* or *posterolateral sclerosis.* About 90 per cent of all cases of pernicious anemia develop after the fourth decade of life. There occurs pathological change in the posterior and lateral columns of the spinal cord. The posterior column involvement produces tingling and numbness of the hands and feet, loss of position and vibratory perception, and an unsteady gait. Secondary to lateral column disease are muscle weakness and spasticity in the extremities. Dysfunction of bowel and bladder may occur. There may also be associated degenerative changes in the white matter of the brain and in the peripheral nerves.

With adequate therapy employing liver or liver substitute preparations there will be no progression of the neurological involvement if present, and no development of neurological disorder if not present. Once the neurological component of the disease is well established, the neuropathology is not reversible.

TRAUMATIC DISORDER

It is commonly known that direct trauma to the spinal cord results in a catastrophic loss of function, since there is extremely limited capability for regeneration of the neuronal elements within the spinal cord. However, improved understanding of the altered metabolic, skin, bone, neurological, and genitourinary function and improved surgical techniques have resulted in markedly increased life-span which can be productive. Trauma to the spinal cord may be categorized as concussion, contusion, compression, laceration, puncture, and physical transection as a result of penetrating wounds, vertebral dislocation, or fracture-dislocations. Not infrequently, the injury results from diving into a shallow body of water and striking the head against the bottom, from a direct blow to the upper back inflicted by a falling object, or by falling from a height landing feet first with subsequent conduction of the impact force upward and production of sudden violent flexion of the low back.

Concussion is temporary, with brief loss of spinal cord activity, including loss of motor and sensory function along with loss of bowel and bladder function. This is an extremely rare occurrence that results from a direct blow to the spinal column or entire body. The transient loss of function may be due to altered circulation of spinal fluid. It is a completely reversible phenomenon; the establishment of this diagnosis is made only after an adequate period of observation following the trauma. Treatment is entirely supportive; no surgery is considered for this type of spinal cord dysfunction.

The remaining categories of spinal cord lesions may run the gamut from small areas of hemorrhage and swelling of the cord to complete severance and maceration. Between these two extremes may be found varying degrees of pathological change. Fracture-dislocations of the vertebral column are in a great number of instances accompanied by compression of the cord that results in a physiological transection, in that the physical continuity of the cord is not disturbed. However, transmission of impulses can no longer occur across the site of injury.

Early exploratory surgery (decompressive laminectomy) has become an acceptable procedure to assist in more complete assessment of the trauma, to correct the dislocation, to remove bone or disc fragments that may be pressing on the cord, and to surgically cut the denticulate ligaments in order to reduce the angulation of the cord that may be present. Such surgical intervention may be able to assist in the resolution of some or all of the reversible pathological changes by relief of extrinsic pressure. Operative exploration is further justified by the low incidence of morbidity and mortality. Currently, opinion differs on the need for operative fusion at the site of the vertebral fracture. The fifth and sixth, and to a lesser extent the fourth and seventh, cervical vertebrae in the upper vertebral column, and the vertebrae from the eleventh thoracic to the second lumbar in the lower column are most commonly involved in traumatic fracture-dislocations.

The degree of motor and sensory loss depends on both the level of injury in the spinal cord and the extent of damage at that level. As explained previously, the level of spinal cord injury does not correspond with the level of the vertebral injury. Injury at or below the first lumbar vertebra spares the cord but damages the cauda equina. Hereafter, any level of injury stated will refer specifically to the spinal cord segment and not the site of vertebral injury. From a standpoint of normal function remaining in body segments, all those that receive innervation from the cord above the site of injury will be assumed to have normal function. Those body areas innervated from the site of injury and below will have impaired function. Transections of the cord or cauda equina resulting in complete lesions produce immediate motor and sensory paralysis, loss of reflexes, generative function disorder, and loss of voluntary bowel and bladder function.

It is the rare individual who survives complete injury to the third or fourth cervical cord segments, since respiratory difficulties secondary to loss of function of the diaphragm ensue. Damage at the fifth cervical segment spares the diaphragm for respiratory function; the only significant motor functions remaining are neck muscle function and the ability to shrug the shoulders. No other voluntary motion is present in any of the four limbs; the functional level is that of the fourth cervical segment.

The following list is related to the critical levels of spinal cord functioning following injury. The level as presented is consistent with intact function at this cord segment and all those proximal to it, and loss of function to a greater or lesser degree in the distal segments. Each level includes all function of previous levels in addition to the increment stated.

C 5   Partial strength of all shoulder motions and elbow flexion.

C 6   Normal power of all shoulder motions and elbow flexion, wrist extension
         which indirectly permits gross grasping by the fingers.

C 7 Elbow extension, flexion, and extension of fingers.

T 1 Completely normal arms and hands.

T 6 Upper back extensors, upper intercostal muscles.

T 12 All muscles of thorax, abdomen and back.

L 4 Hip flexion, knee extension.

L 5 Partial strength of all hip motions with normal flexion, partial strength of knee flexion, partial strength of ankle and foot motion.

The sensory loss may be readily appreciated from the dermatome drawing (Figure 14).

REHABILITATION

The physical rehabilitation of individuals with spinal cord disorders is essentially treatment of the symptoms and signs, since the capacity for regeneration of spinal cord neural elements is virtually nonexistent in the confines of current medical knowledge. An important consideration in the planning of the therapeutic program is the nature of the pathology in terms of its being progressive, static, or possibly subject to remission.

QUADRIPLEGIA AND PARAPLEGIA

The impairment is described as quadriplegia when there is motor deficiency in all four extremities, and paraplegia when it involves both lower extremities only. The paralysis is flaccid in the presence of muscle hypotonus, while that with increased muscle tone is termed spastic. Sensory loss is manifested when there is involvement of the sensory elements of the cord.

Patients with spina bifida involving neural elements, with viral transverse myelitis, with traumatic lesions, and with space-occupying lesions that have produced irreversible damage to the cord and spinal nerves, though having diverse pathology, may all manifest similar impairment and complications.

Knowledge of the level of cord involvement permits, in the absence of complications and given a well-motivated individual, a prediction of functional potential:

C 4 Completely dependent for all needs.

C 5 Dependent for dressing and hygiene activities as well as transfer to and from wheel chair, able to propel wheel chair for short distance on level, able to manage feeding with specially adapted utensils as well as handwriting or electric typewriter.

C 6 Added increment permits activities of C 5 with more ease and with simpler adaptive devices. Wrist motion provides a grasping mechanism to hold large objects.

C 7   Manages transfer, dressing, and hygiene activities with minimal assistance. Able to write and use electric typewriter without adaptive apparatus.

T 1   Able to accomplish all manual activities. Requires only minimal, if any, help in transfer, dressing, and hygiene activities. May manage automobile with hand controls.

T 6   Able to achieve complete independence in transfer, hygiene, and dressing activities. Complete independence in use of automobile with hand controls. Ambulation with braces for physiological purposes is a reasonable goal.

T 12   Complete independence in all phases from wheel chair. Ambulatory on level or stairs with bracing of knees and feet.

L 4   May be able to manage without wheel chair. Bracing required for loss of function in ankles and feet.

The quadriplegic patient will always require some attendant care. Though the majority are homebound, a significant number, especially those with low cervical levels, will be able to function outside of the home if private transportation is available. A few achieve ambulatory skills. However, because of the energy requirements and limited respiratory reserve, ambulation contributes little to functional ability.

The high paraplegic (first thoracic) has limitation in ambulation similar to the low quadriplegic. In sedentary activities there are no manual deficiencies. The low paraplegic patient has few limitations in sedentary work. Though the paraplegic with a fourth lumbar level is fully ambulatory with proper support, his major activity limitation would be apparent in repetitive stair climbing and getting into and out of chairs.

The measures for achievement of optimal function include therapeutic exercise for prevention of contractures, for attaining optimal power of uninvolved musculature, and for exploiting any function in the involved areas when present. When medically indicated, the patient is started on weight bearing using a tilt table or splints. This contributes to improvement of vascular and renal function.

Training in *activities of daily living* is that aspect of therapy where the patient is taught to take care of his physical needs, within the limits of his function, by increased mechanical efficiency. These include eating, dressing and undressing, hygiene, ambulation, communication, and travel.

One of the major considerations in the treatment of the quadriplegic or paraplegic patient is the development of efficient, socially acceptable bowel and bladder function. The goal of the former is the establishment of a regular pattern of elimination, which can be achieved by virtually all patients. Satisfactory bladder function is defined as complete or nearly complete evacuation at regular intervals without episodes of incontinence. This may require limiting fluid intake to certain parts of the day. Some 60 per cent of patients with complete cord transection develop automatic micturition; with partial transections this may be on the order of 85 per cent.

Spinal cord injury itself does not preclude fertility. It is felt that erection and ejaculation may be possible when there is no destruction of the sacral segments of the cord, the cauda, or the parasympathetic plexus. The latter function can be affected by an extensive lesion between the sixth thoracic and third lumbar segments or by damage to the sympathetic components on this part of the cord. In the female with spinal cord injury, pregnancy can be established and completed, though menstrual periods may be irregular.

COMPLICATIONS. Though a spinal cord lesion is a local phenomenon, previous portions of this section have already explained that the manifestations are systemic. Thus it may be appreciated that complications can occur in diverse areas.

Skin. Continued localized pressure on skin areas, especially over bony prominences, results in necrosis and decubitus ulceration. In spinal cord dysfunction there is inability of the more superficial circulation in the involved areas to adjust to increase in external pressure. The sacral, trochanteric, ischial, heel, and ankle areas are most prone to this complication. Regular changes in position, both day and night, can do much as preventive measures. Once developed, decubiti require prolonged periods away from regular activity with special positioning and possibly plastic surgery.

Spasticity. Spasticity of the involved extremities, especially the legs, may reach a level of severity where it prevents exploitation of the patient's residual function. Minor degrees of spasticity can be successfully overcome by exercise. There are currently no oral pharmacological preparations that have stood the test of providing more than transient relief. Remedial procedures that may become necessary are:

1. Local injection or surgical section of peripheral nerves that supply the offending muscle groups.
2. Injection of alcohol or phenol into the spinal canal.
3. Cutting of appropriate spinal nerve roots (rhizotomy).

Urinary Tract. Infection is the most common of several complications to which the urinary tract is prone. An inefficient bladder is the source of bladder infection as well as infection throughout the remainder of the urinary tract, including the kidneys. Bladder and kidney stone formation is another complication common during the first two to three years of the disorder. Altered metabolic function coupled with urinary infection predisposes to stone formation.

Training to improve efficiency of bladder emptying, including a plan of fluid intake, and use of chemotherapeutic agents can do much to minimize infection and stone formation. Bladder function may be hindered in the presence of spasticity, so that measures similar to those described for limb spasticity may be indicated.

Pain. Intractable pain in the numb areas still present on arising several months after the injury is not fully understood and may pose a special problem. The improvement following additional surgery is disappointing in patients addicted to narcotics or where the pain has a psychogenic component.

MULTIPLE SCLEROSIS

The elements of rehabilitation of multiple sclerosis are not fixed because of the natural history of the disorder, that of exacerbations and remissions. Therapeutic exercise *per se* does nothing to alter the course of the disease. However, it may play a strong role in preventing joint contractures and deconditioning and in enhancing skills in activities of daily living.

Incoordination due to proprioceptive disorder is helped by use of vision as a more important source of sensory input. When incoordination is secondary to interruption of cerebellar connections, coordination exercises are indicated.

Bracing can be of help not only for support of weakened joints but also for control of spasticity. Gait-training measures are considered in the light of existing muscle power, spasticity, sensation, and coordination. Hydrotherapy has been of limited value, since the increased temperature fatigues the multiple sclerosis patient.

Attention may be necessary to maintain acceptable bowel and bladder function. Bladder dysfunction in multiple sclerosis is often amenable to drug therapy.

SPINAL ATROPHY AND DEGENERATION

In the degenerative disorders of spinal muscle atrophy, lateral sclerosis, and amyotrophic lateral sclerosis, treatment is palliative. This includes measures to maintain uninvolved musculature at optimal levels of strength, minimize spasticity, prevent joint contractures, and improve gait.

The subacute combined system disease accompanying pernicious anemia may be helped by instruction in using visual cues for reinforcement to compensate for proprioceptive loss. The motor weakness is helped by muscle reeducation; specific measures for the spasticity may be indicated in some instances.

POLIOMYELITIS

The early phase of care in paralytic poliomyelitis is related to relief of muscle spasm and its complications and the therapeutic exercise for regaining all potential muscle power. Virtually all motor power that will return has done so within 12 to 18 months of conservative medical management.

Subsequent to the early phases, treatment is directed to:

1. Prevention of deformity as a result of muscle imbalance.
2. Reconstructive surgery for joint fixation and muscle transfer.
3. Orthotic appliances for support.
4. Development of skills within the limits of available muscle power to improve functional ability, with adaptive devices when indicated.

Long term follow-up is required to ensure maintenance of optimal function and in children to minimize growth deformities such as scoliosis and inequality of leg length. In the sedentary individual a modified program of therapeutic exercises may be indicated over a prolonged period beyond the convalescent stage.

ASCENDING POLYNEURITIS

Ascending polyneuritis, or Guillain-Barré syndrome, in severe form may require a program of care not unlike that of poliomyelitis. The flaccid quadriplegic with respiratory involvement demands, in the acute phase, lifesaving measures related to maintenance of nutrition, hydration, respiratory exchange, normal temperature, and prevention of superimposed bacterial infection of the pulmonary and genitourinary systems.

BIBLIOGRAPHY

Goss, C. M. Gray's Anatomy of the Human Body, 27th ed. Philadelphia: Lea and Febiger, 1959.

Rusk, Howard A. Rehabilitation Medicine. St. Louis: C. V. Mosby Co., 1958.

X

DISORDERS OF HEARING

It has been estimated that there are as many as 8 million people in the United States who have a hearing problem; to some of these the hearing loss is merely a nuisance, but to countless others it is a major handicap.

Since the problem is so great, it behooves us to consider its medical background.

STRUCTURE AND FUNCTION OF THE EAR

The ear is a primitive organ found in lowly forms of animal life. Fish—for example, the dogfish—possess a primitive ear. Along the side of the body they have a row of tiny pores that communicate with the water that surrounds them. These pores contain sensitive nerve endings which respond to water-borne vibrations and may serve as part of an "early warning system."

Since man does not live in a watery environment, the ear must be able to respond to air-borne sounds. This requirement makes the human ear relatively much more complicated than the primitive ear of the fish.

It is well known by many fishermen that air-borne noise does not reach fish but is reflected from the surface of the water. However, the vibrations of a pebble dropping into the water may scare fish away. Since more than 99 per cent of the energy of air-borne sound waves

By M. STUART STRONG, M.D., Chief, Otolaryngology, Massachusetts Memorial Hospital; Professor, Otolaryngology, Boston University, School of Medicine; and CHARLES W. VAUGHAN, M.D., Assistant in Otolaryngology, Massachusetts Memorial Hospital; Assistant, Otolaryngology, Boston University, School of Medicine, Boston, Massachusetts.

is reflected in this way, force is required to drive the sound waves into the fluid of the human inner ear. As we shall see, this force is supplied by the eardrum and the special bones of the middle ear.

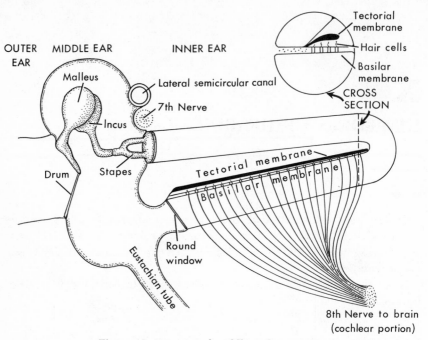

Figure 15. Diagram of middle and inner ear.

INNER EAR

Basically the inner ear is similar to that of the fish. It is a bony tube, contained within the temporal bone of the skull and coiled upon itself two and a half times, called the cochlea. The function of the inner ear can be most easily understood if the cochlea is visualized as a straight tube. This tube contains fluid, suspended in which is a membranous tube containing a dissimilar fluid. The outer tube has two windows facing the outside world: the oval window containing the footplate of the stapes bone (or stirrup) and the round window which is closed by a thin membrane.

The inner membranous tube contains the sensitive nerve endings, the hair cells of the organ of Corti. These hair cells have the capacity to generate an electrical current when the fluid that surrounds them causes them to vibrate against the overhanging gelatinous tectorial membrane. These electrical impulses are transmitted via the eighth cranial nerve to the auditory cortex of the brain.

The fibers of the basilar membrane on which the hair cells rest vary in length and thickness rather like the strings of a piano. In this way when a sound wave of a certain frequency forces the fluids of the inner ear into vibration, only those hair cells that rest on the fibers capable of resonating to the particular frequency are stimulated so that the brain can appreciate the pitch of the sound. The hair cells that respond to high tones are at the base of the cochlea near the windows, whereas the low tones are received by the hair cells at the apex of the cochlea.

AUDITORY CORTEX

The centers for hearing are located in the cortex of the temporal lobe of the brain; each ear has connections with both sides of the brain so that damage to one temporal lobe may not be associated with a hearing loss.

MIDDLE EAR

The middle ear is an air-containing space that houses the ossicular chain, consisting of the malleus (hammer), incus (anvil), and stapes (stirrup); it transforms the air-borne sounds into water-borne vibrations. The middle ear communicates anteriorly with the back of the nose via the eustachian tube and posteriorly with the mastoid air cells.

It is necessary for the eustachian tube to open occasionally (for example, when swallowing) to replenish the supply of air in the middle ear; if the tube becomes obstructed, air is absorbed into the blood stream, and a partial vacuum is created, pulling serum into the middle ear. Under these circumstances the drum and ossicular chain cannot vibrate normally.

The malleus, which is attached to the drum, transmits sound waves through the incus to the stapes. When the stapes moves inward, the round window moves outward, and vice versa; as the fluid of the inner ear is set into vibration in this manner, the inner ear nerve endings are stimulated.

The force necessary to drive the sound waves from the air of the ear canal into the fluid of the inner ear is supplied by the drum and ossicular chain. Because the vibrating surface area of the drum is so much greater than the area of the footplate of the stapes, the drum amplifies the sound by a factor of 17. In addition, the ossicular chain is so arranged that it constitutes a simple lever system with a mechanical advantage of 1.3 to 1. The combined effect of these two factors is an amplification of 22 times.

Loss of ossicular chain continuity or part of the drum surface does not, therefore, cause total deafness but rather a moderate hearing loss which usually interferes with the listening process in conversation.

EXTERNAL EAR

The outer ear affords protection for the eardrum, which is set at the bottom of the ear canal, and may also serve to reflect the sound waves toward the drum in the same way that a cupped hand held behind the ear will perceptibly help the hard of hearing.

HEARING TESTING

The purpose of hearing testing is to determine the extent of the loss in comparison with average hearing and to locate, if possible, the site of the defect.

LIVE VOICE

A very useful impression of the hearing status of a person may be gained by using a whispered voice, a conversational voice, and a loud shout to one ear with the other ear occluded.

Whispered numbers should be audible at a distance of 20 feet in a reasonably quiet room. If a whisper cannot be heard at 3 feet, it is probable that the patient has a moderate loss of hearing and has trouble with ordinary conversation.

If a conversational voice cannot be heard at a distance of one foot, the patient has a severe loss which interferes markedly with person-to-person contact.

The use of a loud shout with mouth to ear is a convenient way of determining the presence or absence of useful hearing. In using the test it is necessary to mask the opposite ear by applying a distracting noise of high intensity to it if the hearing loss is predominantly on one side. Inability to hear a loud shout with mouth to ear indicates a profound loss and that the ear is no longer useful.

TUNING FORKS

Whether a given hearing loss is due to a defect of the middle ear (*conduction or impedance loss*) or of the inner ear (*neurosensory loss*) can be determined by the use of a tuning fork.

Ordinarily when a vibrating tuning fork (for example, one that vibrates at 500 cycles per second) is held close to the ear, it sounds louder than when it is pressed against the mastoid bone behind the ear. In middle-ear deafness, however, the relationship is reversed. When the difficulty is located in the inner ear or nerve, the patient may hear the tuning fork when it is alongside the ear, but the sound is absent when pressed against the bone.

A tuning fork placed in the midline of the skull will be heard equally in each ear under normal conditions; if one ear is obstructed (an impedance loss) the fork will be heard more loudly in that ear because it receives no interference from the ambient noise. In cases of neurosensory loss, the fork will be heard in the better ear.

AUDIOMETER

An audiometer is an electrical instrument that can deliver to an earphone pure tones of variable pitch and variable intensity or speech of variable intensity.

The pitch varies from 125 to 8,000 cycles per second, and intensity varies from the faintest sound the average normal ear can just hear to a sound 10 billion times as loud. This range of loudness can be conveniently represented by the use of a decibel scale in which zero is the smallest sound the normal ear can hear, 10 decibels is 10 times louder, 20 decibles, is 100 times louder, and so on in logarithmic progression up to a maximum of 100 decibels. If an ear cannot hear the test sound at the 100-decibel level, the ear is useless.

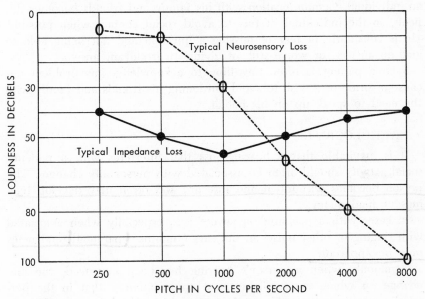

Figure 16. Audiogram.

Each tone is delivered to the patient, and the level at which he can just hear it is recorded graphically on the audiogram. The frequencies at 500 to 2,000 cycles per second are the important ones for understanding speech and must be recorded with great care.

Frequently the curve of the audiogram will be characteristic of an impedance loss in which all the tones are equally affected and the curve is flat or of a neurosensory loss in which the high tones may be more involved than the low tones.

In certain types of neurosensory loss there is a much greater loss of speech discrimination than a pure tone audiogram would suggest. This is the situation when the person can hear the voice but cannot understand the words. For these patients speech audiometry is necessary. Specially selected lists of words are delivered to the patient until the level (in decibels) is found at which he can understand most of the words. This is the speech reception threshold. In a similar way, his discriminative ability can be measured by delivering the words well above the threshold until the maximum score is achieved—his discrimination score.

Significance of Hearing Loss

SOCIAL

When a hearing loss is such that the better ear is below the 30-decibel level on a pure tone audiogram, it is a significant handicap to an individual. Communication with his family and friends becomes difficult, so the individual prefers to avoid social contact when possible. He is constantly in fear of missing a question and not being able to give an answer, or worse still, of giving an irrelevant answer.

Such a patient is often unwilling to acknowledge his problem because of pride or a wish to avoid burdening his friends and family with the need to speak up on his behalf.

PSYCHOLOGICAL

It is inevitable that a hearing loss that interferes with a patient's social activity should often be associated with personality changes. The person becomes withdrawn and insecure and often may develop feelings of inadequacy.

In cases with a profound or severe loss, especially when associated with ringing or other noises in the ears (tinnitus), paranoid tendencies may be apparent.

Commonly when a person's hearing has been improved, the one change for which the family is most appreciative is that in the personality of the patient. The patient is no longer withdrawn and tends to enter into normal social activity.

ECONOMIC

There are a few jobs in which perfect hearing is mandatory. In most jobs, however, perfect hearing is not so critical, but employers tend to look askance at a potential employee who has a hearing defect, especially if the employee will be in contact with the public. Subconsciously many people today still equate hearing loss with stupidity.

On occasion, a person who is well suited to his profession, for example, a schoolteacher, may find it impossible to continue teaching should he develop a hearing impairment.

A hearing defect is certainly an economic handicap to many individuals who, because of it, cannot be employed to the maximum of their capacity.

VARIETIES OF HEARING LOSS

IMPEDANCE LOSS

SEROUS OTITIS MEDIA. Obstruction of the eustachian tube during respiratory infections, during airplane trips, and while skin diving is often followed by the transudation of fluid into the middle ear. In children, the condition is especially common because of the presence of adenoids which tend to obstruct the tube.

The presence of fluid in the middle ear interferes with sound transmission from air to the inner ear; much of the sound energy is reflected by the fluid, and the capacity of the drum to vibrate is greatly impaired.

If the eustachian tube opens spontaneously, the fluid escapes and the hearing returns. In children, this happy outcome does not always occur; because the eustachian tube is often obstructed by a mass of adenoids and the fluid does not escape, the child is left with a significant hearing loss which may account for his grades beginning to deteriorate. Such a hearing loss is often first detected by a routine school hearing test.

MIDDLE-EAR INFECTION. There are several ways in which middle-ear infection may contribute to an impedance loss:

1. *Acute otitis media.* In all cases of acute middle-ear infection there is some degree of loss of hearing because of the presence of exudate in the middle ear. This interferes with the vibration of the drum and ossicular chain. As the infection responds to treatment and the exudate escapes down the eustachian tube or through a perforation in the drum, the hearing usually returns.

2. *Perforation of the eardrum.* Frequently acute otitis media is followed by rupture of the drum; usually the perforation heals spontaneously and leaves no demonstrable hearing loss. Occasionally the perforation does not heal, and the hearing loss persists because the round window of the cochlea is not protected from the sound waves reaching it directly; in this way the effect of the sound waves reaching the inner ear from the drum via the ossicular chain and the oval window is partially cancelled out.

3. *Damage to the ossicular chain.* In cases in which the middle-ear infection becomes chronic, skin may grow in through the eardrum

perforation and form a cyst, a *cholesteatoma,* in the middle ear. A choles-teatoma is very destructive and is a common cause of loss of ossicular chain continuity. Most commonly the long slender process of the incus which normally articulates with the stapes is eroded, so that sound transmission from the drum to the inner ear is greatly impaired by loss of continuity.

4. *Adhesions in the middle ear.* In response to repeated infections, scar tissue is often laid down in the middle ear. On occasion, this scar tissue becomes calcified, so that the ossicles and drum are im-mobilized and unable to transmit sound vibrations.

OTOSCLEROSIS. The hearing loss in otosclerosis is due to a formation of abnormal bone around the edges of the footplate of the stapes, so that it becomes fixed in the oval window. In this way vibrations reach-ing a normal eardrum cannot reach a normal inner ear.

Most often patients with otosclerosis are found to have an audiogram in which the threshold for pure tones is in the range of 40 to 60 decibels. Occasionally the disease invades the inner ear as well as fixing the stapes in the oval window, so that a profound neurosensory loss is encountered.

Otosclerosis is the commonest cause of bilateral hearing loss occurring in young healthy adults. The cause is unknown although it does appears to run in families as a recessive characteristic, and it is commoner in women than men. The hearing loss may appear in the early twenties and in women may be noted to progress during pregnancy. It has been estimated that 1 per cent of the adult population is affected by otosclerosis.

NEUROSENSORY HEARING LOSS

CONGENITAL. Hearing loss at birth may be severe but is rarely com-plete. It may be due to a variety of causes.

Specific infections—for example, German measles (rubella) or syphilis occurring in the mother during pregnancy—may result in a hearing loss in the newborn. The developing embryo is most susceptible to injury during the first three months of the pregnancy.

Certain drugs, if given to the mother during pregnancy, may damage the developing inner ear; streptomycin and some of the less commonly used antibiotics are in this category.

Anoxia (oxygen lack) occurring before, during, or immediately after delivery may damage the inner ear or its central nervous system connections. Complicated and tedious deliveries may be associated with anoxia in the infant and result in irreversible neurosensory loss.

Rh incompatibility between the mother and the infant producing *kernicterus* may be associated with damage to the inner ear.

Familial neurosensory loss in which the child may inherit the same type of loss possessed by the parents is not common. Possibly some of the instances that have been reported may represent an inner-ear variety of otosclerosis.

VIRAL ORIGIN. The common viral diseases of childhood—measles, mumps, and chickenpox—are occasionally followed by neurosensory damage. Curiously, German measles in the child does not appear to affect the inner ear.

During the course of a respiratory infection, patients will occasionally notice a profound hearing loss associated with earache and vertigo; this appears to be due to a virus similar to that causing shingles. Fortunately, the hearing frequently returns after the infection has cleared.

HEAD INJURY. Fractures of the base of the skull involve the inner ear and destroy its function completely. On other occasions the blow on the head causes a concussion of the cochlea with the resultant damage to the hair cells; this type of damage is usually associated with loss of high tones rather than a complete loss of function. The so-called whiplash of the head on the neck may also produce similar cochlear damage.

ACOUSTIC TRAUMA. Prolonged exposure to loud noise will result in damage to the high tone area of the cochlea in susceptible individuals; the hair cells that receive 4,000 cycles per second are usually first affected. Later the damage may extend to involve the speech frequencies of 500 to 2,000 cycles per second.

Gunfire, trip hammers, pneumatic drills, steel presses, sheet metal work, paint chipping on ships, and jet engines are associated with the noise level of 100 decibels or more. Prolonged exposure to such noise constitutes a hazard to the inner ear of many normal individuals; if the relationship of the noise exposure and the early hearing loss is not recognized, profound loss of hearing may ensue.

DRUGS. Certain antibiotics, notably streptomycin, vancomycin and kanamycin are known to be ototoxic. Of these drugs, however, only streptomycin is frequently needed in the treatment of infections, and the variety of streptomycin now commonly used is not as prone to damage the hearing as the balance mechanism.

When damage does occur it is often in a patient who has had kidney disease or in a premature infant in whom abnormally high blood levels of the drug are prone to occur.

VASCULAR CHANGES. Neurosensory loss may occur suddenly in a previously healthy ear in response to what appears to be a spasm of the nutrient arteries of the inner ear. This is often associated with attacks of vertigo and is then spoken of as *Meniere's disease*.

Fortunately the type of hearing loss associated with Meniere's disease is usually unilateral; nevertheless it may affect the involved ear profoundly. Occasionally an inner-ear vessel may be occluded by clot formation with resulting profound and most probably permanent hearing loss.

Presbycusis is the type of hearing loss that comes on slowly with advancing years affecting both ears in approximately symmetrical fashion. The high tones are first involved, and later the conversational tones are affected in addition.

Presbycusis appears to be part of the aging process and is no doubt related to arteriosclerosis and the noise of the environment in which civilized man finds himself.

Treatment of Hearing Loss

SURGERY

Only those varieties of hearing loss that are due to mechanical difficulties with the drum, middle ear, or ossicular chain are amenable to surgical correction. Neurosensory loss is at present beyond the scope of surgical relief, although intensive research is being directed along these lines.

The _impedance loss of serous otitis media_ can be corrected by incision of the drum (myringotomy) under anesthesia and removal of the fluid by aspiration. The incision in the drum usually heals promptly and leaves no residual hearing loss or visible scar. If a precipitating

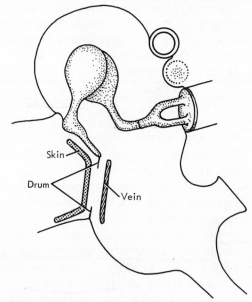

Figure 17. Closure of perforation of drum with graft of skin and vein wall.

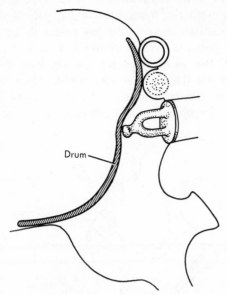

Figure 18. Tympanoplasty. Reconstruction of middle-ear conduction mechanism.

cause such as obstructive adenoids exists, measures should be directed to it in order to prevent recurrence.

A *perforation in the drum* can frequently be closed by grafting a layer of vein wall on the inside of the opening (myringoplasty). If the hole is larger, it may be necessary to apply a graft of skin to the outer surface of the perforation to insure closure. Such an operation is facilitated by the use of the binocular dissecting microscope and is often followed by return of normal hearing.

Defects in the ossicular chain, whether they are due to chronic infection or trauma, can often be repaired by *tympanoplastic reconstruction.* Commonly when the malleus and incus have been destroyed, the drum remnant can be laid directly against the head of the stapes bone to facilitate the transmission of sound from the air to the inner ear. On other occasions a steel or plastic prosthesis may be substituted for an absent or defective incus.

This surgery can only be effectively carried out using the microscope and frequently can be expected to regain useful, though not normal, hearing. A residual hearing loss of 20 to 25 decibels would be a very good result.

Stapes surgery for *otosclerotic fixation of the stapes footplate* is the operation most frequently carried out to correct an impedance loss in adults. Basically this procedure consists of removing part or the whole of the diseased footplate and replacing it by a soft tissue graft or an inert prosthesis. Many surgeons remove the entire stapes (stapedectomy), cover the oval window with a fragment of vein wall, and reestablish mechanical continuity with the incus by using a polyethylene tubular strut or steel wire prosthesis. Some surgeons prefer to use a fragment of fibrofatty tissue or gelfoam instead of the vein graft.

To other surgeons, the placing of foreign material in such close proximity to the inner ear has seemed undesirable; they have found it possible to preserve the posterior limb of the stapes bone and place it over a vein graft, thereby obviating the use of a prosthesis.

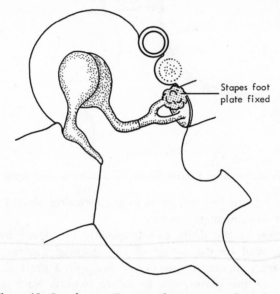

Stapes foot
plate fixed

Figure 19. Otosclerosis. Fixation of stapes in oval window.

In any event, a patient with otosclerosis and good cochlear function has an 85 to 90 per cent chance of regaining and maintaining useful hearing, irrespective of the type of reconstruction favored by the individual surgeon. On many occasions such an operation results in normal hearing for the patient.

HEARING AIDS

A hearing aid consists of a microphone, an amplifier, and a speaker which is fitted into the ear canal. The microphone of the aid picks up many sounds—background noise, noise made by a person's clothing in addition to the spoken voice—amplifies them all, and introduces them into the wearer's ear. This constitutes a problem unless the wearer has maintained good discrimination, so that he can distinguish between the spoken voice and unwanted background noise.

During the past ten years, tremendous progress has been made in the design of hearing aids, so that some are inserted into the stem of eye-

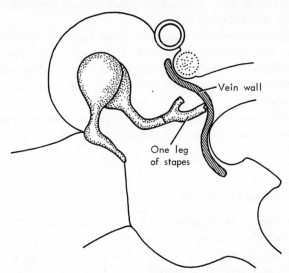

Figure 20. Otosclerosis. Partial stapedectomy and repair with fragment of vein wall.

glasses and others are worn behind the ear. The more powerful instruments require a larger battery and amplifier which must be remote from this speaker and worn on the clothing. A wire connecting cord to the speaker is then necessary.

A person with an impedance loss such as otosclerosis can usually wear an aid very successfully because if the sound merely is made louder he can readily understand. A neurosensory loss, however, often is associated with loss of discrimination, so that an aid, while it makes the sound louder, does not necessarily make it clearer.

AUDITORY TRAINING

Patients who have been hard of hearing for a long time often become discouraged and do not take the trouble to listen any more. When the patients are reintroduced to a world of sound and noise by an aid, they will still be unable to understand unless they learn to listen again.

Recovery of the listening process can be hastened by group instruction; with their aids turned on "low," patients are trained to concentrate and listen intently. Then the aids are turned on higher so that more and more sound is delivered, and in time more accurate discrimination and sound selection are achieved.

SPEECH READING

Many sounds of the English language produce visible movements of the lips, eyes, face, head and shoulders. A hard-of-hearing person who has good vision can be trained to take advantage of these movements;

if he adds what he sees to what he hears, his understanding of speech will increase proportionally.

Instruction in speech reading is of great value to those with a mild hearing loss as well as to those with a profound loss. The greater the loss of discrimination, the more valuable speech reading will be to the person. Commonly patients with presbycusis need speech reading more than amplification.

To reap the maximum benefit from speech reading, patience, perseverance, and concentration are needed on the part of the teacher and the student.

VOCATIONAL IMPLICATIONS

There are certain occupations and professions where it is mandatory to have perfect hearing in both ears—for example, a pilot in the commercial airlines. In other occupations the significance of a hearing loss will depend on a variety of factors.

TIME OF ONSET

A hearing loss that is acquired after a person has completed his education and vocational training may interfere with his performance at work remarkably little.

In contrast, a hearing loss developing during the early years of childhood may, if the problem is not adequately handled, hinder the process of education, so that the vocational opportunities are reduced.

UNILATERAL OR BILATERAL LOSS

For many ordinary jobs a unilateral hearing loss is little or no handicap; a person with good hearing in only one ear does not merely hear 50 per cent of what is going on around him, he hears 80 to 90 per cent of what can be heard with two normal ears.

In a few jobs a person must have at least moderate hearing in each ear. A telephone lineman who works as a splicer must wear a headset with which in one ear he hears the voice of his companion down the line and in the other ear he hears a test tone.

IMPEDANCE OR NEUROSENSORY LOSS

Patients with an impedance loss have little trouble working and concentrating in a noisy environment; in fact, they often indicate that they can hear speech much better against a background of noise.

A neurosensory loss, however, is often associated with recruitment of loudness, so that loud sounds are intolerable and noise in general is confusing; inevitably, performance on the job must suffer.

SUSCEPTIBILITY TO ACOUSTIC TRAUMA

Persons who develop a hearing loss as a result of exposure to loud noise must in the future be protected from such noise or must work where the noise level is not harmful.

Because noise-induced hearing loss is potentially a compensable situation, this is of great concern to industrial management and the insurance industry. It is, therefore, reasonable that potential employees should have preemployment audiometric testing.

SKILL OF THE PERSON

For a person who is skilled in his occupation, an acquired hearing loss may make little difference in his performance. A similar degree of hearing loss in a less skilled and less experienced individual may make it impossible for him to hold his job. The significance of a hearing loss will, therefore, depend to some degree on the capabilities of those involved.

VALUE OF TREATMENT

It is impossible to measure the worth of successful treatment of a hearing loss from a social and psychological point of view. The patient who has been restored to the world of sound is the first to tell what it means to him in terms of happiness and enjoying life; members of the family will often describe in glowing terms what a favorable change there has been in his personality.

The economic value of such treatment can be readily realized from a 1957 Department of Health, Education, and Welfare statistical summary quoted by Canfield:

Twelve hundred deaf people . . . had a combined earning capacity before treatment of $308,200. During the first year after treatment they earned $2,743,000—an increase of 790 per cent.

Twenty-five hundred hard of hearing workers earned $1,610,000, before treatment. During the first year after treatment, their income rose to $5,684,-000—an increase of 253 per cent.[1]

SUMMARY

The ear is the organ of sense by which man perceives sound waves in the air around him; it is essential for proper communication.

The normal function of the ear can be impaired in a variety of ways; a loss of hearing may constitute a social, psychological, or economic handicap.

With adequate treatment and rehabilitation, the handicap can often be removed or at least considerably reduced.

[1] Norton Canfield, *Hearing—A Handbook for Laymen*, New York: Doubleday, 1959.

XI

VISUAL DISORDERS

In the United States of America, there are more than three million people who either are blind in one or both eyes, or have markedly reduced vision. In addition to the incalculable hardship and misery of these people, approximately $85 million per year are expended for their care. Since more new cases of blindness are occurring, especially among the elderly, the costs and complications are constantly on the increase.

Moreover eye conditions, by their visual distortion and discomfort, can and frequently do impede the effectiveness of the individual. Therefore, visual disabilities are not only a disaster to the individual and his family, but also a tremendous economic drain on this country. The prevention and treatment of eye disorders and the social adjustment of those with visual impairment are matters of major significance.

ANATOMY OF THE EYE

The *eyeballs* or *globes* are the receiving sets of the visual system. The eyeball is protected by the lids and rests in a bony pyramid (orbit or socket) filled with fat. The fat absorbs the shock and facilitates movement of the globe. This movement is achieved by four rectus muscles which give upward (superior), downward (inferior), toward the nose (medial), and away from the nose (lateral) motion. There are two obliques which give torsional as well as upward (inferior oblique) and downward (superior oblique) motion.

By DAVID S. JOHNSON, M.D., Associate Professor, School of Medicine, Boston University, Boston, Massachusetts.

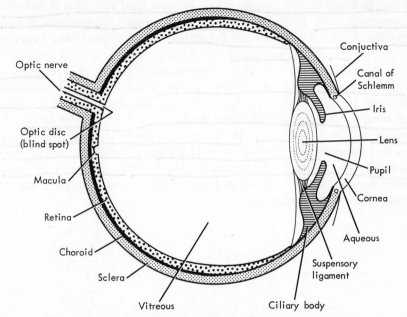

Figure 21. Cross section of the eye. (Courtesy of National Society for the Prevention of Blindness, 16 East 40th Street, New York City.)

The globe has three layers. The strong outermost protective coat is composed of the cornea (clear window and major refractive surface) and opaque sclera (white in color). The medial coat (uvea) carries the blood supply in its three structures: *iris,* giving the "color" to eyes; *ciliary body,* producing the fluid of the aqueous humor and facilitating adjustment for seeing at different distances (accommodation); and *choroid,* with the blood supply for the retina. The inner coat in its front segment contains pigment that prevents light scattering, and in its posterior portion the retina, which is the receptor organ. From the retina, nerve fibers form the optic nerve and carry impulses to the brain. The brain integrates these impulses with other sensory systems and then projects these composite images into space. This projection is termed *vision.*

In the anterior segment of the eye is a watery fluid (aqueous humor) bathing the lens, which in younger people (under 50) allows for distance and near vision. Impinging on the posterior surface and filling the posterior segments is the viscous vitreous humor, which gives form to the globe.

REFRACTIVE ERRORS

The size of the eyeball determines the refractive error, which in turn determines the need for glasses. In the normal eye, distant images come to focus on the macula when the eye is at rest; this is called an emmetropic eye. In the farsighted, or hyperopic, eye the images come to a focus behind or in back of the retina. In other words, the hyperopic eye is an eye that is too small. In order to achieve a clear image, the lens in a hyperopic eye must accommodate the number of diopters (optical measurement of refractive power) that the eye is farsighted in order to bring a distant image onto the macula. In the nearsighted, or myopic, eye the images come to focus in front of the retina; this eye is said to be too large. In astigmatism there is an irregular focus, so that there is more than one area of focus. Astigmatism may be either nearsighted (myopic) or farsighted (hyperopic), or it may be mixed with one of the focus lines in front of the retina (myopic) and the other behind it (hyperopic).

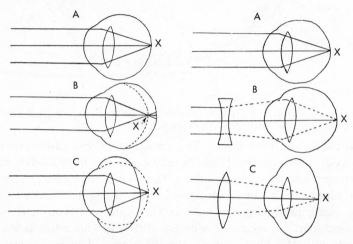

Figure 22. *Left:* Diagrams illustrating rays of light converging in A, normal or emmetropic eye; B, myopic or nearsighted eye; and C, hyperopic (hypermetropic) or farsighted eye. The parallel lines indicate light rays entering the eye; X is the point of convergence, or focus. In A the rays are brought to a sharp focus (X) on the retina. In B they come to focus in front of the retina producing a blurred image. In C they would come to a focus behind the retina. *Right:* Diagrams illustrating the convergence of light rays in a normal eye (A) and the effects of concave lens (B) and convex lens (C) on rays of light. (Courtesy of Diana Clifford Kimber, Carolyn E. Gray, Caroline E. Stackpole, and Lutie C. Leavell, *Anatomy and Physiology,* 14th ed., New York: The Macmillan Company, 1961.)

Extremes of farsightedness and nearsightedness produce their own individual problems. However, the greater the degree of refractive error, the more difficult it is to obtain clear 20/20 vision, even with glasses. The farsighted eye is smaller and this can lead to narrow-angle glaucoma (see section on glaucoma). The nearsighted person has a globe that is too long with stretched sclera, choroid, and retina. In the myopic eye one sees degeneration in the periphery of the retina which in some people leads to retinal detachment (see section on retinal detachment).

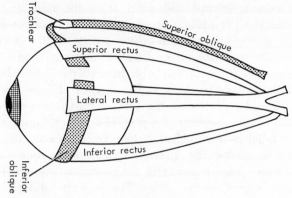

Figure 23. The muscles of the eye (lateral view, left eye). (Adapted from *Alcon Patient Sketch Pad*, courtesy of Alcon Laboratories.)

EXTRAOCULAR MUSCLES

When one considers that there are twelve muscles engaged in binocular vision (six muscles for each eye), and that each globe must be focused within fractions of degrees for accurate visualization and the prevention of double vision, it is truly remarkable that abnormalities of binocular vision are as infrequent (5 per cent of the total population) as they are.

The four rectus muscles attach to the anterior segment of the globe five to eight millimeters behind the cornea. In the straight-ahead position of the eye, the superior and inferior recti control upward and downward movement, but when the globe is turned, they assist in horizontal movement. The horizontally acting recti (medial and lateral)

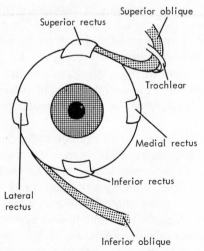

Figure 24. The muscles of the eye (front view, right eye). (Adapted from *Alcon Patient Sketch Pad*, courtesy of Alcon Laboratories.)

control movements toward and away from the nose and have little secondary function. The four recti along with the superior oblique have their origins at the apex of the orbital cavity at the entrance of the optic nerve. The superior oblique travels from its origin to the most anterior superior portion of the orbit next to the nose. Here it passes around a little pulley (trochlear). The inferior oblique arises from the lower inner anterior portion of the orbit almost in a vertical line from the trochlear of the superior oblique. The two obliques then pass in an almost parallel fashion with the globe lying between them, obliquely and posteriorly, under the superior (superior oblique) and inferior (inferior oblique) recti to insert on the posterior temporal (outside and back portion) aspect of the globe. The superior oblique inserts temporally and above the macula; the inferior oblique, below and temporally to the macula. Both obliques produce torsional movements (movements about the anterior-posterior diameter of the eye), thus insuring that the image on the retina maintains a constant spatial relationship as well as elevating (inferior oblique) and depressing (superior oblique) functions.

NEUROPHTHALMOLOGY

The eye and its supporting structures are controlled by a large number of cranial nerves—motor and sensory.

Through the pons funnel all fibers to and from the brain (exclusive of the first and second cranial nerves—motor, sensory, and proprioceptive (receiving impulses from within the body, that is, from intestines, joints, and so forth). The pons contains all the motor nuclei (energizing centers) to the globe and supporting structures. Involvement of nuclei that supply the muscles of the globe produces *diplopia*, or double vision. Since these nuclei are in close apposition to so many other structures, it is little wonder that their pathological involvement produces many other changes. For example, the Millard-Gubler syndrome is an involvement of the sixth nerve muscles producing paralysis of the lateral rectus (this gives diplopia) and paralysis of the opposite side of the body (involvement of the pyramidal tract, the major motor tract for the body).

These nuclei in the pontine area are controlled by programmed commands, similar to computers, from highly integrated systematized supranuclear cortical connections, whose activity controls broad, general movements—for example, both eyes turning to the right. The frontal area (area 8) of the cortex controls voluntary movements of the eyes contralaterally; for example, the right frontal center controls eye movements to the left. These movements are jerky (saccadic) movements. This area is in close relationship with the area that produces turning of the head. The occipital area for conjugate deviation is not localized

OCULAR CRANIAL NERVES CONTROLLING THE EYE

Motor	Extraocular		Intraocular	
	MUSCLES	ACTION	MUSCLES	ACTION
3 (oculomotor)	Superior rectus	Elevation	Muscles of the ciliary body	Accommodation
	Medial rectus	Movement toward nose	Pupillary sphincter	Constriction (miosis) of pupil
	Inferior oblique	Torsion, elevation		
	Levator palpebrae	Elevation of lid		
4 (trochlear)	Superior oblique	Torsion depression		
6 (abducens)	Lateral rectus	Movement away from the nose		
7 (facial)	Facial muscle Orbicularis oculi	Closing of the lids		
Sensory				
2 (optic)		Carries impulses from retina to brain		
5 (trigeminal)		Sensation via ophthalmic and maxillary branches to globe and adnexa		

to any one portion of the occipital cortex. There is some information that tends to point to the fact that there is a direct connection between both occipital areas. These areas tend to control contralateral following movements. These pursuit movements are largely involuntary and do not develop in children until well after birth. Lesions of the cortical areas do not produce diplopia. Because of this, patients are not aware of their deficit if it is produced slowly, as in tumors. This is in contradistinction to pontine lesions where diplopia is an immediate presenting symptom.

Subcortical centers are not well localized for coordinated movements. There is a multiplicity of contradictory and fragmentary knowledge concerning these subcortical centers, which may or may not extend from the basal ganglion at the base of the brain down to the pontine areas. However, the superior colliculi, which are at the most superior portion of the pontine area, are definitely known to be intimately associated with vertical conjugate movements of the eye.

VISUAL FIELDS IN NEUROPHTHALMOLOGY

The visual field of each eye (monocular) is composed of a small two-to-three-degree central area (macula) of very discrete vision. This fades off rapidly so that approximately five degrees away from the fovea *centralis* (center of vision) of the macula, vision is reduced to around 20/200, and from here it is further reduced to finger counting in the periphery. The greatest portion of the field is on the temporal side; approximately one-half is on the nasal portion. The two nasal areas overlap binocularly to make almost a circle, and it is this area that is called binocular. True binocular or stereoscopic vision occurs only in those areas served by both maculae (bifoveal fixation). As one can see from the diagram, there is a split right down the center through the macula of the binocular field of vision. The right visual field is monitored by the retina temporal to the macula of the left eye and the retina nasal to the macula of the right eye. These nerve fibers pass back through their respective optic nerves to be joined by the nasal fibers crossing over at the *chiasm* to form the left optic tract. The left optic tract passes to the geniculate body where it synapses with the left optic radiations, which then pass to the left occipital lobe. The left visual area is observed by the right temporal retina and the left nasal retina (the macula is the dividing line between temporal and nasal fields). The right temporal retina fibers pass in the right optic nerve to the chiasm where they are joined by the left nasal fibers, which decussate (cross over) to form the right optic tract. The right optic tract passes to the geniculate body and synapses with the right optic radiations, which pass to the right occipital lobe, where they are integrated by higher centers that then abstract those data that are most useful. The most interesting feature of all of this is that these consciously perceived images are then projected into space. This projective imagery normally is the product of past experience modified by the present stimulus. It is this projective imagery that allows one to function effectively; abnormalities cause severe physical and emotional difficulties, and vice versa.

If the optic nerve were cut, all impulses coming from the outside world to that eye would be lost to the brain, and the eye would be said to be blind. If the chiasm were injured, it could result in a multiplicity of different patterns depending upon the area injured; for example, pressure in the center anterior to the chiasm, as in pituitary tumors, produces loss of both temporal fields (bitemporal hemianopsia). If the right tract radiation or occipital lobe is destroyed, the left visual field is destroyed (left homonomous—same side—hemianopsia). When a portion of the tract radiation or occipital lobe is destroyed, that portion corresponding to the defect will be gone in the visual field, giving a homonomous defect. The same applies for the opposite side.

Because of the maze of cerebral connections, disturbances in the brain can be pinpointed when they impinge on the visual area. For example, in temporal lobe tumors, visual field changes are characteristically present in addition to headaches associated with convulsions,

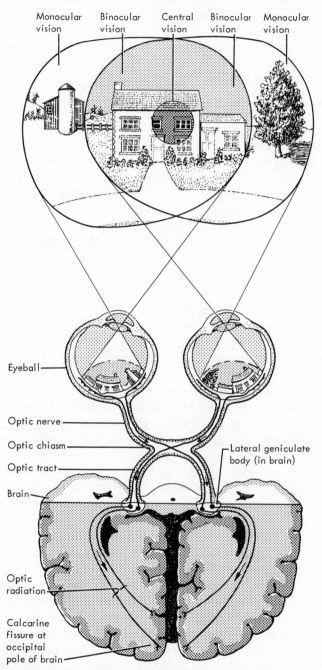

Monocular vision   Binocular vision   Central vision   Binocular vision   Monocular vision

Eyeball

Optic nerve

Optic chiasm

Optic tract

Brain

Lateral geniculate body (in brain)

Optic radiation

Calcarine fissure at occipital pole of brain

Figure 25. Schematic diagram showing monocular and binocular fields of vision. (Adapted from *Vision* by Frank H. Netter, M. D. Copyright CIBA Pharmaceutical Company, Summit, New Jersey.)

abnormal smells, and disturbed hearing. These visual defects involve a complete or incomplete homonomous hemianopsia to the side opposite the tumor.

Strabismus

Strabismus means a crossed or deviated eye. However, strabismus can be present without apparent or cosmetic crossing. In these conditions it is usually associated with loss of vision. Pseudostrabismus (epicanthal folds associated with a broad root of the nose giving an illusion of crossing) has led to the false belief that such eyes will straighten and strengthen by themselves. It is amazing to the author that people will think nothing of having five, six, or seven operations for detachment of the retina, or multiple surgical procedures that may result only in finger-counting vision, but will ignore in their own children reduction in vision due to strabismus. This arises from the mistaken belief that since the globe has no disease it must be normal. However, a blind eye from strabismus is just as blind as one from cataracts, glaucoma, or any other pathological condition of the retina.

The development of strabismus is not well understood. Very often it tends to run in families, and here we say that there is some inherited defect in fusional ability (fusion meaning to use both eyes together for stereoscopic or three-dimensional vision). This may, however, be a myth and some totally unrelated fact may be the cause. Transient nonalignment of the eyes (as in high fevers, bleeding into the globe, transient muscle paralysis, and so on) may result in persistence of this crossing. Such other problems as anisometropia (eyes that have different refractive powers) make fusion difficult owing to the resultant difference in image size. As an example, in a stereoscope if one picture, although similar, is larger, we know that we cannot achieve fusion or stereoscopic vision. Limitation of muscle movements, due to abnormal attachments, have in the past been considered to be one of the basic causes of strabismus.

When one is discussing the cross-eyed child, the terms strabismus, tropia, wall-eyed, squint, cast, "lazy eye," amblyopia, and hypertropia all mean nonalignment of the visual axis.

The type of vision attained is quite different from bifoveal or stereoscopic vision. The vision attained in strabismus is a panoramic picture, which is a composite of both eyes, even though one may have markedly reduced vision when tested alone. Monocular and binocular testing of vision very frequently have no correlation, so that when tested monocularly the vision may be 20/200, but when tested binocularly the vision may be 20/30. The picture obtained in panoramic vision is flat with only monocular clues for depth perception. In the area covered by the two foveas, there is a marked increase in clarity, so that instead of one discrete area as with binocular vision, in panoramic there are two. Suffice it to say that the eye that is being used fixes or determines the visual direction of both eyes; even though images are being recorded within the brain from the deviating eye, these deviated images are so integrated that they appear to the individual as if they were coming from the dominant or fixing eye. This is also true in alternating strabismus where either eye will fix. Here the fixing eye determines the visual direction in space.

It would seem that the deviation of the eyes, if sufficient to be noticeable, creates within the individual emotional problems. Squinters may develop peculiar head-holding positions, lack of "looking you in the eye," and other peculiarities of fixation that only serve to increase psychic disturbances and to impede interpersonal relationships. Surgical correction of this cosmetic defect by operating on the muscles without preliminary and rather extensive eye training (sometimes for years) will result only in cosmetic cure while the amblyopia will still persist. Not only that, but the closer the two pictures come together the greater is the demand for central integration. If the interpretation is imperfect, there is a tendency for certain types of emotional problems to evolve. If there is a strong abnormal retinal relationship (dominance of the fixing eye over the nonfixing eye), very often the eyes return to their original crossed position after surgery, and repeated surgical procedures are necessary to obtain a poor cosmetic cure.

The amblyopic eye, when fixing monocularly, usually fixes with a portion other than the fovea centralis (the 20/20 seeing area) of the macula. This is called *eccentric fixation.* In the past it was felt that by patching the good eye and theoretically making the "lazy" eye work, vision would be restored. This is true, however, only in those people who have strabismus of very recent onset. Professor Bangerter in Switzerland has shown that by patching the amblyopic eye and by teaching it to see under controlled situations monocularly, better results are obtained. The basic technique, *pleoptics,* is to project under direct observation a very bright light onto the retina, so that all the central retina except the macula is dazzled, much as when a photoflash is taken one notices that the vision in the distance has a black image corresponding to the flash in front of it. The patients are then taught to utilize the central clear area (the fovea), and by so doing, macula fixation with resultant visual direction develops.

Since this is a multitreatment daily procedure, carried on for months, there have been attempts to develop many home devices in order to decrease the number of office visits necessary. Such devices include the placing of a nontransparent spot on a light bulb and staring at it, utilizing the afterimage for visual direction, or the placing of a vertical filament in front of one eye and a horizontal one in front of the other (centroscope), utilizing these afterimages for visual direction. These have been of some value in the home treatment of the strabismic patient only when carefully supervised. In the pleoptic school, once central vision is obtained, restoration of fusion is attempted by means of orthoptics.

Orthoptics is a system of visual training whereby similar slides are placed in two arms of a machine, each arm of which is seen by only one eye. These arms are adjusted so that the fovea fixates the central portion of the slide. The arms are moved back and forth in an attempt to see both pictures simultaneously, then to superimpose them and eventually to fuse them for three-dimensional vision. The disadvantage of this technique lies in the use of an instrument where proper visual field and visual direction cannot be appreciated. This results in abnormal relationships between convergence (turning in of the eye) and accommodation. We are dealing with images that do not have the various physical attributes of smell, taste, consistency, and so on. If orthoptics is used prior to the development of visual direction and macula fixation, as in patching of the good eye, one only further ingrains abnormal sensory and muscular relationships.

Panoroptics, which has been used since approximately 1962, attempts to break down panoramic vision and restore proper visual direction and projection in both eyes. In this technique, both eyes are used simultaneously but with different visual clues so that the eyes are seeing monocularly. By repetitive exercise and treatment, there is disintegration of panoramic vision, and normal monocular and binocular visual direction is restored. Fusion is often elicited.

Hypnosis has been used by many with varying degrees of success. Certain tranquilizing agents seem to help stimulate the development of fusion. Drugs applied locally to the eyes (atropine, phospholine iodide, and so forth), by changing accommodative convergence ratios, may also beneficially affect the course of treatment.

Many people confuse cosmetic results from surgery with good fusional results obtained by extensive preoperative and postoperative training and surgery. Surgery should not be attempted until normal relationships between the two eyes have been restored. If the eyes have become binocular with exercise, aligning the eyes by operating on the necessary horizontal or vertical muscles may stabilize fusion. After surgery, very often, exercises are necessary. Although by classic standards anyone beyond the age of five to seven years is considered too old, using these newer techniques there have been occasional patients in their fifties who achieve binocular steroscopic vision.

Diseases of the Eye and Its Structures

LIDS

The lids protect the globe and act as windshield wipers, washing the tears from the upper outer quadrant of the conjunctival sac toward the nose. This constantly clears the cornea of minute foreign particles, which are continually bombarding the cornea. If the lids are rolled under (entropion), abrasion of the cornea by the lashes and the skin occurs. This entropion may be caused by scarring (old injuries, chemical burns, trachoma—a blinding viral disease of the conjunctiva and cornea—and other diseases) or spasm of the muscle. On the other hand, the lower lid may be turned outward so that it extends in a shelflike fashion away from the globe (ectropion). This may be caused by scarring, relaxation of the muscles, or postoperative overcorrection of entropion. With either the ectropion or entropion, infection and even ulceration of the cornea ensue because of exposure of the globe and the introduction of foreign substances (skin, lashes, bacteria, dirt). The lids may be stuck together at their margins (ankyloblepharon); this results in a small contracted conjunctival sac (blepharophimosis). Symblepharon (adhesions of the conjunctiva to the lids) may be congenital or acquired (due to scarring). Blepharochalasis, which occurs in older people, is a fold of loose skin hanging down from the upper lids, oftentimes even over the tips of the eyelashes. Dropping of the upper lid (ptosis) may be so severe as to block the line of sight. Surgical correction here is essential.

Epicanthus is a condition often associated with ptosis in which a fold of skin extends from the lower lid vertically to the brow concealing the inner canthus and caruncle. It is a racial characteristic of Asiatics. In conjunction with a flattened bridge of the nose, epicanthus often gives the optical illusion of crossed eyes (convergent strabismus or esotropia). This disappears with the development of the facial bones.

Blepharitis is one of the most common afflictions of the lid. Dandruff of the scalp is associated with granulations (redness) at the lid margins. This may be compounded by bacterial inflammations, of which staphylocci are the most common. A sty or chalazion—a frequent complication of blepharitis—is an occlusion of the opening of the glands (meibomian) of the tarsus with infection developing within the occluded gland. It may vary from two millimeters to the size of the end of a thumb. When infected, the entire lid may be red and swollen.

The skin of the lid is subject to all the afflictions found in general skin reactions, such as atopic dermatitis or contact dermatitis. Edema (swelling by fluid) of the lids is commonly found in allergies, in hypothyroid, renal, and cardiac disease; it is also found in trichinosis (parasitic infection from eating insufficiently cooked pork). In injuries where the sinuses of the nose are punctured, air escapes into the lid and may give the appearance of edema.

We are all aware of the lashes as a mark of beauty. However, when the lashes do not grow out but rather against the cornea, they become a source of great irritation leading to infection, ulceration, and scarring when left unattended.

LACRIMAL SYSTEM

The lacrimal system (or tear system) is composed of essentially three portions: the lacrimal gland, the conjunctival portion, and the collecting system.

The lacrimal gland is situated in the upper outer anterior quadrant of the orbit. By everting the upper lid, a small fleshy portion can be seen extending into the conjunctival sac. Here tears are continually secreted. Emotion or irritation produces greater quantities of dilute tears. From the gland, they pass by numerous small ducts to the con-

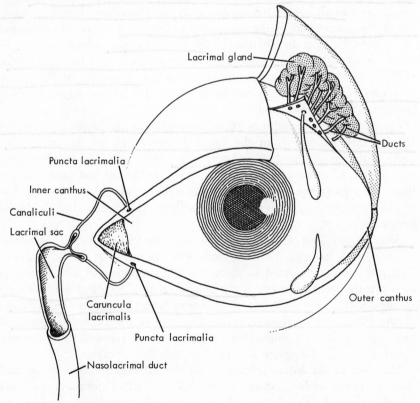

Figure 26. The lacrimal system. (Adapted from *Alcon Patient Sketch Pad*, courtesy of Alcon Laboratories.)

junctival sac. The tears form a thin coat protecting and lubricating the conjunctival and corneal surfaces. At the innermost portion of the tarsal plate on its exposed surface is a small orifice (punctum) which drains tears into the nasal lacrimal sac via small tubes (canaliculi) that lie along the inner lid margins. These canaliculi empty into the nasolacrimal sac which drains into the nose via the nasolacrimal duct.

Inflammation of the lacrimal gland can occur as a primary infection, but usually it is a manifestation of an acute infectious systemic disease such as typhoid fever, mumps, tuberculosis, and many others. Many different types of tumors (from benign to malignant) can develop in the lacrimal gland resulting in the globe being pushed forward (proptosis), downward and toward the nose. The more common type is a slowly growing malignant (mixed) tumor.

The tears contain lubricants and lysozyme, an antibacterial enzyme. Lack of tearing is a very serious problem, since there is no lubrication of the cornea and conjunctival surfaces. This leads to corneal ulceration and scar formation. This lack of fluid may be due to an absence of the gland at birth, scarring of the conjunctiva following inflammations, loss of the normal gland through infection, tumor, and Sjögren's syndrome (arthritis and lack of secretion of the salivary and lacrimal glands).

Tearing (epiphora) is present in certain emotional states due to an excessive production of tears. Irritation or allergies of the conjunctival sac may also produce tearing. Another reason for epiphora is seen in the elderly. In this instance, the tears are able to pour at will over the lid margins, for the glands of the lid are no longer producing enough grease to contain the tears within the conjunctival sac.

Blockage of the collecting system by occlusion of the canaliculi, punctum, or nasal lacrimal duct will cause tearing. With this stasis, the tears serve as a good culture medium, and frequently chronic or acute infections follow. When the nasal lacrimal sac is infected, a draining fistula (a deep sinus ulcer leading to an internal hollow organ and draining on the skin) can occur.

Approximately one out of every hundred newborns has nasal lacrimal obstruction, which may be due to retained debris or failure of the valvelike epithelial structure to open into the nose. Rarely, this may be due to malformation of the nasal bones or congenital absence. If the nasal lacrimal duct is present, a steel wire can be passed from the punctum into the nose, thus restoring the normal patency.

CONJUNCTIVA

The conjunctiva extends from the lid margin under the lid and is reflected onto the globe, back onto the other lid to its lid margin, but not covering the cornea. It is a thin, relatively transparent mucous membrane, avascular in its quiescent state. The three parts are *palpebral* (under the lid), *fornix* (the apogee of the conjunctival sac, which is a transition zone between the palpebral and bulbar conjunctiva), and the *bulbar* conjunctiva (outermost covering of the globe). The conjunctival sac is exposed to a multitude of debris and microorganisms, more so than any other mucous membrane surface. Infection is prevented by the lower temperature due to the direct connection to the outside world, by the mechanical washing of the tears, and by the effect of lysozyme. It is surprising that bacteria that will grow in the nose will oftentimes not grow in the eye, and therefore retrograde infection from the nose is relatively rare. Any irritant to the conjunctiva results in the opening of new blood vessels with the formation of a red eye. When the lids are closed, bacteria multiply at their fastest rate. This accounts for sticking together of the eyelids in the morning.

CONJUNCTIVITIS. Conjunctivitis means infection of the conjunctiva. By far the most frequent type is bacterial conjunctivitis. Acute bacterial conjunctivitis lasts from 10 to 14 days. It is associated with a profuse purulent (pus) discharge which clings to the lashes. The bacteria that produce the acute infection are the Gram-positive and Gram-negative cocci, the bacteria of the *Hemophilus* group, and *Proteus vulgaris.* Nodular ulcerating chronic conjunctivitis is produced by tuberculosis, tularemia, and syphilis. These are rare, but most serious when they do occur, resulting in severe systemic as well as local reaction.

Viral conjunctivitis, on the other hand, is associated with copious tearing and very slight discharge but with marked infection or redness of the conjunctiva. Infections can be seen in all the common viral diseases of childhood (measles, mumps, chickenpox) as well as smallpox and other disease from large viruses. Trachoma and herpes simplex are two viral diseases of great importance for they produce disproportionately large numbers of blind people. Herpes simplex (the common cold sore) produces a dendrite (one or more Roman-numeral-type figures) on the cornea. At first these are only in the epithelium, but they may spread to involve the entire thickness of the cornea (disciform keratitis) with resultant loss of vision. Trachoma (caused by a large virus similar to that causing viral pneumonia) is the leading cause of blindness over the world. This large virus is spread by direct contact and may last for many years. The first symptoms are mild itching, irritation, and photophobia (sensitivity to light). The virus evokes the production of mononuclear cells on the conjunctiva of the upper lid. This process, if not treated successfully in its acute stages with antibiotics, extends downward covering the cornea, producing scarring and quite commonly blindness.

Allergic conjunctivitis is associated with annoying itching and chemosis (swelling of the conjunctiva). Fortunately, it is usually well treated with antihistamines by mouth. Cortisone locally is also very beneficial. Occasionally, specific desensitization to the offending agent is necessary. Vernal conjunctivitis is delineated by swelling of the palpebral conjunctiva, giving a cobblestone appearance. A stringy discharge with a milky pseudomembrane formation is also part of the picture. Another type of allergic conjunctivitis (phlyctenular) is associated with malnutrition or tuberculosis or both. Phlyctenules are small, red, elevated, wedge-shaped lesions at the limbus of the cornea with the apex toward the center. There may be a multitude of them resulting in severe scarring of the cornea with vascularization.

Fungal infections are increasing and are usually associated with a minimum of symptoms and localized inflammation. Tetracyclines and steroids encourage the growth of fungi. Since combinations of these drugs are in frequent use in the treatment of minor ocular infections, it is more than likely that they are the responsible factor.

There are numerous parasitic causes of conjunctivitis, such as roundworms, tapeworms, flukes. Many diseases of unknown cause produce conjunctivitis—for example, pemphigus, psoriasis.

Ophthalmia neonatorum is any inflammation of the conjunctiva occurring in the newborn. Within the first 24 hours this is probably due to the instillation of silver nitrate, which is used as a prophylaxis against gonorrhea. In the second to fifth days, it is caused by staphylococci, pneumococci, or gonococci, and from the fifth to tenth days, inclusion conjunctivitis (virus).

Lymphangiectasis is a localized dilatation of the normal lymph spaces of the conjunctiva; unless cosmetically disfiguring, it is of no significance. A *pinguecula* is extremely common in older people. It is a yellow nodule in the horizontal meridian under the conjunctiva at either the inner or outer canthal area. A pinguecula consists of fat, hyalin, and degenerating yellow elastic tissue. No treatment is indicated unless it becomes inflamed. However, many times pinguecula is misjudged for a *pterygium*, a growth of hyalin and elastic tissue replacing epithelium and Bowman's membrane in its growth across the cornea. Small pterygiums or pterygiums that are not growing need not be surgically removed, as the others do. Patients often equate pterygiums and cataracts; the two have no similarity.

Pigmented spots on the conjunctiva are usually benign; however, some develop into melanoblastoma, a malignant tumor of the conjunctiva which may require the removal of the entire orbital contents for cure. Pigmentation of the conjunctiva is also caused by the use of epinephrine for glaucoma, multiple iron foreign bodies, the prolonged use of argyrol, or by various disease states. Subjunctival (lying under the conjunctiva) hemorrhages are common and may be a manifestation of a systemic blood dyscrasia or emboli coming from vegetation of the heart valves. Most often they are the result of trauma. The bloody appearance of the sclera, although frightening to the patient, has no known deleterious effect on the eye.

Injuries of the conjunctiva due to chemicals or burns require immediate copious washing to remove the causative agent. The prevention of conjunctival adhesions is of paramount importance so that there will be no loss of the conjunctival sac. Conjunctival tears, without the presence of foreign bodies, usually need no treatment other than local antibiotics until they are healed. If foreign bodies are present with or without tear, it is essential that they be removed for the comfort of the patient.

CORNEA

The cornea is the anterior portion of the protective coat of the eye. It is the major refracting surface of the globe and is optically clear. The external surface of the cornea is composed of multilayered epithelium overlying a glassy membrane through which large numbers of nerve fibers pass to end in the epithelium. Because of its multitude of pain fibers, any disruption of the normal epithelium will result in pain and light sensitivity. This foreign-body feeling is augmented by movements of the lid over the cornea. The outermost portion of the epithelium presents an optically smooth surface to incident rays of light. The bulkiest portion of the cornea is the substantia propria— the layered connective tissue so arranged as to be optically clear.

Any disruption of this ordered regularity results in scarring, the density of which will depend upon the amount of damage. This in turn will reduce the optical clarity of the area. The tough inner glassy membrane (Descemet's membrane) is extremely resistant to infection and perforation. On the inner portion under Descemet's membrane is the endothelium. This single cell layer is credited with pumping the water out of the cornea, thus assuring its clarity.

Corneal disease of any type is extremely serious, as permanent visual impairment may result. Corneal disease accounts for about 10 per cent of legal blindness in one or both eyes in the United States.

All corneal ulcers should have cultures taken and scrapings made for staining to determine cell type, bacteria or fungus type. The natural history of a corneal ulcer is increasing ulceration with hypopion (collection of pus in the anterior chamber). This progresses until Descemet's membrane ruptures or perforates. When this happens, the intraocular contents may spill out, and usually endophthalmitis (infection of all parts of the eye) ensues. Perforation is a surgical emergency that requires either a perforating corneal transplant or a conjunctival flap (pulling the conjunctiva down over the entire cornea and suturing it in place).

Ring ulcers (ulcers forming a ring in the periphery of the cornea) are found in staphylococcal infections, phlyctenular keratoconjunctivitis, or Mooren's ulcer. The last is an advancing ulcer with an undermining border leading to loss of the eye for which there is no known cause and as yet no good treatment.

The most common organisms in bacterial ulcers are pneumococci, beta hemolytic streptococci, *Pseudomonas aeruginosa* (*Bacillus pyocyaneus*), diplobacillus of Petit, and Friedlander's bacillus. Viral corneal ulcers are seen with smallpox, chickenpox, and herpes simplex (cold sore). Increasingly, fungi are causing ulceration: monilia, aspergilli, nocardia, and mucor. Facial nerve paralysis produces ulceration by drying of the cornea (exposure keratitis) due to lack of closure of the lids.

The corneal size may be smaller (microcornea)—10 mm or less in diameter—or bigger (megalocornea)—greater than 13.5 mm. These defects may or may not be associated with other ocular abnormalities. However, *buphthalmos* (enlarged cornea secondary to glaucoma in infants) is an outstanding exception. Rarely, the cornea instead of being round is cone-shaped with the apex extending outwardly (keratoconus). Over the years, the apex becomes thinner and thinner; this eventually leads to perforation. Contact lenses are used to give good vision and to prevent perforation. When contact lenses no longer give good vision, or when perforation is imminent, the abnormal cornea is replaced by another cornea (corneal transplant).

Arcus senilis is an opaque white or grayish ring just inside the limbus (demarcation between cornea and sclera). In young people it is called arcus juvenilis and has a fatty appearance. In the young it is significant as a sign of premature arteriosclerosis, but in the elderly it is of relatively little significance. It is not to be confused with band keratitis (a band-shaped opacification that extends across the exposed part of the cornea and contains calcium salts). Band keratitis is present in eyes that are degenerating or that have extensive disease, such as uveitis, or in parathyroid disorders.

Corneal dystrophies are progressive noninflammatory degenerative disorders that result in visual impairment. Many of these have a sex-linked genetic factor. Treatment frequently involves corneal transplantation.

Recurrent corneal erosion is a painful affliction occurring after some relatively insignificant injury of the corneal epithelium, usually with wood or a fingernail. The inciting injury may be several years in the past. The pain is usually greatest in the morning; however, it may awaken the patient from a sound sleep. The use of local anesthetic, while temporarily soothing, prevents healing. Corneal erosions may be associated with visual impairment.

SCLERA

The sclera is contiguous with the cornea. The white sclera is tough and opaque, composed of irregularly interlaced connective tissue fibers, and represents the posterior protective layer. It is much larger and of a different radius of curvature than the cornea. The sclera is perforated by arteries, veins, and nerves. The largest perforation is the *optic disc*, which is where the optic nerve passes through the cribriform plate (holes in the sclera allowing passage of the nerve fibers).

Episcleritis is an inflammation of the superficial layers of the sclera resulting in discomfort and pain which may appear sporadically. It is usually self-limited and easily treated with local steroids. *Scleritis* is inflammation of the deep layers. It is of long duration and often ends with perforation of the globe. Both of these afflictions produce localized redness, but in scleritis the red areas are larger and of a purplish shade. A staphyloma is a thinning or bulging of the sclera giving a bluish gray or violet color due to the underlying uveal tissue. A staphyloma may extend all the way around the globe, and in some cases it too will perforate.

UVEA

The uveal tract is divided into three parts: the iris, the ciliary body, and the choroid.

The iris determines the "color" of the eye by the amount of pigment it contains. The pupil is the variable aperture in the center of the iris. The size of the pupil is dependent upon the amount of incident light—the less light, the more widely dilated the pupil. The iris is the dividing structure between the anterior and posterior chambers of the eye. These chambers contain aqueous humor.

The ciliary body is composed of three muscles—circular, radial, and longitudinal—whose contractions allow for the increase or decrease of the anterior-posterior diameter of the lens (accommodation). This accommodative ability, which allows one to change from distant to near vision, is gradually lost with years until at age 50, accommodation is almost absent (presbyopia), necessitating bifocals.

The choroid is the posterior extension of the uvea and is largely composed of blood vessels whose function is the nourishment of the retina and elimination of its waste products.

Uveitis. Uveitis, the inflammation of the uveal tract, can be divided into two types: nongranulomatous, which is the most common, and granulomatous. Nongranulomatous uveitis is localized to the anterior portion (the ciliary body and iris). It has frequent exacerbations and remissions, the cause being unknown but thought to be due to an allergic autoimmune process (allergy to specific proteins contained within the eye and precipitated by some extraocular infection). After repetitive attacks, nongranulomatous uveitis may emerge into the granulomatous form. The onset is acute with severe pain and light sensitivity. Vision is blurred. On examination, very fine white dots (collection of cells) may be observed on the posterior surface of the cornea. The anterior chamber may contain protein cells and even blood clots. The pupil may be small and irregular, bound down to the lens by scar tissue (posterior synechia). Nodules may be present in the iris, and there may be protein in the vitreous as well.

Granulomatous uveitis has an insidious onset with minimal pain. Vision at first is only slightly blurred. The corneal flush (redness extending from the cornea into the conjunctival area) and photophobia (sensitivity to light) are mild by comparison with acute iridocyclitis (nongranulomatous uveitis). Large "mutton fat" keratitic precipitates (collection of large cells on the posterior surface of the cornea with a greasy appearance) are calling cards of granulomatous uveitis. Similar collection of cells may be present in the iris, forming nodules, and the pupil may be irregular due to posterior synechia (adhesion of the iris to the lens). When the choroid is involved, so also is the overlying retina. When viewed through the ophthalmoscope (lighted instrument for viewing the back of the eye) they have a ·yellowish white appearance with black speckling. The overlying vitreous is usually

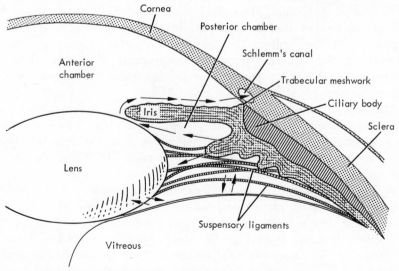

Figure 27. Production and flow of aqueous humor. (Adapted from *Alcon Patient Sketch Pad,* courtesy of Alcon Laboratories.)

hazy. The course is prolonged and the outlook is very poor. Granulomatous uveitis is found in association with toxoplasmosis, tuberculosis, sarcoid, sympathetic ophthalmia (uveitis occurring after a perforating injury of the fellow eye), and other diseases. Uveitis may be seen in association with a ruptured or leaking lens capsule, rheumatoid types of disorders, viral inflammations, Behçet's syndrome (aphthous ulcers and uveitis), and other bizarre disorders. The finding of an etiological agent and the treatment of it may result in a cure of the condition. However, in a high percentage of cases, treatment is ineffective, as no cause can be found.

GLAUCOMA

Glaucoma is a name signifying a complex of diseases that cause blindness by increased intraocular pressure. The one exception is so-called pseudoglaucoma or low-tension glaucoma, in which progressive field changes typical of glaucoma occur, but the tensions are not elevated. This increase in intraocular pressure must obviously be caused by either an increase in secretion (hypersecretion glaucoma, which is extremely rare if it occurs at all) or a resistance to outflow of the fluid.

The fluid (aqueous humor) is produced by the epithelium of the ciliary body which has a selective pattern of production. The aqueous passes around and nourishes the lens; some enters the anterior surface of the vitreous. The rest rushes through the pupil into the anterior chamber, then into the trabecular meshwork (the filtering structure or sieve and the entrance to the canal of Schlemm), and thence to the canal of Schlemm. From Schlemm's canal (an empty space for storage of aqueous that lies just peripheral to the cornea in the sclera which circles the limbus) the flow to the venous system is accomplished by the aqueous veins. In the process of transit, there is a constant exchange of nonelectrolytes and water in and out of the vessels of the iris stroma.

DIAGNOSTIC GLAUCOMA TESTS. *Ophthalmoscopy* is examination of the posterior segment of the eye with an ophthalmoscope, which is a self-illuminated series of lenses for viewing the posterior segment. Here one can detect degeneration of the optic nerve, by either change in the margin or loss of color.

A *field examination* is a monocular examination made with the patient looking at a screen placed perpendicularly to the line of sight. The area that is seen is plotted at one and two meters with various colored test objects ranging from 1 to 15 mm in size. In glaucoma, this test is used for the diagnosis of damage due to increased intraocular pressure. It is also used to follow the course of glaucoma and to determine the effectiveness of medical and surgical therapy.

Tonography is a method for measuring the intraocular pressure of the eye. The tonometer is a weighted device which presses on the cornea. Scale readings from the tonometer are extrapolated from charts to give a reading in millimeters of mercury. A single normal reading certainly does not rule out glaucoma. Conversely, neither does a single high reading mean the patient has glaucoma, but it should suggest the possibility of it.

A tonogram is produced by an electronic tonometer. A continuous recording over a period of four minutes produces a tracing from which an interpretation can be made as to the ability of fluid to flow out of the eye. This, in conjunction with the water loading test, is very diagnostic, when positive, of early open angle glaucoma. It is also useful in following the effect of therapy, as the coefficient of outflow (rate of flow of fluid out of the globe) will change and improve upon treatment.

Gonioscopy is examination of the angle of the eye by means of a special prismatic lens that optically allows one to overcome the corneal curvature and see the back of the cornea, the trabecular spaces, and the anterior surface of the iris. This allows the distinction of open angle from angle closure glaucoma.

In the _water loading test,_ the patient is asked to drink rapidly a quart of water. Tensions are taken prior to the drinking and every 15 minutes after the ingestion of the water. If open angle glaucoma is present, a marked to moderate increase in pressure will occur.

TYPES OF GLAUCOMA. In _primary glaucoma_ there is no antecedent ocular disease. There are three major forms of this disorder—namely, open angle glaucoma or chronic simple glaucoma, angle closure or acute glaucoma or narrow angle glaucoma, and infantile glaucoma or buphthalmos.

Open Angle Glaucoma. Open angle glaucoma (the root of the iris does not obstruct the trabecular meshwork) is the most common form; it is the so-called sneak thief of sight. Its onset is gradual and without pain. Symptoms are minimal until severe visual field constriction is present. The pressure at first may be normal except on rare occasions, but these occasions increase in frequency until finally the tension is abnormal at all times. The onset has been so gradual and insidious that the eye adapts to the increased pressure, and pain is not produced. When one is suspicious of open angle glaucoma, tension tests at different times of the day are important for diagnosis. Gonioscopy insures that the angle is open. Field test and ophthalmoscopy determine the degree of damage.

Although the pathology is poorly understood, it is believed that the degeneration of the collagen and elastic fibers of the trabecular meshwork cause the reduction of outflow.

The treatment in the cooperative patient is usually medical. Miotics (constrictors of the pupil) increase the outflow, and epinephrine normalizes the coefficient of outflow. There are now available many drugs that suppress the secretion of aqueous by the ciliary epithelium. Surgery is used only with recalcitrant patients or refractory glaucoma.

Angle Closure Glaucoma. Angle closure glaucoma (the root of the iris plugs the trabecular meshwork), in contradistinction to open angle glaucoma, is primarily a surgical disease. Acute glaucoma starts with the appearance of halos about lights. Redness of the eye, severe pain with associated nausea and vomiting, and loss of vision quickly follow. This rapid increase in intraocular pressure is caused by the rapid complete blockage of the trabecular meshwork with the iris root. Without prompt treatment, a blind painful eye rapidly ensues.

Subacute or chronic angle closure glaucoma is a disease that may or may not have symptoms. It progresses slowly by permanent iris adhesions to the posterior surface of the cornea closing off the trabecular meshwork. The occasional attacks may cause blurring of vision or halos about light, but rarely pain in the eye. Eventually this leads to an acute attack of glaucoma after most of the trabecular meshwork has been permanently closed. During this time, the course has been similar to open angle glaucoma, as witnessed by the insidious loss of visual field.

The cause is an extremely narrow space between the iris and the posterior surface of the cornea. On dilatation of the pupil by emotion or darkness, the already compromised angle is closed. Physiological iris bombé (pupil held against the lens) occurs when there is a wide margin of contact between the lens and the iris. The aqueous has a difficult time seeping through the pupil and tends to push the peripheral iris forward, closing the angle. With increased size of the lens there is further displacement of the iris forward, which is further accentuated by accommodation. Precipitating factors may be severe emotional tension, watching television at night in a darkened room, and other unknown factors.

Sometimes acute glaucoma is difficult to differentiate from secondary glaucoma in that the anterior chamber is filled with protein and cells, some of which may be deposited on the posterior surface of the cornea simulating keratitic precipitates (collection of large mononuclear cells on the posterior surface of the cornea). However, in acute glaucoma, the pupil is mid-dilated, the tension is hard, and the cornea is edematous, so that it is difficult to see beyond the anterior chamber.

If the attack is of recent origin (24 to 36 hours), a small surgical hole in the periphery of the iris is frequently sufficient for normalizing tension. This allows the aqueous to enter the anterior chamber and break up the physiological iris bombé. However, if the attack is of greater duration or if gonioscopy shows extensive closure of the angle, then a filtering operation (a hole in the sclera allowing a communication between the anterior chamber and the subconjunctival space) is necessary. When the tension is not lowered by medical therapy, surgery must be performed. This is undesirable, for surgery in the presence of an elevated tension may produce malignant glaucoma.

Malignant glaucoma is a marked postoperative tension rise with the iris and lens in contact with the cornea. It only occurs in surgery of angle closure glaucoma with an elevated tension. Dilatation of the pupil may be helpful in treatment, but the lens, with or without intentional vitreous loss, may have to be extracted.

Infantile Glaucoma. Infantile glaucoma occurs within the first three years of life. One of the first signs is tearing, another is photophobia (sensitivity to light). As the pressure increases, the corneas become larger (buphthalmos). Diagnosis should be made with the patient under general anesthesia so that adequate tension measurements may be taken. The treatment is primarily surgical. An incision is made in the trabecular meshwork (goniotomy) under direct visualization with the gonioscopic lens. Sometimes perforation through the sclera is performed (goniopuncture).

Secondary Glaucoma. Secondary glaucomas are those in which preexisting ocular disorders are present. They may be produced by pupillary block or plugging of the trabecular meshwork, or they may be secondary to cataract surgery.

Pupillary block occurs when the lens is either dislocated or swollen and plugs the pupil, thus preventing aqueous from entering the anterior chamber. Uveitis causes another type of pupillary block; the iris at the pupil becomes bound down to the lens due to inflammation.

The trabecular meshwork may be plugged by *blood,* as in trauma or surgery, *pigment* secondary to degeneration of the pigment epithelium, *lens capsule* (pseudoexfoliation of the lens capsule), *leaking lens substance,* or *increased protein* in the aqueous from uveitis.

In cataract surgery the vitreous may bulge forward and plug the pupil, causing pupillary block glaucoma. When the anterior chamber has not reformed after extraction of the cataract, the iris may become adherent to the posterior surface of the cornea (peripheral anterior synechia). The trabecular meshwork may also be plugged by an ingrowth of conjunctival tissue into the anterior chamber. This produces a highly incurable glaucoma.

RETINA

The retina is the photographic film of the eye. The rest of the structures exist only to protect, to nourish, or to focus the rays of light on it. The retina is the posterior portion of the inner tunic. The inner tunic of the eye starts as the posterior epithelial layers lining the under-surface of the iris. The pigment layer determines the color of the iris. The pigment epithelium then extends over the ciliary processes, producing the aqueous humor. From here the epithelium extends over the pars plana (that portion of the ciliary body closer to the back of the eye). At the ora serrata (junction of pars plana and retina) the anterior layer becomes the retina and the posterior layer the pigment epithelium, which rests on the choroid, where it is said to be the energy storage area (battery) for the rods and cones.

Since the retina and the optic nerve are outgrowths of the brain itself, they do not regenerate when injured. The macula, which is the size of the head of a common pin, and specifically the fovea centralis (greatest concentration of cones), is the only portion of the retina that has discrete or completely clear vision (20/20). The light rays pass through the clear innermost portions of the retina (excluding the opaque blood vessels on the surface of the retina) to the outermost portion, the rods and cones. These are light receptors, which convert incident light rays or energy (photons) to nerve impulses by photochemical means. These nervous impulses are modified by the body of the retina (the inner portion), which is a complex network of nuclei and connections for augmenting, suppressing, and coordinating these nervous impulses, which are then passed to the ganglion cells at the innermost portion of the retina.

Long fibers or axons extend from these ganglion cells, forming the inner fiber layer of the retina. These fibers funnel through the optic disc to form the optic nerve.

On the surface of the retina are blood vessels that undergo changes in various disease states. In the early stages of hypertension there are narrowing and irregularity in the caliber of the arterioles. In the very far advanced disease there may be hemorrhages, exudates (collections of cells), and edema. In the terminal stages, edema of the optic disc takes place. There is a gradual reduction in the color of the arterioles in hardening of the arteries (arteriosclerosis). When very severe, the arteries become occluded and totally white.

Hypertension and arteriosclerotic changes are present in the veins and arterioles in diabetes. The major change, however, is new vessel formation. At first small outpocketings (microaneurysms) from the blood vessels are noted. The veins becomes dilated, then exudates and hemorrhages follow. The hemorrhages finally become so severe as to completely block vision or cause production of scar tissue (glial tissue) with new vessel growth extending into the vitreous. This, in turn, pulls the retina away from the choroid (retinal detachment) into the vitreous space with resultant loss of vision.

Occlusion of the central retinal artery causes immediate painless loss of vision. If blood flow is not restored within 20 to 30 minutes, blindness follows. On the other hand, occlusion of the central retinal vein results in backup of blood into the rest of the eye. Visual loss comes slowly, and is caused by the multitude of hemorrhages, some even into the vitreous. Approximately one-fifth of these patients develop near normal vision after venous occlusion.

DEGENERATIVE DISEASES OF THE RETINA. *Retinitis pigmentosa* is a bilateral degenerative genetically determined disease rarely associated with hypogenitalism, obesity, and deafness. The onset is in early life; it is more common among men than women. Loss of night vision (nyctalopia) is the first symptom. Gradual progressive constriction of the visual field eventually produces legal blindness. Degeneration of the rods with overgrowth of scar tissue and migration of the pigment about vessels is the basic defect. The disease process starts at the equator and moves toward the disc and macula. Although 20/20 vision may be preserved, people are incapacitated by their restricted visual field, which prevents orientation in their surrounding visual space. To date, there is no good treatment. Macula degeneration results in a loss of central precise vision. Depending upon the severity, vision may drop to counting fingers. A full peripheral field, however, is maintained. Changes in the macula are seen more frequently with drüsen (yellowish colloidal tissue located in the posterior pole in the choroid). Disciform degeneration, central serrous retinopathy, senile macula degeneration, heredodegeneration of the macula, are all disorders producing macula loss with slightly different clinical pictures. Common as they are, the cause of these is not known, nor is their treatment.

DETACHMENT OF THE RETINA. Separation or detachment of the retina occurs when the retina comes off the choroid and floats in the vitreous space. Since the choroid is the nutritive source of the rods and cones, any prolonged detachment results in permanent visual loss after reattachment. The exact amount of this loss is a function of time. If the macula is off for more than one week, good central vision is doubtful. Detachment of the retina is caused by either tumors (malignant or cysts), fluid underneath the retina without hole formation as in toxemia of pregnancy, glomerulonephritis, or strands of vitreous attached to the retina which contract and pull it off, as in diabetes.

Detachment of the retina from unknown cause (idiopathic) is not uncommon. In idiopathic detachment, holes occur in the periphery of the retina, either at the site of cystoid (breakdown in the peripheral retinal structure) degeneration, by vitreous traction, or from a cause unknown. Through these holes vitreous flows, stripping the retina from the choroid much as one steams old wallpaper off a wall. If the detachment extends into the macula area, it is very important to insure rapid retinal reattachment, or all central vision will be lost. The method of reattachment is to locate all the holes in the retina and close them by means of diathermy (heat machine), applied either via light (photocoagulator) or by electronic machine. Pieces of plastic are sewn into the sclera over the holes, pushing the choroid into contact with the retina. Subretinal fluid is released by puncture, and the retina settles back in a high percentage of cases. Approximately 60 per cent of people with detachment in one eye will develop it in the other eye. Untreated retinal detachments usually result in blindness, secondary glaucoma with pain, or phthisis bulbi (death of an eye) with resultant enucleation (removal of the eye surgically).

In adults, tumors producing retinal detachment are either metastatic (spread from other organs of the body) or malignant melanomas. Malignant melanomas can occur anywhere in the uveal tract. They almost never occur in Negroes. Initially, they cause no symptoms. When the tumor is of sufficient size to produce glaucoma or visual changes due to pushing forward of the retina, patients seek treatment which requires enucleation. The tumor may extend outside of the globe or spread by the veins to other organs. With malignant melanoma there is increased pigmentation in the iris. Metastatic tumors to the eye are less pigmented and occur in the posterior pole. Not infrequently the fellow eye is involved.

A retinoblastoma is a malignant tumor of the retina itself. There is a strong genetic factor. Most of these malignant tumors occur prior to the age of five and are frequently bilateral. The tumor usually arises in the posterior portion of the retina and gives a yellow color to the pupil (cat's eye). If only one eye is involved with this highly malignant tumor, it is removed. However, if both eyes are involved, the treatment of choice is enucleation of the more severely involved and treatment of the less severely involved eye by x-ray, intravenous or intra-arterial antimetabolites (anticancer drugs), diathermy, and photocoagulation.

Retrolental fibroplasia can mimic retinoblastoma. Retrolental fibroplasia is almost always a disease of both retinas found in children whose birth weights are generally under five pounds. In the past, it was associated with an excessive amount of oxygen. Certainly decreasing the amounts of oxygen within the incubator of children with birth weights less than five pounds has markedly lowered the incidence of this disorder. The disease starts with edema of the retina. This is followed by dilatation and tortuosity of the vessels with detachment of the retina peripherally. In later stages, scar tissue replaces the retina. This contracts, giving total detachment of the retina lying behind the lens. A rare disorder that mimics retinoblastoma and retrolental fibroplasia is persistent primary hyperplastic vitreous, which develops during the uterine existence of the fetus.

Coats' disease is a rare disorder mostly affecting young, healthy boys.

Usually unilateral, it is formed by a hemorrhagic exudative mass with dilated vessels, inflammatory cells, tissue debris, and cholesterol.

Color blindness is probably the most common affliction of the retina. Color blindness is classified by the perception of two of the basic colors (dichromatic) or one of the three basic colors (monochromatic). Males outnumber females ten to one; approximately 4 per cent of the male population has some degree of it. There is no danger to sight. There is no pathological change that can be demonstrated. It is present from birth, and no treatment is of any value.

LENS

The lens is a biconvex relatively transparent avascular structure. It is suspended between the ciliary body by delicate connective tissue (zonules), and posteriorly, the vitreous holds it in place. The lens in youth is plastic, clear, and transparent with a tendency to assume a spherical shape. As years pass, the malleability of the lens decreases. The lens is the other major refracting surface of the eye and is the only one that is movable, thus accounting for accommodation. Its dimensions are 9 mm in diameter and 5 mm in thickness; the latter is the anterior-posterior diameter, which varies with accommodation. Its layered protein structure is increased over the years by continuous fiber production by the equatorial lens epithelium. This epithelium starts slightly behind the equator under the semipermeable lens capsule to cover the entire anterior portion of the lens. Through this capsule comes the nutrition from the aqueous humor, which surrounds the lens except at its most posterior aspect. Here the lens rests within the anterior surface of the vitreous.

CATARACTS. Cataracts are opacifications of the lens. They may be congenital, toxic, developmental, senile, or traumatic. The site of the opacity determines the name (for example, nucleus–nuclear cataract). To date there is no way of preventing cataracts or impeding their progress once they develop. Certain drugs, diseases, and chemicals will produce them, and intraocular inflammation favors their development.

When a cataract is of sufficient density to interfere with the activities of the individual, the lens is removed surgically. A cataract extraction may be intracapsular or extracapsular. Extracapsular cataract extraction occurs when the anterior surface is removed and the lens substance is expressed from the capsule and out of the eye. The posterior membrane remains. This often necessitates the further surgical procedure of incising the thickened posterior capsule. In intracapsular extraction, the entire lens is removed.

In the aphakic eye (eye minus its lens), a lens of equivalent power is placed in the spectacles. This magnifies and moves objects closer to the patient. Gaze through the periphery of the spectacle lens is markedly distorted. Under these circumstances, it is not wise to operate on a cataract until the other eye has shown marked progression of its lens opacity so that it soon will be ready for extraction. If the patient is willing to wear a contact lens, binocular vision can sometimes be achieved in monocular aphakia. Contact lenses in these instances minimize the peripheral distortion and decrease the magnification sufficiently to allow fusion.

VITREOUS

The vitreous is a highly viscous, colloidal, collagenous material that maintains the form of the globe. When the fibers coalesce, they produce spots (floaters) that wander across the field of vision. Cholesterol soaps may infiltrate the vitreous and also cause floaters, but these also are of no great significance. At times the vitreous pulls away from the retina (detachment of the vitreous), producing spots. These spots demand that the periphery of the retina be checked in order to rule out retinal hole formation and impending detachment of the retina.

OPTIC NERVE HEAD

The optic disc is the only portion of the posterior pole where rods or cones are not present. This, therefore, forms a blind spot that normally is found in the field of vision. At the optic disc, the retinal nerve fibers pour in to form the optic nerve. The optic nerve is an outpocketing of the brain and has the same coverings as the brain. There is a direct extension of cerebrospinal fluid along the bottom of the optic nerve. Therefore, infections or increased pressure of the cerebrospinal system are transmitted to the nerve head. Swelling of the nerve head may be due to increased intracranial pressure (papilledema) or localized inflammation (papillitis). The physical findings of these two conditions ophthalmoscopically make them difficut to distinguish from each other, but history, field examination, and other neurological findings will help make the diagnosis. In optic atrophy, the disc changes from an orange-red to a white or gray-green color. This may be caused by toxic substances such as lead, arsenic, or quinine, increased intracranial pressure, demyelinating disease (for example, multiple sclerosis), trauma, glaucoma, and many other disorders.

REHABILITATION

The principles of rehabilitation are fairly constant for the various visual disabilities; the specifics will vary somewhat, depending on whether the individual is congenitally blind or was adventitiously blinded, and on whether he is totally blind or partially sighted. The individual who was born blind faces the tremendous task of learning how to get along in a sighted world. The person who becomes blinded at a later age faces the equally tremendous task of switching from a sighted adjustment to a sightless one. Each type of blindness poses its own adaptive problems. The partially sighted individual may respond more slowly to certain rehabilitative procedures than the one who is totally blind, because there is a tendency to cling to old—and now often unsatisfactory—sighted ways of doing things. For this reason, the partially sighted individual in a rehabilitation center may be required to wear occluders that cut out all vision and force him to learn new methods of travel, communication, self-care, and so on.

Individuals classified as blind, and eligible for services as such, may have some degree of vision ranging from light perception through motion perception to travel vision. The definition of legal blindness varies somewhat in the United States, but the usual definition is central visual acuity of 20/200 or less in the better eye with correction, or a field defect in which the widest diameter of the visual field subtends an angle no greater than 20 degrees.

As with other disabilities, the goals of education and rehabilitation should include acceptance of, or psychological adjustment to, the disorder, social adjustment to family and community, self-confidence, maximum function and self-sufficiency, and a meaningful role in life as a worker, homemaker, student, and so on, whenever possible. Blindness poses many complications and limitations for the individual; on the other hand, the rehabilitation potential of the blind is amazing. This is reflected in the wide range of skilled, professional, and managerial occupations in which blinded individuals have been successful.

The following areas are basic to the rehabilitation process:

Mobility. This would include physical conditioning, developing good spatial orientation, teaching the use of other senses, and learning a method of travel. For those who require guidance in travel the alternatives are the use of human guides, dog guides, or canes. The use of human guides as the major form of travel is highly limiting and therefore not too satisfactory. The choice between a dog and a cane depends upon a variety of factors, including the availability of training (both require training), living arrangements, motivation, cost, and so on. In either case, virtually complete independence in travel is possible for the well-trained and well-motivated individual.

Communication. With the possible exception of some partially sighted, the blinded individual should learn to read and write Braille. The ability to use a typewriter is invaluable. Even the congenitally blind individual can learn handwriting, at least to sign his own name. Use of talking books and recording equipment, use of sighted readers, and ability to use a dial telephone are important aspects of communication.

Techniques of daily living. Included here would be various aspects of self-care, housekeeping and use of household devices, use of tools, recreational activities, and so forth.

Optical aids. Special lenses may increase functional vision in certain cases of partial sight. Many special devices such as Braille watches, slide rules, adapted insulin syringes, sewing aids, measuring devices, and tools can be extremely helpful.

A wide range of professional services—medical, psychological, social, vocational, educational, and recreational—is needed in the rehabilitation process. Where blindness is complicated by another disability such as a hearing loss or mental retardation, special rehabilitation procedures are needed. Special classes, schools, and rehabilitation centers are available, but not in the amount needed. National agencies such as the American Foundation for the Blind and the National Society for the Prevention of Blindness are available for technical information and educational services. Many communities provide a wide variety of services through public and private agencies for the visually disabled. In each state, through the cooperation of the United States Vocational Rehabilitation Administration and the state agency for the blind, a broad range of rehabilitation services is available for blinded individuals who may thus be helped to enter gainful employment. Welfare services, special taxation provisions, and veterans services are also available.

XII

NEOPLASMS

Over the past several decades, cancer has assumed an increasingly important role as a cause of mortality and disability among civilized people. This last phrase is of some significance inasmuch as many forms of cancer appear to be far more common among the more affluent societies than among primitive people. This may be due in part to the constantly increasing life-span of man in countries where adequate public health advances have occurred, and due in part to the relative lack of statistical data among primitive peoples. Nevertheless, cancer has been found in all population groups where studies have been conducted. In areas where the life-span is relatively short due to malnutrition, prevalence of infectious disease, or other socioeconomic factors, cancer is not an important health problem. It is an unhappy paradox that as public health improves, the problem of cancer increases. Today, in the United States, as well as in many other countries, cancer is the second leading cause of death, being exceeded only by cardiovascular diseases.

Since 50 per cent or more of cancer is found in persons over 65 years of age, the importance of age in the changing significance of cancer as a health problem becomes apparent. In this age group, too, other illnesses associated with chronic disability become more frequent, thus intensifying the problem of health and rehabilitation.

Another aspect of this problem comes to light when we consider the

By PETER J. MOZDEN, M.D., Assistant Professor of Surgery, Boston University School of Medicine; Cancer Coordinator, Boston University Medical Center, Boston, Massachusetts.

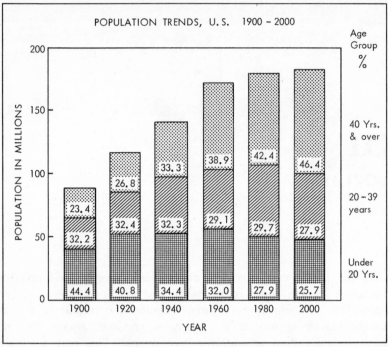

Figure 28. The changing population patterns in the U.S. It is noted that the age group 40-plus years, in which most cancer occurs, has become the predominant group, almost doubling its percentage within the over-all population in the space 100 years. (*Source of Data:* U.S. Bureau of the Census and the American Cancer Society.)

age group 25 to 65, our working population. About 45 per cent of all cancer occurs in these more productive years, causing serious economic loss.

United States Public Health statistics reveal that in 1955 some 500,000 persons in this country developed cancer, and some 250,000 persons died of this disease. Another way of looking at this information, however, is to realize that each year, in the United States, a quarter of a million people will have survived their initial encounter with the disease cancer; the majority of these will remain cured, while the remainder will succumb to recurrence of the disease at a later date. In both groups, however, an element of disability will often be present, since even curative surgical or radiotherapeutic procedures may result in the loss of a limb or radical alteration of some body function.

In brief, then, as the health of our nation has increased, cancer has assumed a significant role in planning our total health economy. It is estimated that in our lifetimes, one in every five men and one in every four women will develop cancer. While the data presented have been based on United States Public Health figures, it should be remembered that this is a world-wide problem, and wherever the standard of health care roughly parallels that in this country, essentially parallel problems exist. This has been true of England, Wales, Scandinavia, and many other European and some Far Eastern countries, where adequate data have been obtained.

THE MEANING OF CANCER

Cancer is currently thought of, not as one disease, but rather as a group of diseases having basic similarities in terms of development and effect upon the host, and also having separate distinctive characteristics that may result in quite different outlooks or prognoses for the person harboring the disease. Thus, over a hundred types of cancer are defined today, each with its own life history, and each in turn acted upon by the host's resistance to a greater or lesser degree. Not all types of cancer have the same meaning. Thus, *basal cell* cancer of the skin, one of the most frequent types of skin cancer, is almost always kept in a localized form within the patient, so that it can be cured in most instances; whereas *melanoma*, another form of skin cancer, fortunately far less common, is often difficult to eradicate even when treated early. The biological nature of *lung cancer*, which is increasing rampantly, or of *stomach cancer*, which appears to be on the decrease,

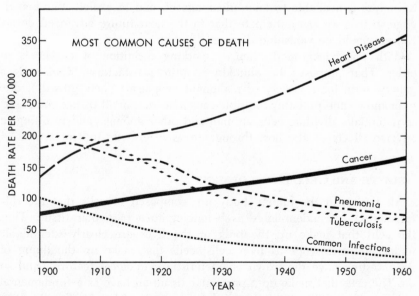

Figure 29. Relative change in the importance of cancer as a cause of death in the United States. It is now the second leading cause of death in the United States (1960). (*Source: Vital Statistics*, U.S. Bureau of the Census and the American Cancer Society.)

is such that we can predict with accuracy that relatively few patients will be cured, despite treatment as soon as symptoms become manifest. The outcome for *breast cancer*, on the other hand, is difficult to predict. The biological nature of this type of cancer is such that cases are frequently seen where the history is of short duration, and yet the cancerous growth is advancing rapidly and cannot be stopped by currently available therapeutic means. In other instances, a patient will have a cancer of several years duration or a growth that appears far advanced, and yet many such patients are alive and free of disease five years or more after standard therapies are employed.

Among this brief spectrum of cancer types, cancer of the cervix, or "mouth of the womb," deserves special mention. Here is a type of cancer in which the time factor, or early stage of the disease, may be all important. This very common type of malignant growth in women is usually seen only when the disease is at least moderately far advanced. In this situation only about half of these women can be cured. If the disease is far advanced (Stage IV), very few are still curable. On the other hand, a relatively simple screening technique, based on the Papanicolaou vaginal smear test ("Pap" smear), is capable of detecting this cancer at the earliest stage of its development (*in situ* cancer). At this stage, cancer of the cervix is at least 99 per cent curable! Thus, in this form of cancer, we are able to appreciate clearly the importance of the time factor in relation to disease curability; a simple and practical technique is available to take advantage of, and to exploit, this knowledge so that we can anticipate that in the near future advanced cervix cancer should be vanishing disease.

With this background, then, a working definition of cancer is in order. That proposed by Shimkin is quite satisfactory: "Cancer is a generic term for a variety of malignant neoplasms (new growth), due to unknown and probably multiple causes, arising in all tissues composed of potentially dividing cells, in man and other animals, and resulting in adverse effects on the host through invasive growth and metastases." [1]

GROWTH AND CELL DEVELOPMENT

All tissues in the human body are composed of cells that are differentiated and indentifiable as belonging to a particular tissue. Thus the cells that make up the bulk of the liver are clearly identifiable under the microscope as liver cells; cells that make up the lining of the intestine have their own characteristic cytological features, and so on. The cells that make up a particular tissue all have as a fundamental property the ability to divide and form similar "daughter" cells. It is

[1] M. B. Shimkin, "Epidemiology of Cancer," Symposium on Cancer, *Modern Medicine*, 28:7 (April 1, 1960), 81-87.

through such an ordered and "disciplined" system of cellular division that tissue or body bulk is maintained and that further growth and development occur, or cease, as the need may be. This ordered and biologically regulated process of cell division is called *mitosis*. Through this process, one cell becomes two, each a mirror image of the other, with an exactly equal complement of cytoplasm, protein content, chromosomes, and so forth. We simply do not know the mechanisms that bring about this orderly growth, although this is a fundamental life process. Therefore, it is no surprise that we possess even less knowledge about those mechanisms or stimuli that cause a disordered growth pattern of cells, which appears to be essentially what cancer represents. The cancerous process is one in which the cells appear to have "escaped" any regulatory or inhibitory influence, and are capable in time of autonomous growth, *even away from the tissue of origin*. Such independent growth at distant sites is called a *metastasis,* and this represents one of the primary ways in which cancer injures or even destroys the host. The damage caused by uninhibited and rapid growth of cancer cells in multiple tissues and organs of the body can readily be imagined.

THEORIES ON THE CAUSES OF CANCER

What is it that stimulates an apparently normal cell to become cancerous? The theories of cancerogenesis are many. Only a brief discussion of the most prevalent theories will be attempted here. We can begin by reiterating that there is probably no single cause of all cancer. Further, it is likely that ancillary factors or perhaps "predispositions" due to heredity, a preceding illness, or other unknown factors may play a role in the development of cancer in a given individual. Thus, age, sex, heredity, and environment have all been shown to be linked in the chain of events that may ultimately conclude with the establishment of a clinical cancer state.

THE CHRONIC IRRITATION THEORY. For many years chronic irritation has been incriminated as a primary factor in the development of some forms of cancer. For example, pipe smokers are much more likely to develop cancer of the lip than the individual who does not use a pipe. This fact is strengthened by the observations that when cancer of the lip does develop in pipe smokers, almost without exception the lesion appears in the area where the pipe is habitually held between the teeth or gums. Here it is felt that the irritative effect of long-continued heat, perhaps coupled with the rubbing of the pipe stem, is the operating mechanism.

Another example may be cited. A custom called *kangri* in Kashmir, and *kairo* in Japan, consists of holding a heating pot against the abdominal wall. Cancer of the skin of the abdominal wall is quite common in this population group, which is quite startling when one considers that cancer of the abdominal skin is most unusual in all other populations.

TRAUMA THEORY. Traditionally, trauma is often referred to as a possible cause of cancer. Much concern has been caused among women that a blow to the breast may lead to cancer, or that accidental trauma in a body part may subsequently lead to cancer in that region. Suffice it to say that a cause and effect relationship here has been most difficult to establish. In most cases cited, examination of the facts does not sustain the claimed relationships. Often the trauma calls attention to a mass that was already present. It is extremely unlikely, then, that malignancy may follow a single trauma.

On the other hand, the relationship between cancer and long standing and repeated trauma is somewhat clearer. Cancer is occasionally seen on the lips in certain occupational groups, such as cobblers or carpenters, who characteristically hold nails and other sharp objects between their teeth and have a recurrent history of cuts and ulcerations in this area. Cancer of the skin has also developed in scars resulting from severe trauma or burns, usually many years after the episode causing the scar.

THEORY OF HEREDITY. There is abundant evidence that the development of some malignant growths in experimental animals is influenced by hereditary factors. In humans, however, noncontroversial evidence establishing this relationship is scant. Nevertheless, a few neoplasms in man have been shown to have strong hereditary factors, such as *retinoblastoma,* a malignant growth of the retina of the eye, and *xeroderma pigmentosum,* a form of skin cancer.

Certain precancerous conditions such as *polyposis* of the colon tend to occur in more than one member of a family group. A high percentage of these polyps, benign at first, eventually develop into frank carcinoma. It is customary, therefore, upon discovering and treating this lesion in one member of a family, to screen carefully and continue to observe other members of the family. In other forms of cancer, such as breast, uterine, rectal, and leukemia, the evidence suggests that hereditary tendencies occur, but here the relationship is not as clear.

THE VIRUS THEORY. The theory that viruses are causative agents in the development of cancer has enjoyed several waves of popularity. Currently this theory is on the upsurge again, and with modern techniques such as the electron microscope, which permits visualization of some virus particles for the first time, significant new positive evidence is being gathered. There is no question but that viruses are capable of producing a wide variety of malignant tumors in experimental animals such as the mouse, rat, chicken, other fowl species, rabbits, frogs, and fishes. A recently discovered virus, the "polyoma virus" of Stewart and Eddy, has been found capable of producing over 20 malignant tumors in different experimental animals, and it is exciting to note that the type and form of malignancy produced vary from animal to animal. Here, then, is one virus capable of producing, in experimental animals, many of the diverse malignant growths whose human parallel is well known.

To this date, however, not a single case of human cancer has been established as being virus-caused; this has been frustrating, since most investigators feel that at least some human cancers have a virus as the etiological agent. With time and diligence, much that is observed in laboratories with experimental animals can also be proven to occur in other species, including man. It will be surprising indeed, if in the near future some forms of cancer in man are not shown to be caused by virus. For the first time viruslike particles have been shown to be present in several human neoplasms, such as leukemia, Hodgkin's disease, and rectal polyps.

It would appear, then, that the virus theory of cancer is now on a firm footing and that significant developments in this area will be forthcoming.

THEORY OF ENVIRONMENTAL CARCINOGENS. One of the most fruitful fields in cancer research has been the study of the factors in man's environment that may play a role, dominant or secondary, in the development of malignant disease. Industry has learned many painful lessons from epidemiological studies. These recorded observations started in 1775 with Sir Percival Pott in England, who noted the high incidence of cancer of the scrotum among "chimney sweeps" and correctly attributed this to soot. It was customary for young boys to be employed as chimney sweeps, lowering themselves through a soot-laden chimney and thus coming in contact with masses of soot, which clung to their skin and was most difficult to cleanse or wash away, especially in the scrotal area. Many of these individuals, sometimes years later, developed cancer of the scrotal skin, a rare type of cancer in the remainder of the population. Industry now recognizes many carcinogenic hazards; as these are made known, rigid measures are instituted.

One of the classic examples of industrial or occupational cancer is the story of cancer of the lung in miners in the Erz Mountains of Europe. Silver was first discovered in these mines early in the sixteenth century. For several hundred years it was appreciated that a disease of the lungs was a characteristic trademark of many of these miners, and that this disease, when it occurred, almost always terminated fatally. After some 300 years it was finally shown that this illness was actually lung cancer, arising in the bronchi. Extended investigations were then undertaken to track down the carcinogenic agent in the environment of the mines that was responsible for the high incidence of lung cancer. It was soon appreciated that miners elsewhere did not show the same high incidence of pulmonary cancer. These mines had been worked at various times for different ores, starting with silver, but also including nickel, copper, iron, bismuth, arsenic, cobalt, and radium. Each was suspect in turn until, finally, it was demonstrated that inhalation of radium particles was the carcinogenic factor.

Nowadays, stringent rules are employed to protect workers against this industrial hazard. Even with the current increased activity in mining uranium ores, no case of lung cancer has yet been reported in the United States among workers with radioactive substances.

The list of carcinogenic agents in our environment is a long one. Arsenic can cause skin and lung cancer in workers exposed chronically to these agents; the tar and oil industries are keenly aware of the carcinogenic substances present in these basic raw materials. Creosote oil, anthracene oil, and carbon black have all been incriminated as causing cancer of the lung; and various radioactive chemicals have caused leukemia and bone cancer.

Even the rays of the sun may be carcinogenic; witness the comparatively very high incidence of skin cancer among North American cowboys, Argentine gauchos, and sailors everywhere. Skin cancer, if it develops in these individuals, characteristically occurs primarily in those areas of the body that are habitually exposed to sunlight.

A variety of agents, then, has been shown to be potential causes of cancer. These vary from factors brought about by cultural customs and habits, to living organisms (viruses) capable of causing fundamental changes in body cells on a submicroscopic level, to physical agents in our environment that we accept as part of the process of daily living, to a wide variety of inorganic and organic chemicals present in our foods, our fuels, and in many of the basic raw materials that are vital to a highly organized industrial society.

TUMORS, BENIGN AND MALIGNANT

In the original and general sense, a tumor can mean any localized swelling, be it caused by inflammation, new growth, or any other cause. For our purposes this ancient usage of the term must be discarded, and we shall imply specifically that a tumor is synonymous with a neoplasm or "new growth." A tumor, then, is an abnormal mass of tissue, the growth of which exceeds and is uncoordinated with that of the normal tissues (after R. A. Willis). It should be appreciated at the outset that tumor does not necessarily mean a cancer. Another way to state this is to say that tumors may be benign or malignant. Only the malignant tumors represent a form of cancer.

BENIGN TUMORS

What are benign tumors, and how do these differ from the malignant variety? In brief, a benign tumor is an abnormal mass of tissue, which may develop virtually anywhere in the body, is not associated with a lethal potential except in exceptional instances, and is characterized by certain gross and microscopic features that enable a surgeon or pathologist to distinguish it from its lethal counterpart, the malignant tumor or cancer. Very common examples of benign tumors are the soft, spongelike growths, referred to as *lipomas,* that occur as moundlike swelling beneath the skin of certain individuals, and are microscopically shown to be composed of adipose tissue. Sometimes these tumors may occur within the chest or abdominal cavity, and their benign nature cannot be ascertained except by surgical removal and histological diagnosis.

In general, benign tumors tend to be circumscribed and, even when multiple, can be clearly delineated from the surrounding tissues. This is in sharp contrast to a malignant tumor—that is, a cancer, which often tends to invade neighboring tissues with no plane of separation between the malignant growth and adjacent structures. Benign tumors, then, tend to be circumscribed and do not invade. Under the microscope, the benign nature of these tumors is readily apparent to a trained pathologist. The individual cells tend to be uniform and symmetrical, the ratio of the cytoplasm to the nucleus tends to fall within normal ranges, and the cells are well differentiated—that is to say, are clearly identifiable as to the tissue from which the tumor arose. Benign tumors, although capable of rapid growth, do not metastasize; they are not capable of autonomous growth at a site distant from the point of origin. This is a most important consideration that clearly separates benign tumors from the malignant variety, which sooner or later may develop the ability to metastasize and destroy the host.

Benign tumors often cause symptoms, chiefly because of location or size, whereby pressure may be brought to bear in a nearby organ, producing pain or other symptoms. Benign tumors may grow to enormous size before they become evident and the patient seeks medical attention. For example, some benign cystic tumors of the ovary may closely resemble a full-term pregnancy when first seen. Nevertheless, the removal of such tumors is highly successful, usually resulting in a cure.

As already noted, some benign tumors, chiefly because of their location, may harbor a lethal potential. For example, benign tumors of the brain, spinal cord, or within the chest cavity, by their gradual enlargement and expansion, may place intolerable pressure on vital structures. If not removed early, they may produce a severe deficit, or even cause loss of life. In these instances, severe disability may follow in the form of hemiplegia or loss of form or function in some part of the body. Except for these instances, however, the disability factor associated with benign tumors is quite low; if troublesome, these tumors can usually be removed with a high degree of success.

MALIGNANT TUMORS

When one uses the term "malignant tumor," one really means a type of cancer. Perhaps the expression "cancerous tumor" would be more accurate, although physicians have learned to avoid using the term "cancer" in discussing a patient's disease with him, because of the serious and lethal connotation that the word has come to have, often unnecessarily, as any physician who treats cancer knows.

Malignant tumors also are abnormal masses of tissue, although here almost all similarity with a benign tumor ends. Certain gross and histological features help to define a tumor mass as "malignant." Even grossly, a malignant tumor often imparts to the examiner the appearance of rapid growth. Surrounding structures are invaded, so that the malignant tumor often cannot be removed except by also resecting considerable amounts of normal tissues or structures to which it is attached. If a malignant tumor arises in a peripheral location, such as a muscle or extremity, this lends itself to successful removal even though a large muscle mass or even an extremity needs to be sacrificed. However, when a malignant tumor arises in a body cavity such as the chest or abdomen, invades, and is inseparable from, surrounding structures such as lung tissue, loops of intestine, or major blood vessels, then the problem can be quite formidable.

Under the microscope, too, malignant tumors have histological features that permit a pathologist to state with a high degree of accuracy that the tumor is of the malignant variety. Evidence of rapid cell growth and division is usually present in the form of numerous mitotic figures, which indicate that rapid cellular division is occurring. Microscopic evidence of invasion of small blood vessels or surrounding capsules may be evident, thus revealing the true nature of the tumor. Various degrees of dedifferentiation are present—that is, the individual cells begin to lose their original identity. This factor can often be used as a guide to the degree of malignancy present. A generalization may be made that the more malignant a tumor becomes, the less the degree of differentation. Tumors of a high order of malignancy may often show bizarre microscopic architecture with all resemblance to the tissue of origin having been lost. Finally, malignant tumors possess the property of "metastasis"—autonomous growth at distant sites. This often occurs through the process of embolization. The tumor invades a small blood vessel or lymphatic channel, then a small cluster of cells, or even a single cell may be desquamated into the blood or lymphatic stream, whence it travels in the circulation until a site favorable for a new growth is reached. The tumor cell or cells then implant themselves on an appropriate area, voraciously invade the local host tissue, cause a blood supply from the surrounding tissues to be formed for their primary use, and begin to multiply rapidly, outstripping the growth pattern of the normal tissue so that this becomes displaced as the bulk of the malignant tumor tissue increases. Since the lungs and the liver act as filtration areas, circulating tumor tissue often stops and implants at these sites.

Not all malignant tumors metastasize; some produce disability and symptoms due primarily to wide local growth and metastasize only when very far advanced. Other malignant tumors, however, characteristically metastasize early; and deposits of malignant tumor may already be developing in many areas of a host patient, even though the "primary" site may still be rather small and innocuous in appearance. Certain breast, lung, and gastric tumors, as well as the melanoma of the skin, characteristically may metastasize quite easily.

It is of some interest to note that this characteristic of autonomous growth, or metastasis, indicates that these cells have reached a degree of autonomy that permits them to "take" even in another heterologous host. Dr. Harry Green, of Yale University, some years ago demonstrated that several human tumors that had already metastasized could be transplanted and grown successfully in heterologous species, such as the rabbit and the guinea pig. Malignant tumors, however, that have not yet metastasized—that is, still have some restriction to their autonomous growth—could not be similarly transplanted.

Types of Cancer

The classification of tumors presents the medical student or scholar in this field with a puzzling array of terms based, in a rather haphazard manner, on various factors such as etiology, embryology, histology, behavior, or regional anatomy. As a result, considerable confusion in the terminology confronts the physician who attempts to learn a practical system of classification. Persons involved in classifying scientific or other fields of inquiry can themselves be divided into either the "lumpers" or the "splitters." The lumpers tend to place as much as possible under one roof; they tend to see the similarities between diverse objects. As such, they have often been accused of oversimplification. The splitters, on the other hand, note the differences, albeit minute, in objects otherwise homogenous; and in order to place these differences in proper perspective, subclassification and further subdivision become the order of the day. In the classification of tumors, the splitters have had their day.

Fortunately, in recent years, a serious attempt has been made by thoughtful pathologists to bring some semblance of order to this field. The following paragraphs will reflect the current attempts at organization which permit even the relatively uninitiated to see the basic relationships among the many types of tumors.

It should be strongly stated at the outset that the only system of classification that has consistently been shown to make sense, and to make understanding easier as one delves deeply into this area, is the system fundamentally based on histogenesis—that is, according to the tissue from which tumors arise and of which they consist. It should be appreciated that in the great majority of instances, tumors consist of a single type of cell, derived from only one of the tissues of the body. Dr. Mallory has aptly stated that "the type of cell is the one important element in every tumor, and from it the tumor should be named." [2] In other words, tumors are classified on a histological basis, like other tissues.

One rather simple yet informative way to think about tumors is to divide them into two main groups, the solid tumors and the malignancies of blood-forming tissues. Thus, in the first category are all those tumors whose presence is manifested by the appearance of a neoplasm or a new growth somewhere in the body. The vast majority of tumors, some 85 to 90 per cent, are of the solid tumor variety. The remainder, or about 10 per cent of all malignancies, are those cancers derived from elements of the blood-forming tissues. Thus, all the leukemias, or blood cancers, as well as the malignancies arising in lymphatic tissues, are of this variety.

In order to gain some insight, however, into the significance of the various types of individual tumors, it is necessary to consider these under five histological groupings; (1) of epithelial origin, (2) of mesenchymal origin, excluding hematopoietic tissue, (3) of hematopoietic tissues, (4) of neural tissue, and (5) miscellaneous.

TUMORS OF EPITHELIAL ORIGIN

As the term implies, this group of tumors includes all those arising from epithelial surfaces of the body. It should be remembered that even internal structures have an epithelial lining. Therefore, in addition to tumors of the skin and external surfaces of the body, this group will include all tumors arising from the gastrointestinal tract epithelium, breast epithelium, and so forth. Since these epithelial surfaces of the body also contain glands, often minute, the glandular or adenomatous tumors are included here.

As with tumors elsewhere, tumors of epithelial origin may be either benign or malignant. Benign tumors that arise from surface epithelium— that is, of the stratified squamous variety—are usually referred to as *papillomas*, a descriptive term denoting their histological appearance. Benign tumors arising from glandular tissue are referred to generally as *adenomas*, indicating that histologically these tumors tend to appear as glandular or gland-forming elements. Thus, benign adenomas may be

[2] F. B. Mallory, *Principles of Pathologic Histology*, quoted in R. A. Willis, *Pathology of Tumours*, London: Butterworths, 1960, p. 9.

found arising anywhere from surface epithelium, such as a vocal cord adenoma, adenoma of the stomach, ovarian or rectal adenoma, and so on.

All malignant tumors of epithelial tissues, however, are referred to as carcinomas. Characteristically, carcinomas are of two types, either an *adenocarcinoma*, indicating a malignant epithelial tumor of glandular origin, or an *epidermoid* or *squamous cell* carcinoma, indicating again a malignant tumor of surface epithelium, but not of glandular origin. Thus, we have the terms adenocarcinoma of the stomach or adenocarcinoma of the colon, the pancreas, and so forth, indicating a malignant epithelial tumor of glandular origin and identifying the organ in which the malignancy arose. On the other hand, epidermoid carcinoma of the lung or of the skin or of the vagina indicates again a malignant tumor of stratified epithelial surface, and adds the organ of origin for further identification. The word carcinoma is often abbreviated simply as *Ca*, resulting in terms such as adenoca or epidermoid ca. Other descriptive terms are often tacked on, such as *scirrhous ca*, indicating a "hard" ca, or *mucinous adenoca*, indicating that this glandular malignant tumor shows evidence of mucin production.

TUMORS OF MESENCHYMAL TISSUES

This group of tumors arise for the most part from the "supporting" or connective tissues of the body, such as bone or cartilage, fibrous tissue, blood vessels, muscles, and tendons. Again, these tumors may be either benign or malignant. The benign tumors are identified by carrying the name of the tissue of origin. Thus, a benign tumor of the bone becomes an *osteoma*, derived from the Greek *osteon* for bone, a benign tumor of the cartilage is a *chondroma*, one of fibrous tissue is a *fibroma*, of fatty tissue a *lipoma*, of muscle a *myoma;* if the muscle is skeletal then the term used is *rhabdomyoma;* if the muscle is "smooth" then the term is *leiomyoma*. Various combinations may be listed, such as osteochondroma, meaning a benign tumor containing both the elements of bone and of cartilage.

The malignant variant of tumors of mesenchymal origin is referred to as a *sarcoma*. An osteogenic sarcoma indicates a malignant tumor of bone, a chondrosarcoma indicates a malignant cancer of cartilagenous origin, a fibrosarcoma indicates a malignant tumor of fibrous origin.

The *carcinoma* of epithelial origin and the *sarcoma* of connective tissue or mesenchymal origin, therefore, are the two principal types of cancer of the solid variety. At times, because of extremely rapid growth, most of the cellular differentiation is lost, and the pathologist may be unable to state clearly whether the tumor is of the carcinomatous or sarcomatous variety. In such instances, the term "anaplastic tumor of unknown origin" or "undifferentiated malignant tumor" may be used.

On the other end of the scale, the term *carcinoma in situ* is used to describe the earliest possible stage of definite malignant change in cells of epithelial origin, even though local invasion has not yet occurred. This is the most favorable time to find and destroy a potential cancer, for if a lesion is in the *in situ* stage when found and treated, the cure rate approaches 100 per cent.

TUMORS OF HEMATOPOIETIC TISSUES

This group of tumors includes all those malignancies that occur in the blood-forming elements of the bone marrow, and those arising in other tissues or organs that may give origin to blood cells, such as the lymphatic system, and the reticuloendothelial system, including certain elements of the liver, spleen, and other organs.

The common term for malignancies of the blood, or "blood cancer," is *leukemia,* after the Greek *leukos* for blood. Leukemias are characterized by an overproliferation of the leukocytes, or white blood cells. These cells appear to have broken free of the factors controlling and regulating their growth and proliferation, and are present in vast numbers in the blood stream, often in very bizarre and immature forms. The leukemias are further described after the predominant cell type present. Thus the *monocytic* leukemia indicates that the monocyte is the characteristic cell present.

Lymphocytic leukemia and *myelogenous* leukemia indicate that the predominant cells present are the lymphocytes and the myelocytes of the bone marrow series respectively. Each of these types of leukemia is associated with a characteristic life history; each may respond differently to various therapeutic measures. Therefore, clear-cut identification is important.

Leukemia may be of the acute or chronic variety. Acute leukemia indicates a rapid onset and rapid progress of the disease. "Chronic" leukemia is characterized by an insidious onset and a course that sometimes stretches over many years, even with no specific therapy. Acute leukemia occurs most frequently in children in the first five years of life. Leukemia is the most common form of cancer in children. Chronic leukemia usually occurs in adults in the age group 45–60 years.

TUMORS OF NEURAL TISSUE

As the term implies, this group of tumors includes all those arising from neural or nerve tissue. Thus, brain tumors, as well as tumors of the spinal cord and of the peripheral and autonomic nervous system, fall within this category.

Here the terms employed tend to follow the particular histology identified. Thus, the *gliomas,* such as the *astrocytic glioma* or the *oligodendroglioma,* indicate a tumor of central nervous system tissue in which the predominant cell is the *astrocyte* and *oligodendrocyte* respectively. The *pinealoma* is a malignant tumor of the pineal gland. The *retinoblastoma,* a tumor of the eye, is one of the few tumors in which a hereditary aspect is acknowledged to be present. Many other descriptive names can be included in this category. The listed ones are indicative of the general nature and nomenclature of tumors in this group.

MISCELLANEOUS TUMORS

In any classification there always remain a few misfits that do not belong clearly in any category. Such is the case with tumor classification as well. A few of the more common of these may be noted.

The *melanoma* is a malignant tumor that arises from pigment cells in our body, the melanophores. These cells characteristically are present in our skin where they impart a definite brownish hue; they are also present in the choroid of the eye, the anus, the meninges, and perhaps the adrenals. The origin of the melanophore is still a histological controversy. Some experts consider them to be part of the epithelial tissue of our body, and accordingly, the term *melanocarcinoma* is sometimes used.

A significant feature of melanomas is that these tumors may arise from the benign pigmented "moles" so numerous in humans. The term "black mole" has come into common usage to indicate the type of melanoma that has a particularly malignant outlook. It also reflects the idea that the so-called benign moles, which suddenly darken or become black, should be regarded with suspicion. Early excision of any mole undergoing such a change is of the utmost urgency, despite the fact that they may have been quiescent for 30 to 40 years or longer. A change in any mole or pigmented area of the body is one of the seven danger signals of cancer as noted by the American Cancer Society.

The *chordoma* is a malignant tumor of the vestiges of the notochord, an early embryonic structure. Remnants may persist and in later life give origin to tumors that are characteristically located at the base of the brain or in the sacral area. The exact histology of these tumors is disputed so their clear classification is not possible.

The *teratomas* are an academically fascinating group of tumors that basically are composed of more than one tissue or origin. Traditionally, these tumors have been thought to arise from "multipotential" or "totipotential" cells—that is, cells that represent an early embryological stage before any specific differentiation toward tissue types occurred. These tumors are usually found in the ovaries and testes and in the retroperitoneal areas, in general where embryological rests are frequently found. The theories of origin are legion. They are fascinating to study and to diagnose because of their bizarre nature. Being derived of multi-potential cells, these tumors often contain elements of hair, teeth, bones and cartilage, and abortive attempts at glandular formation. Despite the volumes of print the teratomas have stimulated, they remain poorly understood.

METHODS OF DIAGNOSIS

At the present time, no test is known that permits early diagnosis of all forms of cancer. A great deal of scientific effort and hard work have gone into the many attempts to develop a simple screening procedure for the detection of cancer, but no real success has yet been achieved. The one exception to this general statement is the recent wide application of the "Pap smear" or vaginal smear test, which is turning out to be a remarkable advance in the detection of cancer of the uterine cervix. Further, no uniformly successful treatment exists for managing cancer in the advanced stages, although in recent years the advent of new classes of chemotherapeutic agents, or anticancer drugs, has produced some remarkable, although limited, results in some forms of cancer. The cure of cancer today, then, depends almost completely on surgical extirpation or x-radiation. It is important to remember that both of these modalities are "local" forms of therapy, capable of cure only when the neoplasm is localized or in an early stage. Early diagnosis remains the cornerstone of successful treatment. The American Cancer Society has done the public a significant service by intensive efforts to teach this fact.

Two ingredients appear to be essential to establishing an early diagnosis of cancer. These are the prompt seeking of medical attention by any person who has developed a suspicious sign or symptom, and a high index of suspicion on the part of the examining physician toward the disease cancer. Ideally, cancer should be discovered while it is still in the asymptomatic stage at the time of routine check-ups or when examination is carried out for other causes. Studies have clearly shown that cancer detected under these circumstances is cured significantly more frequently than when discovered because symptoms clearly indicate that something is wrong. For some years the American Cancer Society has distributed informative booklets and widely circulated the knowledge that there are seven danger signals to warn the patient about the possible presence of cancer. The information imparted by these signals, listed below, is vitally important:

1. Any sore that does not heal quickly, especially about the mouth
2. Any unusual bleeding or discharge from any natural body opening

3. Any painless lump, especially in the breast, lips, tongue, or soft tissues
4. Any persistent indigestion or unexplained weight loss
5. Any progressive change in the color or size of a wart or birth mark
6. Any persistent hoarseness or cough or difficulty in swallowing
7. Any unexplained change in regular bowel habits

Other diseases besides cancer can cause these signs and symptoms to appear. Therefore, the appearance of one of these danger signals does not necessarily mean that cancer exists. However, the physician, on obtaining such a history from a patient, is committed to consider and to rule out the presence of malignant disease. The primary methods employed in a medical examination to establish a diagnosis of cancer may now be noted.

THE HISTORY

Taking a careful and detailed history remains the cornerstone upon which a medical diagnosis is established, not only for cancer but for most diseases as well. The physician probes into many areas about which patients are surprisingly reluctant to talk freely. It is remarkable how often a patient will state that a lesion of the breast, for example, has been present for "only a few weeks" when it is perfectly apparent to a trained examiner that the process may be of many months or even years duration. Symptoms of bowel disorders are also notoriously difficult to obtain clearly, although here the patient is often sincere in stating that a real change in habit has only been present for a month or so. Skillful questioning, however, will often raise the likelihood that lesser symptoms have actually been present for many months but have been discounted as a "little diarrhea" or constipation.

A history of an environmental exposure to a carcinogenic hazard may be uncovered about which the patient may be entirely unaware. Such information often points a finger at the correct diagnosis even in obscure situations. Careful history taking, then is essential to early diagnosis of cancer.

PHYSICAL EXAMINATION

The next part of the physician's approach to diagnosis is a careful and searching physical exam. Peripheral areas that tend to harbor evidence of cancer "inside the body" are carefully checked. These include such areas as the neck, looking especially for signs of unusual glandular activity, the breasts, armpits, groins, and abdomen. For aesthetic reasons, and often because of the patients' reluctance, two particular areas are often not examined as a matter of routine, unfortunately. These areas include the anorectum in the male and female and the pelvis in the female. No examination for cancer is complete without a careful screening of both these areas. Patients should request that these areas be checked if the examining physician passes them by. The price of losing the chance to diagnose an early asymptomatic lesion of the rectum or female pelvis is far too high to pay in order to maintain a prudish outlook toward a truly innocuous procedure.

X-RAY STUDIES

The x-ray is often used by the physician as a means of probing into areas "where the hands cannot reach and the eyes cannot see." Yet one must not be misled into thinking that the x-ray is an infallible diagnostic tool. Its primary importance lies in its ability to discern disease in the lung fields, most of the gastrointestinal system, and the bones of the body. Here the x-ray study can be a valuable asset indeed. Nevertheless, there are many so-called blind areas where the x-ray must not be depended upon to rule a tumor in or out. The last six or so inches of the rectum, for example, are often obscured by the overlying hip bones, so that this area becomes relatively blind. Yet cancer in this area, within the reach of the examining finger, is notoriously common. Tumors within the abdominal cavity, but outside the intestinal tract proper, are also difficult to see by x-ray. Tumors of the "soft" tissues such as muscle or breast are likewise difficult to visualize, although recent advances in x-ray techniques suggest that it may now be possible to examine breasts by the x-ray with a high degree of success. Needless to say, tumors of the blood, the various leukemias, also cannot be demonstrated radiologically until far advanced changes in more solid parts of the body have occurred.

BLOOD STUDIES

The hope has been that a simple blood test could be developed to indicate that a given individual may be harboring cancer. None has been successful so far, although many physicians feel that changes are present in the blood of any individual harboring cancer, if only we knew how to detect them. Some progress along these lines has been made in recent years with the demonstration that certain of the body enzymes and some of the protein constituents of our plasma are altered in the presence of neoplastic disease. The urine, too, is being carefully reexamined biochemically, for there are indications that certain tumors, as a result of their presence, produce changes that may be detected in the urine by appropriate methods. These procedures, however, are quite complex and can be performed with reliability only in a highly controlled research laboratory. What is badly needed is a detection test of a high order of reliability, one so simple to perform that its practical application on a very wide scale will be possible. Such a test has not been found thus far.

SMEAR TESTS

Over the past two or three decades, it has become widely appreciated that cancerous tissue tends to shed surface cells and that these cells, if appropriately collected, can be identified and serve to indicate the presence of cancer, often at a very early stage of its development. Thus, cancer cells have been found circulating in the blood stream of some cancer patients, and smears of body surfaces such as the vaginal epithelium, oral, or bronchial surfaces have also yielded telltale cells, desquamated from the surface of tumors located in these areas. One of these smear tests, the vaginal or "Pap" smear (named after its discoverer Dr. George Papanicolaou), has shown striking effectiveness in detecting cancer of the cervix at an early stage. Moreover, the procedure of obtaining and preparing the smear is simple enough to be done in any physician's office, by either the physician or his nurse. Statistical data already collected have shown that cancer of the cervix, if detected and treated at the earliest stage, should be almost 100 per cent curable. Cancer experts feel that this goal is actually within reach through the wide application of the "Pap" smear test, done in the course of routine check-ups of all female patients.

BIOPSIES

Establishing a definite diagnosis of cancer finally rests with the demonstration, under the microscope, that the tissue under question possesses those identifiable histological features that enable a trained pathologist to state with a high degree of certainty that the cells are malignant. In order to do this, a tissue sample must be obtained, via a minor surgical procedure, which is then appropriately prepared and stained for analysis. This is referred to as a "tissue biopsy." Only in exceptionally rare instances would surgeons remove a breast because of a "lump" or tumor mass before removing a small biopsy specimen for pathological confirmation. In other words, the diagnosis of cancer is a histological or tissue diagnosis. It cannot be established with certainty by any other means, although a smear test may indicate that cancer should be suspected, or the gross appearance of the growth may be such that there is relatively little doubt about what the histological diagnosis will be. A biopsy also serves to indicate to the surgeon or physician responsible for the patient's care the nature, characteristics, and prognosis for this particular type of cancer. After judging these facts, the physician can best decide the course of treatment to pursue. This involves deciding whether a cure is potentially possible with adequate surgery or x-ray therapy, or if the malignancy is now too far advanced to permit a cure. In the latter case various hormonal or chemotherapeutic modalities are employed in an attempt to arrest or control the growth of the tumor and palliate the patient.

TREATMENT OF CANCER

The therapy of cancer today, as it has for many decades, depends on three modalities—surgery, various forms of irradiation, and drug treatment. Significant changes in each of these methods, however, have occurred over the past 10 to 20 years. Surgeons today are performing operations routinely that were considered to be wild and dangerous dreams as little as 25 years ago. The development of supervoltage techniques and of radioactive isotopes, a by-product of World War II research, has permitted far wider application of irradiation, even to tumors hidden within the body. The development of new anticancer drugs has been the most exciting and fruitful area of cancer research in the past 10 years. The hope that a chemotherapeutic agent might be found that would cure cancer has been dim for many years. Suddenly, within the past 10 years, a host of new compounds have been developed that have been shown to possess anticancer activity. In experimental animals, where their action can be exploited fully without great concern for their other possibly harmful future effects, some of these agents have shown remarkable effectiveness. In man, these agents must be employed with great caution, so that at the present time they are used chiefly in very far advanced cases. Under these conditions, the results so far have been less spectacular. Nevertheless, in at least two tumor types ordinarily almost uniformly fatal when in an advanced stage—the choriocarcinoma of the uterus and Wilms' kidney tumor in children—the equivalents of five-year or more "cures" have now been recorded in a significant percentage of cases. Although on a limited front, this virtually amounts to a breakthrough in the cancer field and lends encouragement to the hope, which has never been brighter, that drugs may be the ultimate weapon against this disease.

In considering the therapy used in the treatment of cancer today it is well to know something of the philosophy and the jargon of the medical profession in this area. Thus, when a patient presents with a tumor problem, the necessary data have been gathered, and the diagnosis of cancer established, the physicians then must decide whether the patient is to be treated for "cure" or for "palliation" only. A decision to treat for cure signifies that the available data indicate that the malignancy is still in a curative stage; that is, there is no evidence of widespread dissemination or metastases. In these instances, physicians call upon those modalities of treatment that are capable of completely eradicating a localized cancer, chiefly surgical resection or, in a few tumor types, localized x-ray therapy. In some cases, however, where the tumor appears to be moderately advanced, or where the tumor is developing rapidly but still without evidence of distant spread, the decision as to whether to try for a cure or aim for palliation is tremendously more difficult to make. In these borderline cases, the surgeon or the "team" concerned with the therapy for this particular patient is prepared to take even serious risks with extensive surgery as long as the chance for a complete cure is present. Actually, it is the patient who "takes the risks" and who must adjust to any resultant disability if this is part of the price for cure, but current medical jargon would imply that the physician "takes the risk." This is partly true in a sense, inasmuch as it is the qualified physician who must make the decision, on the basis of the facts gathered, whether or not to try for a cure in difficult cases. While patients should be informed of various factors involved, it is unfair to present the patient with the facts and then to ask him to make the decision in borderline cases; the trained cancer surgeon or oncologist is the one person qualified to make a reasonable and objective decision. This responsibility cannot or should not be avoided by requesting an emotionally involved and often frightened patient and his family to comprehend and then to decide the best course to follow.

Surgical treatment, in those instances where the cancer is extensive although still localized, often must be of a "radical" nature if the hope for a cure is to be realized. Every last malignant cell must be removed along with a margin of normal appearing tissue to insure that local invasive elements are completely extirpated. It has been amply documented that such an aggressive attack is capable of still curing a patient's cancer, whereas more standard and conservative procedures are doomed to subsequent recurrence and failure. Radical approaches, however, are not without their price. The loss of an extremity or the urinary bladder or the total stomach or the larynx with resultant loss of the voice mechanism, while willingly borne to permit a cure, is associated with definite disabilities to which a patient must adjust after the cancer is cured. Hand in hand with radical surgery, however, have been the developments in rehabilitation techniques and facilities for restoration of normal or near normal function. Without these advances, surgery, no matter how successful, would result in a pyrrhic victory, leaving a patient minus a bladder, minus a voice, or, to his mind, minus everything.

Recent years have seen the development of combination techniques, utilizing more than one therapy simultaneously or in planned sequence to permit a higher percentage of cures, especially in difficult cases. Thus, surgery and x-ray therapy are often employed in sequence, and more recently surgery combined with adjuvant chemotherapy has shown promise in the treatment of selected tumors.

In summary then, treatment "for cure" of cancer differs in certain fundamental respects from treatment for palliation. Although a cure can often be achieved simply and by conservative measures, there are also many instances in which a cure can be attempted only at considerable risk to the patient.

Current medical philosophy tends to balance the various factors involved and to favor acceptance of added risks as long as the chance for success is still present.

When the evidence indicates, however, that a cure is no longer possible, a marked temperance of therapeutic aggressiveness follows. Conservatism is the fundamental approach, with all efforts directed at keeping the patient comfortable for as long a period as possible. Significant advances have been made as well in the area of palliation during the past one or two decades. Various forms of x-ray therapy and of drug therapy are the mainstays of treatment here, with surgery playing an important but subdued role.

Thus, radium applied to a nonresectable cancer of the uterus or bladder may alleviate symptoms significantly and for prolonged periods, even though it is accepted that after a period of time, which may be months or years, the disease will reactivate and the symptoms recur.

Similarly, external x-ray therapy, applied to certain tumors that may produce severe symptoms due to their size or location, may result in sufficient shrinkage of the mass for a time so that a comfortable period for the patient is obtained. In some forms of cancer, especially of the breast, prostate gland, or cervix, metastases to the bones, producing painful pathological fractures or collapse of vertebrae, are common in the natural history of these tumor types. Here, too, external irradiation therapy, skillfully applied, may result in very gratifying relief of symptoms and restoration of a more normal functioning state. Advances in the past 10 years in the tumor irradiation field have been significant. The advent of supervoltage techniques, employing one million or more volts, has resulted in technical benefits that permit the administration of effective amounts of x-ray in a shorter time and with far less discomfort to the patient. Certain hormonal and other chemotherapeutic agents are proving of considerable worth in palliating patients with advanced cancer. Thus, various forms of estrogen or female sex hormone therapy can keep a patient with advanced carcinoma of the prostate gland comfortable, working, and functioning for many years with minimal disability. Many patients with breast cancer, advanced and incurable, are nevertheless able to remain at home and continue to care for their families under the palliative effect of androgens or male sex steroid or other hormonal therapy. In those tumors that are responsive to hormones, some of our most worthwhile palliative effects have been achieved.

The advent of drugs or chemotherapy has been regarded with extreme interest in the cancer field. During World War II it was noted that individuals or animals accidentally or experimentally exposed to the effects of mustard gases suffered from leukopenia, a sharp reduction in the number of circulating white blood cells. It was logical, therfore, to try out a derivative of this compound, nitrogen mustard, for its possible therapeutic effect in human leukemia, a condition characterized by an overwhelming overabundance of white blood cells that in time becomes lethal. The dramatic result of this therapeutic attempt was a marked reduction in the white blood cell count, with striking improvement in the clinical condition of patients who were often moribund. With greater experience it was learned that this improvement, although striking to observe, was only temporary, and in time the white blood cells would again rise to lethal numbers and destroy the host. Often, a second course of nitrogen mustard was again effective, but sooner or later, the malignant cells become resistant to this particular form of treatment. Nevertheless, this was the first real demonstration that a drug could actually cause a malignant condition to regress significantly in more than isolated instances. The enthusiasm engendered by this discovery has caused a great influx of scientific interest in this field, resulting in the development of many thousands of agents with potential anticancer activity. With two agents thus far—*methotrexate* in the treatment of choriocarcinoma of the uterus and *actinomycin D* in the treatment of Wilms' tumor of the kidney in children—complete remissions, equivalent to surgical "cures" in that the complete absence of any apparent residual disease has lasted for five years or longer, have been produced in a significant percentage of cases so treated.

In all other instances to date, however, the available anticancer agents have been able to exert only a temporary restraining effect on the malignant growth, when they have been effective at all. At this time, therefore, these agents are used for palliative purposes only, and never in place of surgery or x-ray therapy when a possibility of cure exists. It is logical, however, that they be used simultaneously with surgery or with x-ray in the hope that combined effectiveness may ensue, and this hypothesis is being actively pursued in many medical centers in the world today. Cancer chemotherapy is one of the newest fields of medical endeavor. Although widespread application of these new drugs has been limited because of their simultaneous toxicity to tissues of the body other than tumor tissue, nevertheless it is appreciated that as more effective and less toxic compounds are developed, significant further palliation and perhaps even cures may be in the offing.

In brief summary then, when a malignant tumor is no longer curable, therapeutic attempts are focused on palliating the patient. The philosophy here is characterized by a conservative approach, aimed at maintaining the well-being of the patient for as long a period as possible, and this can be successfully achieved in many cases. Surgery plays a lesser role in the palliative treatment of tumors than in curable situations, being employed palliatively for such reasons as to remove large bulky masses, to relieve obstruction through bypassing procedures, and in some cases to obviate pain by selective resection of nerve pathways containing the pain fibers. X-radiation techniques, hormone, and anticancer drug therapy are the mainstays of the palliative treatment of cancer.

DISABILITY DUE TO SPECIFIC TYPES OF CANCER

CANCER OF THE LUNG

The most significant aspect of current thinking about lung cancer revolves around its changing incidence and its relationship to cigarette smoking. Lung cancer alone accounts for more fatalities annually in the United States than do all traffic fatalities, even though both figures are sadly rising. Lung cancer is increasing more rapidly than any other form of cancer in the body. Currently this disease is causing some 41,000 deaths annually, and it is important to appreciate that the death rate from lung cancer is now 10 times what it was 30 years ago. That this increase closely parallels the marked increase in the smoking habit during this same period is generally appreciated, although the significance of this is hotly disputed by the tobacco industry. It is interesting that lung cancer in women, once rather rare, is also increasing markedly, paralleling the increasing use of tobacco by women. Results gathered from many sources and in many countries have shown that the difference in lung cancer between smokers and non-smokers is striking indeed. The degree of the smoking habit appears to be of direct importance; the half pack a day smoker has a likelihood 15 times greater of dying from lung cancer than the nonsmoker, whereas the smoker using two packs or more each day increases his chances of dying from this disease to 64 times that of the nonsmoker. Many of the arguments raised against the validity of this statistical relationship are being answered as time passes. It has been pointed out for many years that cigarette smoke or its products have not been able to produce cancer in experimental animals. Recently, however, this has been accomplished by painting the skin of mice with cigarette smoke condensate, thus demonstrating clearly the presence of a carcinogenic agent in cigarette smoke. Further, it would appear that cigarette smoke condensate also contains co-carcinogens—that is, chemicals that in themselves do not cause cancer, but that may markedly increase the cancer-producing qualities of carcinogens present.

It has also been pointed out that certain other causes of lung cancer have been demonstrated and therefore cigarette smoking should not be incriminated as the cause. This is certainly partially true, since other substances such as radioactive ores, nickel, and chromates have been shown capable of causing lung cancer. The most convincing evidence indicates that while cigarette smoking is not the only agent causing lung cancer, it nevertheless is probably the major cause of this disease at this time. It is certainly evident to anyone who deals with cancer that malignancy of the lung in a nonsmoker is quite uncommon.

One of the primary symptoms of lung cancer is the development of a cough. Since cigarette smoking in itself often produces this symptom even in noncancer patients, this symptom is often ignored. Chest pain, weight loss, and hoarseness are also produced, but usually these indicate an advanced stage of the disease.

The diagnosis is then usually easily established via x-ray, a "needle" biopsy, or at time of bronchoscopy (which consists of visualizing the bronchial tree with a slender telescopic instrument).

The primary treatment of lung cancer today is early and adequate surgery. That this disease is usually not picked up early is reflected in the overall cure rate, which continues to be depressingly low, between 5 and 10 per cent. However, when resection is still possible, usually at the cost of removing a lobe of a lung or the entire lung on one side, then the cure rate may be at least tripled to around 30 per cent five-year cures. The use of supervoltage x-ray is being actively explored as a possible way of increasing the five-year cures.

The disability resulting from surgery or x-ray therapy for lung cancer usually manifests itself as pulmonary insufficiency, which produces symptoms of shortness of breath. The degree of this depends on how much lung tissue was destroyed, excised, or is replaced with tumor. If tumor is still present these individuals rarely live beyond two or three years; therefore, the chief problem resides among those individuals who are cured. If only a lobe of a lung needs to be removed, the pulmonary insufficiency will be minor; however, if an entire lung is removed, then such an individual, while appearing quite normal when at rest, will experience varying degrees of shortness of breath when he exercises or attempts to work. No satisfactory treatment for this disability exists at the present time. All efforts are directed toward maintaining the remainder of the lung tissue as functional as possible. Even minor repeated upper respiratory infections take their toll of the remaining lung reserve by diminishing this reserve each time by a small amount. The important consideration here is to recognize and appreciate the disability and then to plan one's activities and work within the functional capacity of the remaining lung.

CANCER OF THE STOMACH

Cancer of the stomach, similar to cancer of the lung, is usually in an advanced stage when first treated. This is because the symptoms caused by an early stomach cancer are very mild. Many patients will have noted only a minor degree of vague indigestion, which is easily passed off inasmuch as most persons experience indigestion at one time or another. Loss of appetite, nausea, weight loss, and finally obstructive symptoms and vomiting are usually indicative of an advanced stage of the disease. Sometimes, a little bleeding may result from an ulcerating tumor, just as from a peptic ulcer, and the bowel movement will become dark or black. This may occur early in the disease process; therefore this symptom always demands a thorough investigation.

The diagnosis is usually established when the symptoms bring the patient to the physician and x-ray dye studies of the upper gastro-intestinal system are carried out. About 10 to 15 per cent of the time, x-rays will fail to reveal the tumor even when symptoms strongly suggest that all is not well.

Surgery again offers the only hope of a cure, but unfortunately, as in the case of lung cancer, exploratory surgery often indicates that the disease is advanced and nonresectable. Therefore, the overall cure rate for stomach cancer is again quite low, in the region of 8 per cent only. However, when the lesion is in an early stage at the time of operation, the cure rates goes up fivefold to 40 per cent or higher. New techniques for diagnosing stomach cancer early are badly needed.

The disability associated with gastric cancer usually occurs in those individuals in whom a total or near total gastrectomy was performed in an attempt to cure the cancer. Patients with lesser (subtotal) resections, in the order of 50 to 70 per cent of the stomach removed, usually experience little difficulty after a brief rehabilitative period and are able to assume a pretty normal role in family affairs and in their work capacity. However, patients who have lost their entire stomach suffer from loss of appetite, severe weight loss, and easy fatigability, leading to varying degrees of chronic disability.

Careful dietary management and an understanding by the patient of the altered physiology with which he now must live may accomplish a great deal in keeping these persons functioning. They must be taught to eat small meals frequently and to avoid rapid intake of food. Sometimes it helps to omit fluids at mealtimes inasmuch as fluids may wash the food into the intestine too rapidly. In brief, individuals who have lost all or a large part of their stomach have lost a major portion of their digestive ability. They must learn to alter their eating and drinking habits considerably if they are to avoid the sequelae of significant weight loss, anemia, and gradual debilitation which are frequent concomitants of this disease.

CANCER OF THE INTESTINES

The average length of the intestinal tract in the adult is about 30 feet, of which about four-fifths is in the "small intestine," where most of the digestive and absorptive functions are carried out, and the remainder, about one-fifth, is in the large intestine, or colon-rectum, where chiefly functions of storage and evacuation are performed. It is a puzzling fact, known for many years, that cancer of the small intestine is very uncommon, whereas the large intestine, or colon-rectum, is one of our most common sites of malignant disease, even though this area accounts for only a small portion of out total intestinal system. Cancer of the small intestine, then, poses no problems of practical importance in this discussion since it is so infrequently seen. Malignant disease of the large bowel, however, becomes increasingly common after 40 years of age and accounts for much of the problem of disability and rehabilitation related to the digestive system.

The diagnosis of cancer of the large bowel is usually made after certain symptoms call attention to trouble in this area and appropriate x-ray studies are made. These symptoms are usually a change in bowel habits or the appearance of blood in the stool. In persons whose bowel habits are very regular, even a minor change may be significant. In most persons, however, the changes may be sufficiently subtle so that these are often overlooked or attributed to a "little irregularity." Blood in the stools, however, is always an indication of disease and demands further investigation. Sometimes, the presence of free blood in the intestinal tract manifests itself as unusually dark or even black stools due to the chemical changes occurring in blood pigment after a few hours time.

The diagnosis of a mass in the lower bowel is usually established by an x-ray study referred to as a barium enema, which consists of instilling a little barium "dye" via the rectum, which then opacifies and outlines the lining of the colorectal area.

About three-quarters of all malignant tumors of the rectum are located sufficiently close to the anal area so that they can easily be felt on digital examination. This points up the importance of this diagnostic aspect already stressed before—namely, that routine rectal examinations are capable of picking up most of the tumors in this area, and often at an early and asymptomatic stage of their development.

The primary treatment of tumors of the large intestine is surgical. If the tumor is sufficiently extensive, the entire large bowel may need to be removed; the distal end of the remaining bowel is then exteriorized to the skin surface of the abdominal wall for excretory purposes. This new opening, or stoma, on the abdomen is called a "colostomy" if some part of the large intestine is exteriorized, or an "ileostomy" if the entire large bowel is removed and the distal portion consists of

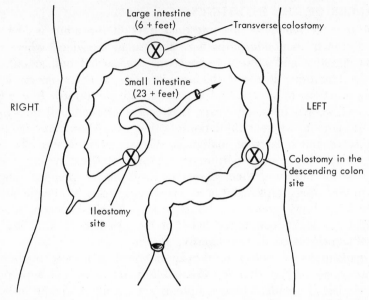

RIGHT

LEFT

Large intestine
(6 + feet)

Transverse colostomy

Small intestine
(23 + feet)

Colostomy in the
descending colon
site

Ileostomy
site

Figure 30. Diagram showing the most common sites of colostomy and ileostomy. A colostomy located in the descending colon is easiest of all to manage; the ileostomy presents the most problems in management.

ileum, or small intestine. Another aspect of this same problem obtains in cases where the tumor is very low in the colon—that is, in the anal or low rectal area. Here, although a large portion of the large bowel remains, still the distal sphincter or voluntary control mechanism is removed and, again, a colostomy needs to be fashioned.

It is in the management of the colostomy or ileostomy that the great majority of disability problems occur following therapy for tumors in this area. The fundamental problem with a colostomy or ileostomy is that these "artificial" stomas are not subject to voluntary control. The sphincter mechanism is lacking. As a result the patient is never quite sure when a bowel movement may occur, and, therefore, it is necessary to wear a small plastic or rubber bag type of appliance to safeguard against unexpected evacuation. Needless to say, much anxiety is engendered in a patient with such altered function, and basic adjustments in the pattern of living need to be made. Nevertheless, a great many patients are able to make these adjustments quite satisfactorily and resume a fairly normal way of life. It is not at all unusual to find professional persons such as lawyers, physicians, and teachers, or persons in the mechanical trades or in hard labor areas, performing their usual daily tasks despite a colostomy, without their colleagues being aware of this fact.

Several general statements apply to the colostomy-ileostomy group of patients. In general, the lower in the intestinal tract that a colostomy can be made, the easier it is for the patient to manage. Thus, when a colostomy is made in the lowest two or three feet of the colon, the fecal residue in this area tends to be fairly solid and lends itself to easy management. Many patients with such a descending or sigmoid colostomy find that after irrigation daily or every second day with tap water to produce a scheduled evacuation, there is no further discharge or evacuation until the next irrigation. Indeed, many of these patients find it unnecessary to wear any appliance. On the other hand, when the new terminal bowel stoma is fashioned in the more proximal portions of the colon, the disability or problem in management becomes enhanced due to the partial liquid nature of the bowel content in this region. This becomes most marked when an ileostomy, or small intestine stoma, is constructed, as occurs when the entire large bowel is sacrificed. Patients with an ileostomy have considerably more difficulty in management than do colostomy patients, inasmuch as an ileal evacuation is usually semisolid at best, and an appliance or collection apparatus needs to be worn constantly.

The cornerstone of successful management of an ileostomy or colostomy is proper dietary intake and regular irrigations. The person soon learns which foods to avoid to forestall unexpected evacuations, and also what kind of irrigation routine is best suited for him.

Considerable advances have been made in recent years in the field of ileostomy and colostomy appliances, so that patients are usually able to find an appliance that is especially suited to them. In recent years, too, a number of clubs or organizations have spontaneously arisen, in which the members, usually harboring a colostomy or ileostomy themselves, meet frequently in groups and open sessions to discuss their

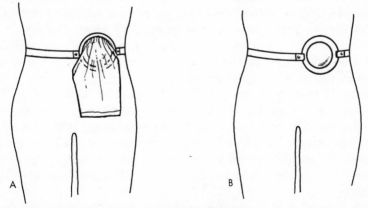

Figure 31. Sketch showing the wearing of an ileostomy or colostomy type appliance (A). The lower portion provides an opening for controlled emptying of the appliance which can be worn several days without a complete change. Often, in the case of a descending colostomy, no appliance need be worn. Sometimes a protective disc is simply worn for added security (B).

respective problems and the solutions to these problems. Members
of the medical and allied professions often work with these organizations in a supportive way. From personal experience with such groups
I can state that such organizations, where they do exist, are a remarkably effective way of improving the status and lessening the disability
among persons with an ileostomy or colostomy.

CANCER OF THE BLADDER

The problems encountered with bladder cancer, as related to disability, parallel those for intestinal cancer. Here, too, in cases of advanced cancer, where a cure is still possible, it may be necessary to
remove the bladder completely and to divert the urinary stream. Up to
a decade or so ago, it was customary in such cases to deliver the
ureters—small tubelike structures that deliver the urine from each
kidney to the bladder—to the skin surface, where again a collective
device had to be worn. More recently, however, it has been found possible to construct "artificial" bladders utilizing a segment of intestine
isolated from the remainder of the intestinal tract and to transplant
the ureters to this new bladder substitute. In general, the results using
bladder substitutes have been considerably more satisfactory, inasmuch
as these bladder substitutes permit some storage of urine to occur.
Nevertheless, none of the bladder substitutes developed to date provide
any element of voluntary control. The urine still leaves its new "bladder" in more or less constant fashion all day long; therefore, an appliance of some sort needs to be worn constantly so that the urine
can be collected and the patient remain dry. In general, the appliances for this purpose are quite similar to those employed by
the patient with a colostomy or ileostomy. Patients tend to manage
the problem of a substitute bladder quite well, and no irrigations or
special dietary precautions are necessary. The chief disability results
from the necessity of constantly wearing an appliance. No completely
satisfactory substitute has yet been developed, although investigative
efforts in this area are quite active.

Another approach to the problem of a bladder substitute has been
to transplant the ureters to the rectum, and thus to have the urine
pass out through the rectum and anal area along with the regular
bowel movements. At other times, a colostomy is made proximal to
the point where the ureters are made to join the rectum or sigmoid,
and in this way the lower bowel is "reserved" exclusively for urinary
excretion.

At first hand this would appear to be desirable, since this would
permit some measure of urinary control via the anal sphincter. However, it has been found that patients with such an altered physiological
mechanism tend to experience repeated bouts of infection ascend-

ing into the kidneys from the contaminated rectal area, and this in time can lead to serious impairment of kidney function. Also, this type of hook-up tends to result in stasis of urine in such a rectal segment with considerable reabsorption of urinary constituents, especially the chloride ion, leading to serious problems in electrolyte balance in the body.

In general then, the disability problems encountered with bladder cancer are similar to those of intestinal cancer. Patients with artificial bladders manage their appliances and altered physiology somewhat more easily, inasmuch as irrigations and careful dietary restrictions are not necessary. However, a satisfactory bladder substitute still needs to be developed.

CANCER OF THE BREAST

Cancer of the breast is the most common form of cancer in women, accounting for about 20 per cent of all cancer seen in the female population. It is estimated that about 5 per cent of all women will develop cancer of the breast at some time in their lives. Cancer of the male breast, which also occurs, but far less commonly than among women, needs only to be mentioned here. While x-ray therapy, hormones, and chemotherapy all play roles in the management of breast cancer, surgery remains the primary treatment in this country when a cure is possible. The standard surgical therapy employed for breast cancer is the so-called radical mastectomy, which consists of the total removal of the affected breast, the underlying muscles down to the ribs of the chest wall, and a complete dissection of the axillary contents. This operation has been devised to attempt to remove not only the primary cancer, but also the most likely areas of early spread of the cancer as well. In general, it can be stated that if there is no evidence of spread of the disease in the resected tissue beyond the primary focus, then a cure is achieved in about 75 per cent of the cases. However, when examination of the removed tissue discloses that cancer has already spread to the axillary lymph nodes, the commonest site of initial spread of this type of cancer, then the cure rate drops down to about 35 per cent. In other words, early diagnosis and treatment are essential here as in other forms of cancer. Since the breast is easily accessible for examination by either the patient or her doctor, it is disconcerting to know that even today almost two-thirds of all patients with breast cancer, when operated upon, will already show evidence of spread of the disease to the axilla.

Following a radical mastectomy, assuming that a patient is cured of the disease, a fairly complete recovery can be anticipated in most instances, and no significant disability is anticipated, in the physical sense of the word. About 25 per cent of patients will experience some difficulty with arm swelling on the operated side, and in a few instances this may reach massive proportions, in which case the arm becomes virtually useless. Some impairment of strength of the arm on the operated side is often noted, although usually this is not great, and these patients can continue to take care of their homes and their children as before.

In losing a breast, however, a woman loses a great deal, and the emotional disability that follows may be far more significant than the physical problem. In general, married women with a reasonably understanding spouse tend to adjust quite well. In unmarried women, however, or in the young woman just beginning to raise a family, the problem resulting from breast cancer and the necessary loss of the breast can be a severe one. The physician and the related professional personnel in this area have serious responsibilities in helping such patients to adjust. With time, most patients do adjust satisfactorily, although they require considerable support during the early stages. Frequent follow-up visits to the physician during the first year or two serve a dual purpose—to check on possible tumor recurrence and to allay the patient's anxieties in this regard, while providing her with the emotional support and encouragement she badly needs at this time.

In patients in whom a cure is not possible much can nevertheless be done. Many of these patients are able to live for several years or longer despite the continued presence and gradual spread of the disease. Disability becomes increasingly severe with time. Initially, virtually all of these patients return home to their usual responsibilities and pattern of living. Hormonal therapy, chemotherapy, and x-ray therapy can accomplish a great deal in securing for these patients many additional months, and often years, of worthwhile life, often while their families are still young and require parental care most. Eventually, however, the disease spreads to the lungs, the bones, and other areas with gradually increasing disability from pathological fractures, shortness of breath due to pulmonary insufficiency, and progressive anemia. In time total disability ensues, although fortunately life expectancy is then of brief duration.

In brief then, the disability of breast cancer is more often in the emotional sphere rather than due to physical or physiological impairment. Even in those patients in whom a cure cannot be achieved, much can be done currently to allay symptoms, prolong life and well-being, and permit significant rehabilitation in terms of economic and family needs.

CANCER OF THE UTERUS

Under the term cancer of the uterus we really must consider two distinct types of cancer, that of the uterine cervix and that of the uterine body. Patients who develop a malignancy of the uterine body are the more fortunate of the two in that cure rates of 75 per cent or over have frequently been reported in this disease. It is capable of cure about equally well both by radiotherapy and by surgery, and happily, in either instance, cure is obtained without resorting to radical procedures. Therefore, the resultant disability is relatively low. In cancer of the uterine cervix, however, such is not the case. Here the biological nature of this disease is such that spread and invasion of contiguous structures, such as bladder or rectum, may occur by the time that symptoms bring the patient to a physician. In order to offer such a patient a chance for a cure, the disease must be removed in its entirety, often necessitating the removal of the invaded bladder or rectum or even both of these structures. Such a procedure is one of the most formidable in all cancer surgery and is referred to as a total pelvic exenteration. It is also performed in those instances where radiation therapy is employed as the initial attempt and fails to eradicate the disease. Fortunately, it is necessary to carry out this extensive procedure only in far advanced cases; most patients can be given a chance for cure by lesser procedures such as x-ray and radium therapy and by the so-called Wertheim radical hysterectomy, which consists of an extensive resection of the uterus and cervix, but which spares the rectum and bladder.

The disability resulting from cervix cancer, then, is seen in two groups of patients—in those in whom a cure is not possible because of far advanced disease, and in those in whom an extensive exenteration procedure is carried out. In the first instance, the problem is one of chronic and progressive debilitation with gradual anemia and weight loss developing in a lingering fashion. Distant metastases, which may claim life rapidly, occur in only a small percentage of these patients. In most, the disease develops by gradual infiltrating spread from the point of origin until urinary tract obstruction and uremia develop or the intestinal tract becomes obstructed. In these instances, diverting colostomies or bladder substitutes are usually not performed, inasmuch as this might only prolong a painful and miserable existence without producing any fundamental improvement. Medical and even religious concepts in such cases do not favor a vigorous attempt to prolong life for the sake of life alone.

In those instances, however, where an exenteration procedure is carried out because it is felt that this is the only way in which a cure may be achieved, the resulting disability is formidable. This stems from the need to construct, for these patients, a substitute bladder, or a colostomy, and often both of these maneuvers are necessary. The problem is essentially the same as already described under intestinal and bladder cancer, except that here it may be compounded. On the whole, this group of patients presents a stirring example of human resourcefulness in the face of most exacting vicissitudes. Being keenly aware that they have had a serious encounter with the disease cancer, and grateful for the chance to be cured and to be alive, these patients display remarkable adaptability to their major physiological alterations. Recently such a patient, with both an artificial bladder and a high colostomy, returned from a cross-country trip by automobile, including a side trip to Alaska, during which she did all the driving, and following which she was already enthusiastically planning her next trip. The disability, then, in such cases, is partly an individual problem. Proper support and guidance from the concerned medical, nursing, and other professional personnel can rehabilitate many of these patients to the point where useful and happy lives may be led.

This discussion on cancer of the cervix, however, should not be concluded with a description of the tribulations that face a patient requiring extensive surgery in this area. Rather, it should be stressed again that techniques are now at hand, through a periodic vaginal smear test, to detect this disease at a very early stage in its development. If the early cancer is detected in such a manner, the therapy required is far, far less; moreover, at this stage, the chance for cure approaches 100 per cent. Widespread recognition of this fact, and the application of this simple technique, should make advanced cervix cancer a vanishing disease, and the necessity for doing ultraradical pelvic surgery in women should rarely, if ever, arise.

CANCER OF THE LARYNX

Cancer of the larynx, or "voice box," presents a number of unique problems in terms of rehabilitation, inasmuch as this area is intimately concerned with the three important body functions of phonation, deglutition, and respiration. If the malignant focus occurs superficially on one of the paired vocal cords, then highly successful treatment can be carried out by x-ray therapy, especially since the advent of supervoltage techniques. In such cases, a satisfactory voice almost always returns, sometimes to quite normal levels.

In certain areas of the larynx, however, surgery has been found to be the better modality of therapy in terms of offering the patient a maximum chance for cure. In the surgically treated cases, the resultant disability depends largely on the extent of the surgery that is necessary. If a lesser procedure can be safely done, such as a "laryngofissure" or a partial laryngectomy, then only slight impairment of the voice or swallowing mechanism results, and the disability element is not great. However, in those instances where the cancerous growth in the larynx is extensive, or where radiation cannot be adequately carried out, a total laryngectomy must be done. In such instances the trachea, or "windpipe," has to be divided below the larynx and the end of the windpipe brought out to the skin level, low in the midline of the neck, just above the superior part of the sternum. This usually does not result in any severe respiratory problem; the patient adjusts quite readily to breathing through the new opening, or stoma, in the neck. This is easily kept discreetly hidden by the collar of a man's shirt or by a woman's wearing a dress with a moderately high neckline.

The chief problem in rehabilitation following total laryngectomy is

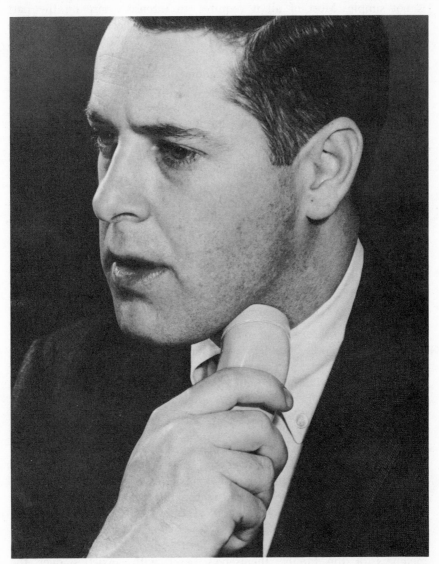

Figure 32. The electronic artificial larynx developed by the Bell Telephone Laboratories. The unit contains a diaphragm which is made to pulsate by an electromagnetic stimulus. The vibrations thus produced are transmitted from the side of the neck to the oral cavity. (Courtesy of American Telephone and Telegraph Company.)

The Cooper Rand Electronic Speech Aid (not illustrated) contains a minute tone generator; the sound produced is carried to the oral cavity via a small plastic tube.

the loss of the voice. Formidable as this unhappy situation is, much can be done today to improve it and to permit communication again. The best solution lies in voice retraining—that is, the development of an "esophageal" voice. By this mechanism the patient is taught to swallow or to aspirate air into the upper esophagus which can then be "regurgitated" to produce sound. Learning to develop an esophageal voice is not simple. Most of all it requires an intense desire on the part of the patient to achieve this goal. Although speech therapists are prepared to help in this training, it has been found that introducing such a patient to a person who had the same disability, and has mastered the esophageal voice technique, is the most successful way of getting a new "trainee" to believe that the technique can be mastered and that the results can be highly satisfactory.

In those patients who cannot develop an esophageal voice despite conscientious effort, an artificial larynx may be tried. Several different types of electronic devices are now available which emit tones or sounds upon placement against the neck or upon passing a small plastic tube into the mouth; the sound thus produced can be molded into speech in a reasonably satisfactory manner. The Cooper-Rand and the Bell Telephone Laboratories have pioneered in the effort to help these voiceless persons and in recent years have produced much more satisfactory instruments. Nevertheless, if the more natural esophageal voice can be learned, this tends to be the more satisfactory solution.

Family, Social, and Community Aspects of Cancer

In addition to the physical and physiological problems that may face a cancer patient, other problems, on a family, social, or community level, need to be recognized and approached with understanding by personnel engaged in rehabilitating a patient with cancer.

On a family level, it should be appreciated that the members of a patient's family very frequently need considerable support and explanation themselves so that they can better understand the problems of the patient recovering from a bout with cancer. This tends to be one of our neglected areas in cancer management. To assume that a family innately knows and appreciates the fears and anxieties of a cancer patient in their midst, and then proceeds in a reasonable manner to assuage those anxieties, is folly indeed. In fact, if a patient fails to be progressing satisfactorily, even though a cure is anticipated, very often the family relationships will be found to be at least a partial cause of this. The members of the family, themselves beset with anxieties over the "tragedy" that has disrupted their security, and wondering if this illness could be hereditary or infectious, as is very commonly imagined by the laity, do little to establish a tranquil and comforting environment for the cancer patient. He senses their fears, and if the prognosis is uncertain, he senses and suspects that the family knows something that he does not. Thus, the family and the patient often become wary and guarded with one another, at the very time when close union and understanding are most desirable.

Physicians, nurses, and social service personnel must do all they can to enlighten and to prepare the family for the continued care of the cancer patient. This requires a full discussion with the family concerning the outlook, the plan for follow-up care and guidance, and some explanation as to the role and importance of the family in the future needs of the patient. Often, within a family unit, there will be one or more members who themselves are unable to accept the facts of this disease, especially if the outlook for a cure is poor or questionable. In such instances the remainder of the family strive to keep the news from the sensitive members, and often from the patient as well. These factors, though quite understandable as one gets to know the family, nevertheless make adjustments difficult for both patient and family. The persons engaged in the care and rehabilitation of these patients must be aware of the problems within a particular family unit, for ignorance or disregard of these may lead to an inappropriate word or statement that can totally disrupt the balance achieved.

On a social level, one frequently finds that the cancer patient tends to avoid contacts with individuals other than the immediate family and begins to shun public gatherings such as meetings, dances, and the cinema. This is especially true if the patient is left with a colostomy, substitute bladder, or an altered voice mechanism. The dread of an "accident," such as an unexpected evacuation while in a public place, keeps these persons in virtual seclusion if not actively combated. The truth of the matter is that sufficient experience in these areas has now been gained so that it is apparent that virtually all such persons can live essentially normal social lives. The management of a colostomy should offer no real obstacles toward holding down a responsible position or taking part in social events. The loss of voice has been successfully overcome through voice retraining and especially the development of esophageal voice by many individuals who now take pride in being able to address public gatherings without anyone being the wiser. The important factors, in between the loss and the successful adjustment, are education and retraining. This has been the important lesson learned in the past several decades, and fortunately, many advances have been made that facilitate a successful adjustment.

On a community level it is probably most important for the cancer patient, his family, and those professional persons involved in his care and rehabilitation to be aware of the various resources that may already exist in a given community which can be of considerable practical value if exploited. For example, the Visiting Nurse Association, available to most communities, can be most helpful if called upon to assist. The trained nurse can visit the patient in his home daily if need be in the beginning, assist with colostomy care and management, encourage the person through what may be a difficult adjustment period, and in general provide a sense of security by providing continuing professional care after the "haven" of the hospital has been given up. Also, many communities are now fortunate enough to possess a "tumor clinic," often within the framework of the local or regional hospital, where expert advice and consultation are available to the patient and family physician upon request. Such extremely practical matters as transportation to a tumor clinic, financing an artificial limb or appliance, or payment for special medications or procurement of special services need not be a burden for the family to obtain or struggle with, inasmuch as many of these are readily available in average communities. The state, often in cooperation with federal or national agencies, provides many services to cancer patients if only these are requested by the patient's physician or by the social service worker. The state-supported specialized cancer hospitals are an example of this. In these institutions, at nominal cost, one can obtain the finest care available utilizing the latest techniques and equipment.

One last word should be said about the follow-up of a patient with cancer. It is most important that a patient with a diagnosis of a malignant disease be carefully followed for a prolonged period, perhaps for the rest of his life, by appropriately informed medical personnel. After a period of some time, usually five years, if no evidence of recurrent or metastatic disease has been observed, then the patient's chances for a cure become quite good. Nevertheless, especially in some types of cancer, recurrences, developing many years after primary treatment, are part of the natural history of this disease. It is far easier to treat successfully a recurrence of the disease when this is caught early, in the course of a routine check-up, rather than when symptoms bring a patient back to the physician whom he may not have seen for years. Often, during the first two or three years after treatment, the physician may want to see the patient at quite frequent intervals, every two or three months, to be on the lookout for recurrent disease. After this, the intervals may be spaced somewhat longer, until, when a cure is virtually assured, an annual check-up may suffice. The concept of long-continued follow-up care is the important thing, and this must be appreciated by those individuals providing state and community services, as well as by the patient and his family. In many institutions, or within the framework of a personal patient-doctor relationship, the concept of a periodic return for a check-up continues long after a cure has been assured. This is most desirable, for the friendly relationship engendered between patient and doctor or clinic not only provides reassurance for the patient that all continues to be well, but also takes us into the realm of being able to practice a preventive type of medicine, which is, by far, the best way to provide medical care.

BIBLIOGRAPHY

Ackerman, L. V., and J. A. del Regato. *Cancer: Diagnosis, Treatment, and Prognosis.* St. Louis: C. V. Mosby Co., 1962. Chap. 1–5, pp. 1–155.

"Cancer: A World-Wide Menace." Report No. 1009. Committee on Government Operations, U. S. Senate 86th Congress, 1959.

Care of Your Colostomy. A Source Book of Information. New York: American Cancer Society, 1964.

Cigarette Smoking and Cancer. New York: American Cancer Society, 1963.

Trends and Practices in Cancer Diagnosis and Treatment. New York: American Cancer Society, 1963.

Willis, R. A. *Pathology of Tumours.* London: Butterworths, 1960. Chap. 1–12, pp. 1–207.

XIII

AMPUTATIONS

Amputees constitute an appreciable and increasing proportion of the disabled requiring rehabilitation services each year. They appear in all age groups, from birth to old age. The majority of adult amputees can be successfully rehabilitated physically and vocationally. They may be found functioning competitively in every profession, industry, trade, skilled or unskilled job, and most sports.

✓ Amputation is performed to remove a pathological part or all of a limb. The resultant disability is created by the surgical procedure and not by the pathology. Amputation is in a sense a mechanical problem. Amputations following acute trauma occur in otherwise healthy individuals, who, after the amputation heals, have no pathology but are faced with the mechanical problem of replacing lost function. Most upper extremity amputees fall into this category and are more easily rehabilitated than the average leg amputee. This does not necessarily imply that loss of an arm is less disabling than loss of a leg. It does, however, point up the fact that accidental injuries occur in younger people who are subjected to the hazards of working with industrial machinery and engaging in high-speed driving on the highways.

More than 75 per cent of the amputations currently performed in the lower extremities are carried out on people over the age of 60. Amputations on people in the older age group are generally not isolated mechanical problems such as they may be in traumatic cases. The amputation is superimposed upon an elderly individual who is suffering from a vascular problem and other chronic degenerative diseases.

By ALLEN S. RUSSEK, M.D., Director Prosthetic Service, Institute of Physical Medicine and Rehabilitation, New York City, New York.

The vascular patient has impairment in both lower extremities, one of which has been amputated, and it is possible that the limitations of the remaining limb may be more disabling than the amputated limb fitted with a prosthesis. In addition, many of the elderly patients also have cardiovascular disease, a history of coronary disease, and other chronic disabling conditions.

Successful physical and vocational rehabilitation is dependent upon many factors:

- The cause of amputation
- General health and the presence or absence of other disabilities
- Characteristics of the amputation stump
- Personal characteristics of the individual
- Preparation for function
- Prescription for the prosthesis
- The quality of training with a prosthesis
- The nature of the rehabilitation facilities available to the patient

CAUSES OF AMPUTATION

UPPER EXTREMITY

Amputation in the upper extremity is performed predominantly as a result of industrial and automobile *accidents*. A great many of these accidents result in partial hand amputations or loss of one to five fingers. These are severe disabilities. If the thumb alone is lost, the loss of the use of the hand is evaluated at about 50 per cent. Loss of fingers does not necessarily require replacement with a prosthesis but does often require a protective device with which the individual can work. Cosmetic replacements for fingers and partial hand amputations are available, but there are no functioning devices or terminal devices for loss of fingers or partial hand amputations where the palm of the hand is intact. The terminal devices of the prosthesis begin at the wrist.

There are many *congenital deformities* in the upper extremity with which the child survives quite well and with which he remains functional. In adult life, however, this limb may be repugnant to the individual, and the degree of function necessary as an adult is insufficient. A useless limb may be amputated and replaced with a functioning prosthesis. Many such useless limbs, following long-term paralysis, pain, and other neurological conditions where loss of sensation and function are complete, justify amputation. Where there is loss of sensation and function, the limb is subject to injury, ulceration, and burns. Many of these useless limbs follow severe injuries to the brachial plexus. The flail (flaccid) useless limb can be replaced with a functioning prosthesis in most cases by selecting the proper site for amputation, where some shoulder girdle function remains.

Most industrial and road accidents occur under poor conditions wherein the compound wounds are contaminated. Many of these survive the contamination, but other go on to *infection* that spreads and destroys considerable function. Chronic osteomyelitis is extremely destructive, particularly to the hand; when the hand is useless—even after the infection has been overcome—it is better to have it amputated and replaced with a functioning device or functional prosthesis with a hand.

Malignant tumors are not uncommon in adolescence. In the presence of malignant tumors amputation is performed as a lifesaving measure. These amputations are made much higher than one would consider amputating for other reasons. When a bone is involved, the amputation is always performed above the most proximal joint of which the bone is a part. Where soft tissue malignant tumors are diagnosed, amputation must be carried out above the origin of the muscles of the tumor area. Sarcomas involving bone have a tendency to metastasize before they are diagnosed and before amputation is carried out. They also have a tendency toward local recurrence. The life expectancy of the individual who has submitted to an amputation for a sarcoma is always in question, therefore.

Vascular accidents occur in the upper extremity less frequently than they do in the lower extremity. Amputation may be indicated for damage to the circulation through blockage of a major blood vessel by an embolus, rupture, or the presence of an aneurysm that cannot be corrected surgically.

LOWER EXTREMITY

Vascular insufficiency associated with arteriosclerosis or diabetes is a frequent cause of lower extremity amputation. With improved management of diabetes and the perfection of vascular surgery, many people have survived longer with their vascular impairment, but a good many come to amputation. In this category of vascular insufficiency there are vasospastic conditions, such as Buerger's disease and Raynaud's disease, which often terminate in major amputation.

Where sufficient injury has occurred as the result of *accidental violence* to affect the blood and nerve supply of a limb and render it useless, it is often futile to make repairs, and emergency amputation is carried out. When there is a chance to save the limb, however, amputation should be delayed.

Malignant tumors occur in the lower extremity, as in the upper extremity, and require high proximal amputations as lifesaving measures and for the assurance that the amputations have been carried out high enough above the involved tissues.

Acute *infection* that cannot be rapidly brought under control and becomes chronic is highly destructive to functioning tissues. Many episodes of osteomyelitis and other infections in the lower extremity destroy the usefulness of the foot and the capacity of the limb to sustain weight. Many of these cases definitely come to major amputation if sufficient function cannot be salvaged with further surgery.

Thermal injuries—heat and cold—are important causative factors. Amputations often result from extensive burns and contractures causing loss of function in the extremity. Extreme cold and frostbite in the presence of vascular insufficiency not uncommonly lead to amputation.

There are also a small number of cases where amputation is required as an emergency procedure for saving life, such as snake bite, acute vascular accidents, and gas gangrene.

GENERAL HEALTH AND THE PRESENCE OF OTHER DISABILITIES

Advanced age is one factor that may preclude the possibility of offering the patient very much in the way of physical and vocational rehabilitation. Since most of the lower extremity amputees are in the older age group, they often suffer from other disabling conditions at the same time. Most patients who submit to one amputation for vascular insufficiency also have severe impairment of circulation in the remaining leg. A good many of these patients also have cardiovascular disease and a history of coronary occlusion which they have survived. Patients in this category demonstrate low tolerance for activity and function. Hemiplegics often come to amputation, but even when successfully fitted with a prosthesis, their degree of function is seldom at a high level. Other conditions with which patients in the older age group suffer are osteoarthritis, fractured hips that may or may not have healed, genitourinary conditions, and nutritional disturbances.

CHARACTERISTICS OF THE AMPUTATION STUMP

The amputation stump in most cases is the key to determining whether or not the patient will be successful in developing skill with a prosthesis. The surgeon is responsible for creating a stump that will taper from above downwards, and in which he has handled all of the tissues in the proper manner so that it may be fitted with conventional prosthetic equipment. The surgeon encounters all of the tissues in transecting the limb—namely (1) the skin and subcutaneous tissue, (2) fascia, (3) muscle, (4) bone, (5) vessels, and (6) nerves.

Each of these tissues may be responsible for creating a problem at some later date if not handled properly at the time of surgery. Most of the problems amputees have in adapting to a prosthesis can be traced to some defect of surgical management in the operating room. *Flexion contractures* are often created by closing amputation stumps with the proximal joint in acute flexion. *Skin flaps* that are tightly stretched across the end of the stump remain painful and often break down with the use of the prosthesis. The *fascia* should be used as a barrier between the deep tissues and the skin flaps so that they may be freely movable. The *muscles* must be anchored down to, and in some instances across, the end of the bone so that they do not retract upon movement of the stump. The *bone* requires accurate cutting without piling up the periosteum at the end of the bone, since this often results in the growth of new bone forming a cauliflowerlike exostosis (benign tumor). The presence of this amorphous type of bone is likely to create pain with the use of a prosthesis. Control of *bleeding* during and after surgery is necessary. Control following surgery is maintained by proper compressive dressings. Drainage should always be employed to prevent the accumulation of a large clot at the end of the stump underneath the skin flaps. The *nerves* should be pulled down and cut as high as possible so that they are not incorporated in the scar on the end of the stump. All nerves form neuromas, but when a neuroma is in the scar or low in the stump where it will be compressed against the wall of the prosthetic socket, it becomes extremely painful and may preclude the possibility of the amputee developing tolerance for weight bearing.

The degree of function achieved with the prosthesis is directly proportionate to the amount of the functioning limb remaining. There are standard levels of amputation. In the upper extremity the highest amputation is the interscapulothoracic or forequarter amputation. In this case the scapula and clavicle and entire upper extremity are removed, so that no voluntary movement is present at that shoulder. Such a patient is very difficult to fit, but he can be fitted. There is a serious problem in holding the shoulder cap on a woman. It is readily harnessed on men, since their clothing conceals the shoulder cap and the harness. Amputations at that level are known as *disarticulations at the shoulder,* amputations between the elbow and shoulder are referred to as *above-elbow* amputations, *below-elbow* amputations are those that are done between the wrist and elbow; disarticulations are also performed at the elbow or wrist, and the lowest amputations, those through the hand, are called *transcarpal* or *transmetacarpal.* Losses of individual fingers are not considered major amputations.

In the lower extremity the most proximal amputation is the *hemipelvectomy.* In this amputation half of the sacrum and the entire ilium, ischium, and pubis are removed on one side. No bones are left on that side of the pelvis; these are removed with the entire extremity. In recent years it has been possible to fit a hemipelvectomy patient quite successfully. A satisfactory gait is obviously difficult to achieve, but many amputees with hemipelvectomy have been restored to fairly good function and have returned to daily active work. The amputations below that level are known as *disarticulation at the hip, above-knee* amputation which takes place between the knee and the hip, *knee disarticulation* which takes place through the knee joint without cutting bone, *below-knee* amputation between the ankle and the knee, and *partial foot* amputation. Most partial foot amputations are unsuccessful from a functioning standpoint, since many of them do not require a prosthesis and those that do are cosmetically unacceptable, with a tendency to break down.

In general, the ideal length of an amputation stump is through the middle of the segment, referring to either the arm, forearm, thigh, or leg. In the upper extremity, however, more than half can be saved, which is most desirable. In the lower extremity, it is not necessary to make an excessively long amputation stump, since it would be difficult to fit. With respect to the levels of amputation mentioned above, every joint that is removed must be replaced by a mechanical joint. The more mechanical joints in a prosthesis, the less control the individual has and the more evident is his gait that of an amputee. Amputations carried out just proximal to and distal to a major joint, such as the elbow or knee, are difficult to fit with conventional equipment and require specially constructed prostheses to make these joints useful. The use of the joint is so important that special fittings are desirable when such amputations are performed. Elderly patients who have amputations in the lower extremity for diabetic gangrene have a tendency toward slow healing of the scars. The tissues become somewhat friable and have a tendency to break down with the use of prosthesis. Their surgery requires careful planning in order to avoid absorption of the stresses through tight skin or depressed or painful scars.

PERSONAL CHARACTERISTICS OF THE INDIVIDUAL

Many amputees have been known to function quite satisfactorily with a major amputation without the use of a prosthesis for the upper or lower extremity. A good many people work on crutches and one leg, traveling to work every day. There is an extremely small number of people who are required to do this, since prostheses can be fitted to practically any amputation. The exception is where the stump is too painful to tolerate a prosthesis and the patient refuses to have surgical revision.

The patient himself, in relationship to his amputation, is perhaps the most critical factor in the entire process of rehabilitation. When evaluating any patient for physical, prosthetic, or vocational rehabilitation, it is essential to know him well. The personal characteristics of the individual constitute variable factors in terms of basic potential, the type of artificial limb to be prescribed, and the degree of function that may be achieved. From the standpoint of writing a prescription for a prosthesis, one must look beyond the amputation stump and know *who* is being fitted as well as *what* is being fitted. Each of the following individual characteristics must be taken into account:

AGE

If the patient is over 60, it must be assumed that his adaptability for use of a prosthesis will be slow; his goals may not be very high. Patients in the older age group take longer to achieve their best potential; their treatment requires patience.

SEX

The female amputee may be rehabilitated as a homemaker. This requires considerably less function to be successful than for a man who must travel, work on the outside, and perform physical activities for an eight-hour period.

OCCUPATION

Many amputees can be rehabilitated to return to their former occupation, depending upon how skillful they may be after being trained with a prosthesis. When it becomes obvious that the previous occupation is not a practical goal, one must establish an objective that is compatible with the potential function of the individual. The physical demands of the job must be carefully evaluated so that the amputee does not feel that more is expected of him than he can provide.

ECONOMIC STATUS

This is one of the factors that determine whether or not a prosthesis is to be prescribed. It also frequently determines whether or not the patient can be discharged from the hospital. When it is found that the amputee at his best state of training cannot take complete care of himself, he cannot be discharged from the hospital if he lives alone. Amputations are performed on a great many indigent people who are basically homeless and live in furnished rooms provided by welfare agencies. Such individuals need to have a good enough potential to take care of all of their activities of daily living without the assistance of another individual before they can be returned to living alone once more. A businessman who has a family and can afford an attendant may be quite functional if he has enough help. He may require assistance in applying the prosthesis; he can also be helped by the use of a wheelchair for traveling to and from his office. Once he is seated at his desk, he is quite functional in using the telephone, writing letters, interviewing people, and supervising activities in a business.

The majority of the prostheses that are purchased in our present society are paid for by insurance companies and social agencies. A specific determination must be made as to whether or not the individual will be better off with a prosthesis than he is without one. There are many elderly people who are not benefited by its use, since it is too demanding of them and their remaining degree of function is so small that it becomes impractical.

PSYCHOLOGICAL FACTORS

The personal reaction of the patient must be well understood. In the early postamputation phase, most patients are concerned with the cosmetic effect of the loss of the limb and the prospect of concealing it. Many have the idea that a cosmetic limb can be provided for an upper or lower extremity that will be unnoticeable. This is a rather unrealistic attitude, but it is very common. Some education must be carried out with each amputee so that he understands the function and limitations of the prosthesis. It is necessary to have the full co-operation of the patient, just as it is necessary for the patient to have insight into his problems and the purposes of treatment. On the other hand, there are other types of individuals who are quite aggressive and dynamic despite their age. Many of these people have rehabilitated themselves with very little professional help. In view of the many variations in performance and types of individuals who become amputees, very careful evaluation of the personal characteristics should be carried out.

PREPARATION FOR FUNCTION

The ideal patient for prosthetic rehabilitation is one who accepts his disability, is emotionally and medically stable, has insight into his problems, and has an amputation stump that can be fitted with standard prosthetic components. Any amputee who can be described in this manner must have gone through a considerable degree of preparation to reach that state. Preparing the patient to achieve these goals begins as soon as possible following amputation. The patient is gotten out of bed in what may be a matter of a few days after the amputation. As soon as possible, in lower extremity involvement, the patient is encouraged to stand on the remaining limb to maintain its strength and its functional capacity and to support the circulation. The patient's vascular condition, diabetes, cardiac status, kidneys, and nutrition must be brought to the highest level possible. He must be psychologically oriented to the process of measuring and fitting the prosthesis, and should be informed with regard to what he can expect to achieve as an individual. It is an extremely frustrating experience for a patient to hope for more than he can accomplish; when he eventually finds out that he is more severely disabled than he thought, he is deeply disappointed. It is, therefore, important to promise somewhat less than can be delivered rather than more.

The amputation stump needs to be strengthened, shaped, and allowed to shrink under controlled conditions; the range of motion must be preserved so that no contractures develop or are retained. Amputation stumps shrink for about two years. It is possible, however, by beginning proper shrinking about the third week, to achieve in four or five weeks 50 per cent of the shrinkage that will normally occur in two years. For this reason, shape, strength, and volume of the stump should be carefully prepared. When an amputation stump is swollen or has not atrophied and is fitted with a prosthesis, the early use of the prosthesis with the weight of the body in the socket will cause rapid shrinkage. This, in turn, causes the socket to become too loose; shrinkage may be so massive that it is no longer possible to maintain the fit after only a few weeks of use. This is one reason why it is unwise to attempt to fit any patient who is expected to use a prosthesis to an appreciable extent until the stump is prepared. With older people, however, the principle is to fit as soon as possible. Most older patients have flabby amputation stumps, and their muscles have atrophied from disuse prior to the amputation. There is not as much margin for shrinkage in the older person as there is in the muscular young individual. In addition, older people do not use their prostheses extensively, so that the degree of shrinkage from the use of the prosthesis alone is not so great that the socket cannot be continuously maintained in a satisfactory fit.

The preparation of the amputation stump in the upper extremity is not as critical as it is in the lower extremity. All that is necessary is to make sure that the strength of the muscles has been restored by exercise and that, if swollen, the stump is reduced before it is measured for a prosthesis. One reason for this is that shrinkage is slower and occurs in lesser degree in the upper extremity than in the lower. Another reason is that amputations in the upper extremity usually are performed following trauma, and thus they are not performed on diseased limbs. The remaining stump may be quite muscular and strong and may not deteriorate very much if it is fitted with a prosthesis rather early. Shrinkage is necessary, however, when the amputation stumps are very fleshy, as in obese people, since these will shrink to a greater extent than bony stumps.

Every lower extremity amputee should be encouraged and trained to walk in parallel bars or with crutches on the unamputated limb. This not only helps maintain satisfactory circulation in the limb, but preserves its strength and the proprioception with the ground. A patient who has not had his feet on the ground for a long time has poor balance and requires some time to gain assurance, not only that the prosthesis will hold up, but that his remaining limb will also hold up. This is why many elderly patients cling to their crutches for such a long time. In the preprosthetic stage of management it is important to instruct the patient concerning the procedures. He should know that the stump shrinks and will continue to shrink for about two years, particularly when he is wearing a limb.

The function of a prosthesis in the upper extremity is to provide prehension. This is achieved either by approximating two fingers of the functional hand to a thumb or by the movement of one finger of a split hook against or away from the other. The function of the lower extremity prosthesis is to provide stability, comfort, and safety. Without stability and comfort a lower extremity prosthesis is virtually useless.

Every patient is aware of a phantom sensation following amputation; this is not an abnormal phenomenon. When the phantoms are painful or otherwise create distress (they may be found in peculiar positions, or they may be felt as burning or cold), the amputee is upset and has a tendency not to use the prosthesis. Control of the phantom sensation is extremely important; when a phantom is very annoying shortly after amputation, it becomes all the more necessary to fit the patient with a prosthesis and train him to use it as soon as possible. This is one of the quickest ways to eliminate this serious problem.

PRESCRIPTION FOR THE PROSTHESIS

By the time the physician writes the prescription, he must be satisfied that the patient is under control medically and emotionally, that the stump is well prepared and is ready to be measured for the prosthesis. He must have some idea as to the potential of the individual. Those amputees who obviously will derive great function from the prosthesis must be given a prosthesis that can provide such function. Patients who need stability and protection should be given a prosthesis that can provide such stability and protection. The general concept of the prescription is that it is written in terms of the various components required for each individual patient. The prescription is personal for a particular type of individual, with all of the variable factors taken into consideration. In the upper extremity the prescription will provide for a socket that will encase the amputation stump. The prosthesis will be suspended in a way that will allow the amputee to use his moving parts to operate the terminal device. The joints will be prescribed according to individual needs. A wrist unit and terminal devices will complete the prescription. The terminal device, which may be a hook or a hand or a cosmetic hand, is the tool. The arm and forearm are levers. There is a standard prosthesis for every standard type of amputation.

The forequarter amputation and the shoulder disarticulation do not contain a functioning shoulder. The lever of the arm, therefore, is lost but the forearm can be flexed and the terminal device operated within the radius of the movements of the forearm. If the patient has his own shoulder, he will have the benefit of the additional radius of the leverage of the arm as well as the forearm. In this country, wrist joints and wrist rotation units are not used. They are standard parts in many foreign countries, particularly in Germany. These units do have certain advantages, but they are not standard equipment as yet in the United States.

In the lower extremity, similarly, the prosthesis is prescribed by the component parts—namely, the socket, the joints, and the foot. The above-knee amputation, which is the commonest, requires careful consideration of the type of knee to be prescribed. There are many different types, some of which allow the amputee great freedom, others of which may be locked or protected by locking devices or alignment variations that will keep the knee from buckling if the amputee cannot gain control of the limb in any other way. The commonest types of knees are the single axis knee, the friction locking knee, and the polycentric knee. There are also hydraulic and pneumatic knees, which are used by very functional amputees who live active lives. These decrease the effort needed to use the prosthesis and simulate normal movements more closely.

The selection of the proper foot is also important. There are feet that have no ankle joint and no moving parts other than a compressible heel wedge. These are called Sach feet, referring to solid-ankle-cushion heel. The Sach foot is a relatively recent development, although the principle has been known for a great many years. Another standard foot is one that has a single axis ankle that plantar flexes the foot and returns it to the right angle position on a bolt. This is considered to be an ankle joint; changes in the position of the foot are controlled by compressible rubber in the heel, the instep, and in the toe. It is an articulated foot as contrasted with a solid ankle and foot. When the prescription for the prosthesis is written, it is written with a specific objective in mind—the classification of function each individual amputee is expected to achieve.

The classifications of function vary. Class one is the extremely functional amputee who has been fully restored to function, one who has a handicap but no disability. Classification one is *full restoration*.

There are many people who can compete effectively with nonamputees in every activity, including sports, in spite of their amputation. They are few in number, however, and most amputees do not achieve full restoration.

A great many, however, will fall into class two, which is considered to be *partial restoration*. These individuals have a disability with their handicap, but the disability relates largely to personal activities such as dancing, hiking, skating, and other things that are not essential for earning a living. These are very functional amputees who have discontinued many of the activities on the fringes of basic function.

Classification three is considered to be *self-care-plus*. The interpretation is that the amputee, fitted and trained with the proper prosthesis, not only will be able to take care of all of his personal needs and not need the help of another individual, but can do more. Such amputees are able to work and support their families. Despite the fact that they may require the use of a cane or even a crutch at times, these are disabled people who are functioning at a level sufficiently high to permit them to be competitive with nonamputees on a limited basis.

Classification four is considered *self-care-minus*. Such amputees, fitted and trained with the proper prosthesis, fail to achieve the capacity to take complete care of themselves and do need the help of another individual. This help may be slight or considerable. Some amputees simply need assistance in putting the prosthesis on properly; others may need to be helped down stairs or require assistance in walking any considerable distance. These are the people who cannot be discharged from hospitals to live alone. If they get the help they need, they can actually work. They can be assisted to their place of work and, once seated, are quite functional if they are lower extremity amputees. Upper extremity amputees seldom fall into this category, since if one functioning upper extremity remains, the majority of people can travel and take complete care of themselves.

Classification five is referred to as *cosmetic-plus*. Amputees in this category not only are fitted with a prosthesis to replace the missing lower extremity, but can do a little on their own. These are people who can move from one room to another with crutches, move out of a wheel chair to another chair, and, with some assistance, live comfortably in a home among other people. They do not do much walking and require considerable help if traveling is necessary. The economic status will, therefore, determine the practicality of providing a prosthesis for the individual whose best potential does not exceed classification five in terms of function.

With regard to the prescription for the prosthesis, it must be recognized that the uppermost thought in the minds of most people who have lost an arm is to replace it cosmetically. It is important to have them recognize that some function can be restored although not the equivalent of the lost parts. As previously mentioned, the function of an upper extremity prosthesis is to provide prehension. This small function, however, is very important in acting as an aid to the remaining upper extremity so that the individual, to some extent, is once again bimanual. Most upper extremity amputees will eventually accept a functional prosthesis if they have a working life to consider. They may also have a cosmetic hand which may be necessary for the type of lives they lead or purely for psychological reasons. In general, a cosmetic hand is acceptable to all amputees, but most of them will eventually use the functional equipment most of the day.

THE QUALITY OF TRAINING

The training of amputees is best carried out by individuals who have been trained as therapists for this activity. It requires a considerable degree of skill to teach upper and lower extremity amputees to use their prostheses. In the long run more function is derived from an upper extremity prosthesis, but it takes a great deal more skill to teach an amputee with a lower extremity prosthesis to walk. Although training facilities are sometimes available in the home, it is best to conduct the training in an institution equipped with the proper facilities and staffed with personnel trained to get the best results. Moreover, patients seem to do better in groups. The small degree of competition that may occur as an interplay between patients is highly desirable psychologically for maintaining the highest level of motivation and participation in the program. It is somewhat paradoxical that the patients who derive the most from the prosthesis will require the least training, while those who get the least degree of function from the use of a prosthesis will require the greatest degree of training.

An important aspect of the training is that both the patient and the therapist should know what the ultimate objective is. In a lower extremity situation the patient should know what classification of function is considered to be his best potential. If he is considered, for example, a class three potential—self-care-plus—he may still be using a cane and be somewhat unsteady when he achieves this potential, but he is then succesfully rehabilitated as far as the prosthesis is concerned, and the training may then cease. Every patient is not trained to reach classification one with full restoration of function.

From a psychological standpoint, amputees should not be compared with nonamputees in term of how much they can do. Each amputee should be competitive with his own best potential, and when he achieves it, he may be considered highly successful no matter how small the function obtained. It is only when a patient fails to achieve what obviously is his potential that he is an unsuccessful case.

In training the upper extremity amputee, the basic movements of the arm and the restoration of the proprioceptive factors with regard to position and the use of the joint are taught first. When the patient is capable of placing the terminal device in the various positions, he is then trained to operate it against objects in movements that are used for basic living activities such as dressing, eating, and toilet activities. Later these are extended to activities outside the home, including those related to work and earning a living. If considerable function is present, these patients may also be taught to drive a car, operate machinery, perform their hobbies, and even engage in limited sports.

The training is a step-by-step procedure and is not suddenly achieved by the amputee putting on the prosthesis. Training of the lower extremity amputee begins by teaching the patient to balance, to put the prosthesis on the ground, and to try to establish contact with the ground through his proprioceptive capacity. He then is allowed weight shifting to get the feel of the prosthesis holding up his body weight. He then ambulates with the protection of parallel bars so that he may put somewhat less than full weight on the limb until he achieves tolerance. He may then be graduated to crutches or become sufficiently functional within bars to walk without the aid of any mechanical devices. Most amputees, however, will go from the bars to either crutches or canes. Ultimately they may discard them if they can be trained that far.

Diabetic patients tend to use crutches and walk next to a wall because of sensory impairment. Although every diabetic does not have peripheral neuritis, there is an interference with the sensory input, so that the diabetic does not get much sensation from the floor reaction nor have the proprioceptive feeling that the prosthesis is holding up his weight. He may not even have adequate communication with the floor through his remaining leg because of interference with his peripheral sensation. For this reason, he gets more information from the ground by holding a cane in one of his hands, usually opposite the side of the prosthesis, and putting it to the floor. This contact of the cane with the floor is not used for relieving weight from the prosthesis, but physically and psychologically it gives the patient a great deal more security. Severe diabetics should always use a cane. It is an important safety measure.

In the early part of training, one may evaluate the tolerance of the amputee for his prosthesis. This is an extremely important phase of training, since it must be recognized that tolerances vary from person to person. Elderly people have little early tolerance for the use of a prosthesis, but this may later develop. Training must persist for longer periods of time until tolerance is achieved with the patients in the older age group. It soon becomes evident even with young, vigorous, and active amputees that tolerance is something that must be achieved, since overuse of a prosthesis in the early training periods will make the amputation stump sore. Abrasions or ulcerations may be caused by a single period of abuse.

When an amputee demonstrates that he is achieving a reasonably good level of function, he may then engage in those activities that will prepare him for vocational readjustment. Lower extremity amputees can be trained to walk up and down stairs, to travel alone and use trains and buses, to drive cars, and also to tolerate long periods of standing. This is done by weight shifting and to some extent relieving the prosthetic side of continuous weight bearing and pressure. It is easier on the amputation stump for the patient to subject it to intermittent pressure and release rather than continuous standing without changing position or shifting the center of gravity. In the course of training lower extremity amputees, the therapist must be alert to observing the amputee as an individual—the degree of effort necessary, whether or not he becomes short of breath, how long it takes for him to reach the point of fatigue, and whether or not the process itself is painful. The therapist must also remove the prosthesis and observe the amputation stump to determine whether or not the fit of the prosthesis remains satisfactory or whether any focal pressure or friction areas are developing. These should be reported to the physician so that complications may be avoided, since they are easier to avoid than treat once they have been established.

When a lower extremity amputee is really comfortable, even though he may not have tolerance for continuous function on the prosthesis, he may still be able to tolerate wearing it all day without removing it. The variations from standard amputations have a tendency to diminish the capacity to use a prosthesis all day. Patients with flexion contractures also have diminished tolerance. Those with painful scars do not tolerate the use of the prosthesis all day or even wearing it in the sitting position for long periods of time. Patients with excessively long or excessively short stumps in relationship to a joint have diminished tolerance as compared with those with standard amputations through the ideal sites of amputation. It is in the training period that the level of amputation, the kind of surgery, and the kind of preparation begin to show up in terms of complications and retarding progress in the use of the prosthesis.

THE NATURE OF THE REHABILITATION SERVICES
AVAILABLE TO THE PATIENT

When amputees are managed by physicians who have some insight into the relationship between surgery and the future of the amputee and who are familiar with the step-by-step control of the patient through his various phases of preparation and rehabilitation, the entire process is a rather smooth one. It is not too difficult for the patient and not too time-consuming, considering the formidable nature of the disability. There are no short cuts to proper management of an amputee. One cannot eliminate the psychological control or the management of the medical conditions by prescribing a prosthesis at the wrong time. There is an almost mathematical formula in the step-by-step procedure, which physicians familiar with the management of amputees recognize. When this formula breaks down it is often necessary to take a patient off a prosthesis and go back to an earlier phase of his management in order to bring him up to a functional level with the prosthesis at some later date. Many patients with poor amputation stumps require reamputation and revision of the stump in order to make it possible for them to use a prosthesis at all. There are many patients, not physically or psychologically ready for prosthetic or vocational training, who are thrust into the process prematurely. These cases will always be failures, but they should be recognized as failures who can be salvaged if they are brought back to a lower level of management and gradually introduced to new services when they are actually ready for them. In the prosthetic phase of rehabilitation an entire team is needed to manage every facet of the process. Required are a physician, trained therapists, a certified limbfitter, social workers, and psychologists in a setting with proper facilities.

Prosthetic rehabilitation of an amputee is one of the most satisfying phases of rehabilitation medicine. In the general management of amputees the status of the individual is always known, and whenever a complication occurs, its influence on ultimate function is also known, so that by the time the individual obtains his prosthesis and begins his training the entire amputee prosthetic team is aware of the objective. The patient is also made aware of this, so that he knows precisely what everyone is aiming for.

The prosthetist plays an important role in the amputee prosthetic team. He is the individual who carries out the prescription, and he may often assist the physician in the formulation of the prescription. He does not, however, take the responsibility for determining the various components as they relate to any of the medical factors, since he is not expected to have this knowledge. When a prosthesis is delivered, it needs to be checked out. It is first checked out against the prescription for the original prosthesis to determine whether or not the prosthesis itself complies accurately with the prescription. In addition, there are a number of items in the prosthesis that cannot be prescribed. These relate to the general workmanship, the accuracy of alignment and the means of achieving it through alignment devices, and the excellence of the finishing procedures. The use of plastics in recent years has simplified the fabrication procedures and has improved the quality and function of practically all prostheses. In addition, the accuracy of the fit of the sockets is more easily achieved with plastics that can be molded over plaster of Paris models of the amputation stump. These improvements, however, are best achieved through prescriptions being filled by prosthetists who have been certified by the American Board of Prosthetists and Orthotists, indicating that they have qualified as being competent to carry out prescriptions for modern prostheses.

From the vocational standpoint, there must be an assessment of each individual's functioning ability in relationship to his capacity to perform work. When an amputee is trained and actually performs at his best level, he is an effective individual. His functional ability can be applied within the structure of our society to make him productive again despite his disability.

XIV
EMOTIONAL DISORDERS

It is estimated that almost half of all hospital beds in the United States are occupied by mental patients. While the number of patients in state mental hospitals has started to decrease slightly in recent years, this cannot be taken as an indication that the problem is being brought under control, since at the same time there has been a steady increase in the number of patients admitted each year—both new admissions and readmissions. To the number of patients on active records of all mental hospitals, 1,240,897 in 1957,[1] must be added the large number of disturbed individuals treated by outside practitioners or in nonmedical facilities, and the still larger population who, for one reason or another, receive no treatment at all. One source estimated that in 1948 there were 8,500,000 cases suffering from some type of mental disorder in the total population of the United States.[2] While any estimate of this sort must be quite rough, there is no question that the magnitude of the problem is indeed great.

BACKGROUND

Through the course of history, emotional and behavior dysfunction have been attributed to a variety of causative agents—with related

[1] Joint Commission on Mental Illness and Health, *Action for Mental Health*, New York: Basic Books, 1961, p. 19.
[2] J. R. Ewalt, E. A. Strecker, and F. G. Ebaugh, *Practical Clinical Psychiatry*, 8th ed., New York: McGraw-Hill Book Co., 1957, p. 67.

By JULIAN S. MYERS, PH.D., Associate Professor, Coordinator, Rehabilitation Counselor Training, Boston University School of Education, Boston, Massachusetts.

methods of treatment—including divine intervention, evil spirits, and the waxing and waning of the moon. The word lunatic (*luna* means moon in Latin) indicates that this last point of view was taken quite seriously. In more recent years, many schools of thought have developed, but they generally can be categorized in one of two groups, one biological-organic in orientation, the other psychological-cultural. The tendency to dichotomize is unfortunate; both points of view are needed to understand the range of possible emotional reactions and their consequences.

BIOLOGICAL-ORGANIC

The case for *heredity* as an etiological factor is rather weak except for some rather rare forms of brain disorders (for example, cerebral lipoidosis) that are associated with psychotic manifestations. *Infection,* in the form of advanced syphilis, was a common cause of organic psychosis until antibiotics were developed. This one disease probably gave more impetus to the organic school of thought than any other single factor. *Chemical agents* such as mescaline, LSD, and alcohol are known to be capable of producing psychotic reactions. It is not uncommon to see temporary or chronic psychotic reactions in association with *trauma, disease and high fever, arteriosclerotic* and *degenerative changes* insofar as these affect the brain.

PSYCHOLOGICAL-CULTURAL

The schools of thought classified in this category, although they differ among themselves in some respects, generally maintain that the functional or psychogenic disorders represent man's reactions—in terms of his own personality—to the stresses and strains of his sociocultural environment. One school, which believes that the term mental illness is a misnomer, says it makes no more sense to attribute emotional symptoms to mental illness than to evil spirits. Szasz suggests that what we call mental illnesses are really "expressions of man's struggle with the problems of how he should live." [3] A related point of view was developed by Harry Stack Sullivan who sees emotional disturbances as stemming from, and reflecting, difficulties in interpersonal relationships.

The biological-psychological controversy might imply that there is little or no interaction between these two aspects of man. This is just not so. Man's biological functioning, psychological functioning, and social interactions are merely different aspects of the same entity; each strongly affects, and is affected by, the other. Change one and the others are likely to change in some way. Thus, different forms of treatment—psychological, social, chemical, surgical—may be appropriate under a given set of circumstances.

[3] T. S. Szasz, "The Myth of Mental Illness." *The American Psychologist,* 15:2:117, (1960).

This is not to say that all etiological factors are of equal importance and that all forms of treatment are of equal value. The bias of this chapter is that the functional disorders are caused primarily by psychosocial factors, and therefore the primary treatment should be psychosocial in nature. In a much smaller number of cases, organic brain dysfunction is primarily responsible for emotional symptomatology; biologically oriented treatment should be given priority in these cases. In *all* cases, evaluation and treatment should be comprehensive in nature, utilizing the skills and knowledge of multiple disciplines in concert with the facilities of the community.

A FRAME OF REFERENCE

Emotional disorders are expressions of man's inability to cope effectively with the demands, responsibilities, and problems of life. They represent an imbalance between the emotional or feeling aspects of behavior and the cognitive, intellectual, or control aspects, in which the emotions unduly and consistently dominate and warp the rational elements of the mind. Emotional reactions, even those that are quite irrational, are normal and inevitable in the regular course of events. However, in the emotionally mature individual, they are temporary in nature, yielding sooner or later to a more or less intelligent form of resolution or control. The *degree* of emotional-rational balance is an important consideration, since all individuals are guided by their emotions to some extent. A mild degree of emotionally dominated thinking and behavior would be considered normal and probably healthy. A moderate degree would be described as neurotic, while an extreme degree would be considered psychotic. Intense, but temporary, emotional reactions to powerful stimuli are considered to be appropriate; when they are unduly prolonged, or absent, emotional maladjustment is indicated.

Emotional disorders cannot be understood adequately in terms of typical disease processes or illnesses. To a large extent, they are defined by a society's norms, values, and patterns, and represent deviations from these. For example, hallucinations and paranoid thinking are considered to be quite appropriate in some primitive cultures. In our culture, these are considered symptoms of severe disorders. In the same vein, sociocultural factors play an important role in the development of emotional health or emotional disorders. Biological man is affected by his psychological perceptions of his social interactions. Actually, there is a constant interaction of psychological, social, and biological factors, but poor interpersonal relationships and distorted perceptions appear to be basic to psychogenic disorders in our culture. Economic factors such as poverty and deprivation also appear to play contributing roles in many instances.

The sociocultural setting in which the individual operates determines the psychological supports available to him and the pressures that impinge upon him. These environmental factors, particularly during the formative years, help to shape the personality of the individual—his psychological strengths and weaknesses. In turn, the personality of the individual influences and modifies his environment and the people in it.

PERSONALITY DEVELOPMENT

Personality is here considered to be the unique and relatively enduring way in which an individual relates to other individuals and groups and reacts to situations. It consists of learned or acquired factors, the dimensions of which are delimited by biological or constitutional factors. The acquired factors shape, determine, and channel the constitutional factors and are by far the most modifiable one—through experience, learning or psychotherapy.

Personality, which has both an intellectual and an emotional component, is shaped by the interaction between parents or parental surrogates and the child, and to a lesser extent by other individuals and cultural elements that the child meets. This interaction through constant, meaningful repetition sets up certain *patterns* of feelings, thought, and behavior. It is the basis for the child's outlook on life and his later expectations; it is the yardstick by which the child measures himself and others. The earlier relationships—good, bad, or indifferent—are the prototypes of later relationships. Distortions developed in the earlier relationships tend to result in distorted perceptions in the later relationships. The patterns—healthy or unhealthy, constructive or unconstructive—become deeply entrenched, forming the core or structure of personality. Once established, they are consistent and difficult to change. This is due to the emotional or psychodynamic component of personality, a powerful source of motivation which limits the individual's range of response to stimuli. By the age of five or six, personality structure is fairly well formed, although it continues to grow and change at least through adolescence. In a real sense, personality develops through stages, ultimately forming the foundation for all subsequent behavior. Where the emotional structure is weak or immature the individual will have limited capacity to cope with the anxiety-producing responsibilities and pressures of life. The mature personality is less easily threatened, more flexible, and more able to cope with people and situations.

ANXIETY

Like pain, anxiety is a signal to the individual that something is decidedly wrong or unpleasant. Similarly, it is a powerful motivating

force to do something, sometimes anything, to get rid of the presumed cause. Anxiety is the individual's emotional reaction to that which
is sensed as threat. Implied in this is a feeling of being unable to
cope with the threat, a highly subjective judgment. As the sense of
being threatened increases, or as the feeling of being able to cope
with the threat decreases, anxiety increases. In its extreme form it
becomes panic, a frequent prelude to a psychotic break.

Originally, anxiety has a protective function. It mobilizes the individual's resources to either deal with the sensed danger or escape
from it. In its earlier stages it is a powerful adjunct to learning, since
it vividly emphasizes paths and procedures to be avoided, while indicating, by its absence, "safe" courses of action. Unfortunately, learning
based upon anxiety is often as irrational as it is intense. Moreover,
reactions that are helpful in removing the sense of anxiety in childhood, where they might be somewhat appropriate in view of the
child's dependent status, tend to be retained and used in adulthood
where they are quite inappropriate. In this way anxiety becomes a
deterrent to learning since it perpetuates the childhood sense of helplessness, permits of little variation in pattern, narrows perspective, and
distorts reality. Anxiety frequently precipitates or intensifies other emotions such as rage, hate, and frustration; it is probably an underlying
factor in most, if not all, emotional disorders.

In the infant, anxiety and fear are undifferentiated. Anything sensed
as danger produces an emotional and somatic reaction. Even in childhood, the differentiation between the realistic threat that produces fear
and the subjective, irrational threat that produces the same reaction—
now referred to as anxiety—may be difficult to make. In the adult,
anxiety is on a symbolic basis, carried over with little change from
the childish, largely unreal (except to the individual) sense of danger.
In other words, anxiety can be described as irrational fear. Tension is
the somatic concomitant of anxiety or fear.

The relationship between parent and child is of paramount importance in the development of anxiety patterns in the child. The existence
of the child is almost wholly dependent on the care and attention of
the mother and, to a lesser extent, the father. Tender care, warmth,
feeding, closeness, and protection create a sense of security. Neglect and
indifference to the needs of the child, rough handling, inconsistency,
lack of warmth and closeness create a sense of insecurity. The child
brought up in the former way has less anxiety, needs fewer or less
extreme defenses, feels more wanted, develops a greater sense of identity, self-esteem, and self-confidence. As a result, he feels more able
to cope with life, to stand on his own feet as he grows older. The
child brought up in the latter way feels more anxious, is more defensive,
feels unwanted, lacks confidence and self-esteem. Thus he feels—and

therefore *is*—less able to adapt and to cope with life independently. Consequently, he continues to depend on the parents, or others, for his strength. It is noteworthy that a sense of self-esteem, worth, or importance (a positive self-concept) is inversely related to the degree of anxiety experienced.

Environmental factors that influence the parent-child relationship will also affect the level of anxiety in the child. Poverty, to the extent that it produces broken homes, illness, educational deprivation, malnutrition, and so forth, will contribute to anxiety and the emotional disorders that result from it. Affluence, where it produces satiety, overprotection, rejection, neglect, and a diminution of human values, will do the same. However, the affluent family will be able to afford much better treatment and will also have many more resources to draw upon—factors that presumably would affect the outcome of emotional disorders.

Anxiety in its pure state is sometimes referred to as unstructured or "free-floating" anxiety. It is characterized by visceral discomfort, body tension, increased heart beat and respiration, and a vague, generalized sense of threat or foreboding. This threat may be attributed to any individual or any aspect of the environment, with little or no awareness of its actual cause. All anxiety is probably general in nature—the helpless feeling of an unprotected child—even though specific stimuli generate the anxiety reaction or the anxiety focuses on various symbols.

Anxiety has two important characteristics that should be understood. First, it tends to generalize or spread out. As an example, the child who experiences pain when he receives an injection may react with anxiety not only to the sight of a hypodermic needle, but to doctors, to men who wear eyeglasses or white coats like the original doctor's, to medicinal odors—in short, to any object or individual that symbolizes or reactivates the original threatening situation. Second, anxiety tends to incubate or increase with time if it is not resolved or counteracted. Popularly this is depicted by the rider who is thrown from a horse. If he immediately climbs back on again, he should experience no great anxiety the next time he rides. However, if he puts off remounting the horse, he will find that the related anxiety grows greater as time passes.

The most frequent resolution of the sense of anxiety is through the use of defense mechanisms, patterns that bind up or channel the anxiety so that it is no longer free-floating, but rather is expressed in a structured way with altered or disguised symptomatology. These defenses, which are considered to be unconscious or outside the individual's awareness, relieve the conscious *sense* of anxiety to some degree, but they do not resolve the cause or clear the air. Instead, a shield or barrier is thrown up, or the individual makes good a temporary escape, only to find at a later stage that the sense of threat is still present in similar situations, probably even intensified, while his adaptability and confidence in dealing with the threat are diminished because he has already failed to handle it adequately.

Similar defenses are used by "normals," neurotics, and psychotics, as well as by disabled and nondisabled. The difference is one of degree and intensity. The better adjusted individual, feeling more adequate feels less threatened, so he uses his defenses less. By the same token his armor does not need to be so thick nor his flight so distant, and therefore his defenses are not as incapacitating as the more poorly adjusted individual. His defenses take up less of his time, effort, and energy, and these resources can be turned to constructive ways of living rather than being dissipated by tilting at windmills.

Anxiety-provoking situations are probably avoided or circumvented on a conscious level also. For example, some patients make a comfortable adjustment within the protective sheltered atmosphere of the hospital, and prefer to stay there rather than face the pressures, demands, and confusion of the outside world. This is one reason why rehabilitation requires a series of steps, graduated in terms of difficulty, responsibility, and reward, to lead the patients from the hospital to the community.

SOCIOCULTURAL FACTORS AFFECTING PERSONALITY

Anxiety arises as the result of a conflict between two powerful forces to which the individual is subjected throughout life. The living organism has an innate drive to live, grow, and mature. Primary needs stemming from this are involved with security and survival; when these needs are met, the individual has a drive to seek other satisfactions, to explore, learn, experience, and in general to pursue self-realization. From this innate psychobiological drive stems the basic motivation of the individual in the activities of life.

In conflict with this psychobiological drive are certain pressures of the culture and society, interpreted and enforced by the subcultures of parents and family, community, schools, churches, and other institutions and groups. Since the child is highly dependent on these representatives of culture, sometimes for his very existence, the price he frequently has to pay for satisfaction of his security needs is conformance and compliance with these external pressures at the expense of self-respect and self-realization. Unless the internal drives of the child are gently molded to fit in with the external demands of the culture, an imbalance results. Anxiety derives from the feeling that internal drives are not compatible with parental demands or cultural standards. To seek gratification of these drives for satisfaction or self-realization is to run the risk of losing the source of security and survival. Yet, since they cannot be turned off, some realignment or compromise must be made to cope with this threat to existence. The more irrational, authoritarian, and subjective the demands of the culture or the parents, the more they ignore the needs of the individual, the greater will be the individual's anxiety and distortion of reality.

A supportive parent-child relationship provides the child with flexible guidance and nonpunitive discipline which permit the growth of individuality in socially acceptable patterns. Where the child is neglected or abandoned by parents and society, the result, if the child survives, is likely to be antisocial (sociopathic) behavior patterns. In an authoritarian setting, the child has essentially two choices: to fight back or to submit. Although cultural patterns vary, he is usually at a disadvantage and does not choose to fight, at least not overtly. The result is a degree of conformity on the surface with aggressive elements that are covered over but still active on a deeper level. From the authoritarian relationship, then, stem secondary forms of motivation which involve conformity, seeking approval, and going along with the demands of others, or fighting them constantly, or both, with one aspect overt or conscious, the other covert or subconscious. These patterns are carried over into adult relationships as forms of transference where they tend to control behavior, restrict individuality, and build up unnecessary tension, thus lowering the adult's efficiency and adaptability.

In early life, defenses serve an adaptive function in dealing with the environment; in view of the child's relative helplessness they represent realistic and effective reactions to more powerful forces. However, those defenses which are successful in coping with anxiety while establishing a working relationship with the environment are carried over into adult life as a form of overlearned behavior. The defense patterns that were effective in the young, weak child become quite ineffective and inappropriate in the older, stronger adult. Yet, because they represent a form of protective armor in childhood, and because the adult still perceives himself as weak and helpless, he resists any change that would deprive him of his "protection" and leave him naked in a threatening world.

The use of childlike defenses in the adult defines emotional immaturity. These is a direct relation between emotional immaturity and the need for protective armor or a protective environment. The emotionally immature person goes off on a side path on the road of life which leads to a dead end where he expends his energy dealing with anxiety rather than leading a constructive life. In this situation, anxiety has become the major source of motivation, negative and self-defeating in nature.

Emotional maturity is relative, not absolute. Even the most well-adjusted individual has some built-in defense mechanisms for handling anxiety, resulting in a corresponding degree of distortion, irrationality, and inefficiency. These form a part of his personality or character structure (not in the moral sense, but referring to characteristics). They are always with the individual; rather than representing a "symptomatic" reaction to stress and strain they form an integral part of his make-up. To the extent that they are present, we can think of everyone as having a personality or character disorder. In some individuals they are considered minor eccentricities or quirks; in other they become major obstacles to good interpersonal relationships or meeting the standards of society. While personality disorders should not be confused with "symptomatic" disorders, it is important to note that the personality structure of the individual determines to a large extent the nature and direction of a symptomatic disorder—neurotic, psychosomatic, or psychotic.

In summary, it should be noted that emotional disorders are a product of man's perceptions of himself and the world in which he lives. These perceptions reflect his experiences and his interpersonal relationships; they determine his expectations of what is to come. Invariably, the perceptions are distorted; the threat tends to be overestimated, while the individual's worth and his capacity for dealing with the situation tend to be underestimated. The logic of reality is apt to be ignored.

While the following pages present one of many systems of classifying emotional disorders on the basis of certain characteristics or dynamics that are frequently found together, our diagnostic labels are forms of shorthand which gloss over or ignore many important elements that distinguish one person from another. In other words, these disorders have to be understood on an individual basis which takes into account subjective as well as objective factors, the person interacting with his environment.

Psychogenic Disorders

Disorders occurring without apparent structural or organic changes are referred to as "functional" in medical terminology. The term "psychogenic" is a psychological term meaning "of psychic origin." Although both terms may be used to describe the same disorder, they are not necessarily synonomous, since the former allows for the possiblity of an organic cause being discovered. With the exception of disorders associated with brain injury, emotional disorders are here considered to be essentially of psychological origin, with many contributing factors involved.

PSYCHOTIC DISORDERS

A psychosis is a severe emotional disorder involving a relative inability to test reality and characterized by disordered thinking, delusions, hallucinations, and frequently by bizarre behavior. The individual's ability to carry on routine activities and normal relationships is impaired, but not necessarily absent. Varying degrees of personality disorganization may be present, but it should be remembered that psychotic reactions usually occur in individuals with relatively immature personality structures. Moreover, they tend to occur as reactions to periods of change, to discouragement, to stress such as puberty, young adulthood, or the menopause, to personal crises, and to crises in the family situation. There is increasing recognition that most psychotic reactions are reversible in the acute stage with proper care and treatment, leaving little personality disorganization other than the original weak ego. In the chronic stage psychotic reactions can be modified and improved, although the task is more difficult and requires a longer time. Some disorganization is apt to remain, although with improved rehabilitative techniques this may not be so in the future. A chronic psychosis when neglected and mishandled, as was frequently the case in the back wards of some mental hospitals, is apt to enter a deteriorated stage with considerable personality disorganization. This type of case, which generally has had a poor prognosis for improvement in the past, has shown an excellent response to research-oriented rehabilitation programs in hospital settings.

It is important to differentiate between the *symptoms* that arise as a result of pressure and stress (anxiety) and the *personality* in which they occur. The former can improve when the stress and strain are removed in some way, or through the use of somatic forms of treatment; this does not increase the capacity of the personality to cope with stress and strain in other circumstances. On the other hand, psychotherapy and some rehabilitative procedures have as their goal personality growth—that is, increased capacity to handle anxiety and cope with reality—thus equipping the individual to cope with a greater variety of circumstances and situations.

SCHIZOPHRENIC REACTIONS. Schizophrenia, the most common form of psychosis, represents a maladaptive reaction to the untenable stress and anxiety of the external world in which the individual withdraws from interpersonal relationships and reality, substituting in their place an inner, autistic world. It is marked by regressive, more primitive patterns of thought and behavior, reflecting to a large extent the previous personality structure and the experiences of the individual. The clinical picture is quite variable with relatively few cases falling into a clear-cut classical pattern. As a matter of fact, there is about as much variation within diagnostic categories as there is between diagnostic categories.

Diagnostic labels usually reflect the most obvious symptomatology of the disorder; diagnosticians frequently disagree on the most appropriate label. Moreover, these diagnostic labels frequently represent different schools of thought or current vogues. While there are inherent limitations in the use of diagnostic classifications, they offer certain advantages in communication, treatment, and prognosis which are quite important. The reader would do well to become familiar with any variations in terminology and their implications in his or her local setting.

There is a considerable amount of overlapping of symptomatology to be found in the various categories at all levels. Fortunately, it is rare for the entire personality to be engulfed by the schizophrenic process; there is usually some uninvolved or healthy part of the ego which is accessible to the outside world and treatment.

The schizophrenic is usually a shy, sensitive person. This is reflected in the desocialization and withdrawal characteristic of this disorder. He lives largely in a highly egocentric world of fantasy. Since his emotions, thinking, and behavior are dictated by a subjective inner world, uncorrected by external reality and consensual validation (group confirmation), it is frequently difficult to understand him or communicate with him. Thought processes are often confused and disorganized according to usual standards, speech may be garbled and confused (word salad) containing much unshared symbolism and newly coined words (neologisms), behavior is frequently odd or bizarre, while attention and concentration tend to fluctuate in an erratic manner. Emotional reactions are frequently split off or dissociated from thought processes (isolation) so that these reactions may appear quite inappropriate to the situation (inappropriate affect). However, the schizophrenic is understandable from his own frame of reference, particularly in terms of his experiences, his expectations, and his emotions. His reactions reflect his earlier unfavorable relationships, his mistrust of others, and his low self-esteem, plus his anxiety, frustration, and resentment caused by what he views as a hostile or incomprehensible world.

Paranoid Type. The symptoms of paranoid schizophrenia appear to reflect a repudiation of unpleasant reality, a reality that is empty and meaningless. In its place, the individual magically substitutes a fantasy world in which he is important, powerful, or omnipotent. This is done through a delusional *system,* a rationale based upon misinterpretation of reality through intellectualization (rationalization) and projection (attributing one's thoughts, feelings, and impulses to others). The delusions may reflect the distrust and suspiciousness of the individual with a theme of persecution, they may involve grandiose ideas, or both may be neatly combined. Unrelated activities of others are seen as having some special relationship or significance for the individual (ideas of reference). Ritualistic forms of behavior may be used magically to ward off evil and threat.

In the early stages of psychosis, little disorganization or deterioration of thought may be visible to the observer. The individual preserves a good front, his thinking appears logical, and his emotions seem to be under good control. It is only when the individual touches on his delusional system that the paranoid process becomes manifest.

If the disorder moves into a chronic stage, greater disorganization will occur. Hallucinations, largely auditory because of sensitization to authoritarian verbalizations, develop. There is no longer a good façade; symptomatology is more obvious. At some level, the paranoid schizophrenic is a hostile person; for this reason he may occasionally be dangerous.

Simple Type. Instead of withdrawing from reality, the individual with this type of reaction narrows his horizon, and in this way he limits the reality with which he must deal. The disorder is a slowly progressing one that may not be recognized for years, and then only by comparison with earlier behavior. There is a gradual loss of interest in external events, coupled with a reduction in interpersonal relationships. Hallucinations and delusions are quite rare, as are behavior disorders. The individual may seem queer or odd, rather than acutely disturbed. He tends to make an adjustment well below his potential level of ability. His life may be solitary, lacking in assertiveness, giving an external appearance of apathy, blandness, and flatness. He may work at a low-level job or become an idler and vagrant. Over the course of time there is a gradual increase in symptomatology and deterioration of thought if he is permitted to persevere in his isolation; for this reason it is classified as a symptomatic disorder rather than a personality disorder. At times, this reaction may be confused with mental retardation.

Hebephrenic Type. The onset of this disorder frequently occurs in adolescence. Its start is insidious, but it is characterized by a tendency to rapid regression and deterioration. Manifestations include silly behavior and mannerisms, unpredictable giggling, shallow and inappropriate affect, delusions that are frequently somatic in nature but not systematized, and hallucinations. There is frequently an unrestrained flow of speech expressing bizarre ideas and incoherent thought with word salads and neologisms. Paranoid symptoms may develop; with chronicity all the categories of schizophrenia tend to become more similar. Early bowel and bladder incontinence is not uncommon, with some individuals tending to smear feces on the walls or on themselves. In general, socially accepted forms of behavior are abandoned by the individual. However, this reaction can also be an acute phenomenon with a high degree or reversibility.

Catatonic Type. Bizarre motor phenomena are the most obvious characteristics of the catatonic schizophrenic. More frequently this takes the form of motor inhibition including stupor, mutism, negativism, and occasionally staying in positions that others have put them in (waxy flexibility). Periods of stupor may be preceded or followed by periods of extreme excitement involving a maniclike sequence of aimless acts. In phases of catatonic excitement, the individual can be quite destructive and dangerous to others as well as himself. Posturing, gesturing, and grimacing in a repetitive manner are other motor symptoms of this reaction. At times, there may be regression to a vegetative level. Despite this seemingly complete withdrawal, there is evidence to indicate that the catatonic knows what is going on about him. At times he may emerge from his "stupor," engage in conversation, and then return to his stuporous condition.

Catatonia seems to represent the behavior of a superficially compliant, passively resistant person with strong elements of negativism and hostility. The psychological paralysis is a continuation of an earlier pattern in which action or decision on the part of the individual met with criticism or punishment by dominating, controlling adults. Movement and active decisions are anxiety producing; immobility and stupor are forms of superficial compliance and deeper passive resistance. The phase of excitement seems to represent a breaking through of the violent hostility that was engendered by the earlier restrictive control. There is some evidence to suggest that the catatonic reaction is a product of neglect and the hopeless outlook so characteristic of mental hospitals in the past. In more therapeutic settings this reaction is on the decrease.

Other Schizophrenic Reactions. Since schizophrenic behavior takes many forms, the four classical categories described above are not always adequate for diagnostic purposes. Therefore, other classifications, largely generalized in nature, have been developed to cover the cases that are not readily assigned to the above categories. The *schizoaffective* type includes cases combining schizophrenic and affective (manic or depressive) reactions. The *undifferentiated* type, which may be acute or chronic, is used to classify individuals with symptoms that are mixed or not clearly structured. Turmoil states, occurring in adolescents, combatants, and others, periods of panic, of violent and shifting emotional upheaval, usually of short duration, sometimes self-limiting, may be classified as acute undifferentiated reactions. The *residual* type refers to individuals who have improved after a schizophrenic reaction, but still manifest schizophrenic symptomatology. The *childhood* type becomes symptomatic before puberty and the development of any real personality structure. It takes many different clinical forms, but it usually includes poor contact with people, restricted communication, and autistic (highly subjective and unreal) thinking and behavior. Personality growth and psychological development tend to be sharply restricted.

PARANOIA. One of the major subclassifications of psychotic reactions in classical systems is that of paranoia. As described, intelligence is well preserved, there is little disorganization or deterioration, delusions are encapsulated or limited, and there are usually no hallucinations. Other systems of classification see paranoia, which is quite rare in its pure form, as the early stage of paranoid schizophrenia as described above, with delayed development of symptoms of deterioration.

Affective Disorders. Probably all individuals at some time have fluctuations in mood that range from feeling blue and gloomy to feeling gay and elated. In some individuals the gloomy reaction may tend to predominate, others may be more frequently elated, while still others swing from one to the other with neither predominating. While these mood swings may be reactions to external events, there is usually a highly subjective element involved, reflecting an emotional pattern of the individual. Usually these moods tend to disappear as readily as they appear.

A depressive or elated reaction may represent an appropriate response to an external event (situational or transient reaction)—as examples, sustaining a physical disability or getting a promotion on the job. Cyclic mood swings that are overreactions to external events occur in individuals functioning within normal, neurotic, or psychotic limits. They may occur by themselves, or in combination with other emotional and thought disorders. But in all cases, with the exception of situational reactions, there appear to be predisposing personality patterns that influence the nature and intensity of the reaction.

The term *manic-depressive reaction* is used to describe severe affective reactions of a cyclic nature. Where the mood is primarily elated, it is further classified as *manic; manic-depressive reaction, depressed type*, refers to a primarily depressive reaction. Where both manifestations are combined, the classification may be *mixed type*. Where the two reactions consistently alternate, this is known as *circular type*. In some nosological systems (classifications of disease), separate categories —that is, other than manic-depressive—are used for reactions that occur without a previous history of symptomatic affective disorders—for example, *involutional melancholia* or *psychotic depressive reaction*. However, this seems to be a rather arbitrary form of classification, since the likelihood is great that the individual had previous mood swings though they may have been at a subclinical level. While "manic-depressive" refers to psychotic reactions, similar disorders occur at a nonpsychotic level. These need not, but may, progress to psychoses.

Depressive Reactions. Depression is an emotional reaction to loss, bereavement, or misfortune. It combines a sense of hopelessness with a feeling of being rejected, unwanted, or unloved. It tends to occur in individuals who have turned their hostility "inward" and become very self-critical. A strong sense of guilt is combined with feelings of self-depreciation and worthlessness. Depressions are reactions to anxiety; by ceasing to strive, compete, or place value on anything, the person is able to pull back from an anxiety-provoking world. Instead, he becomes inactive, thus avoiding decision-making, responsibility, the seeking of goals (note the similarity to the "paralysis" of catatonia), at a tremendous price. He becomes guilt-ridden, thinks poorly of himself, and everything becomes unimportant and valueless.

At a psychotic level, there may be delusions, hypochondriasis and body preoccupation, and a strong need for self-punishment. The latter seems to reflect our cultural standard whereby punishment or suffering represent a form of atonement. In the psychotic individual, this may take the form of self-mutilation or suicide. It is important to understand that this type of individual, who cannot express his hostility directly, frequently hurts others by hurting himself. In an *agitated depression,* the individual is restless, overtalkative, constantly moving, pacing, moaning, wringing his hands, and so on. Because of his motor activity, he may be more dangerous to himself than the individual with a retarded depression.

The *retarded depression* is characterized by a general slowing down of the psychological and physiological processes. The individual finds it difficult to perform the simplest task, he thinks slowly, reacts slowly, and is markedly unproductive. Appetite is usually poor, insomnia occurs frequently, and there is a constant feeling of fatigue. Constipation is a common problem. Apprehension, a sense of impending doom, perplexity, and stupor are frequent concomitants.

Involutional melancholia or *involutional psychotic reaction* refers to a severe depressive reaction occurring during the involutional ("change of life") period, presumably without previous manic-depressive reactions. It appears to represent the reaction of some individuals, male and female, to passing advanced milestones in life without having fulfilled certain wishes or achieved subjective goals—a recognition that "time is passing me by."

It is not always easy to differentiate between a psychotic depression and a neurotic depression in the absence of extreme symptoms. However, affective disorders are frequently self-limiting, though they tend to recur. These reactions usually occur at a later stage in life then schizophrenic reactions. Even when they are relatively mild, they pose a problem to the health, economic status, and well-being of the individual and his family. Moreover, mild depressions, often unrecognized, interfere with constructive motivation in educational, vocational, and rehabilitative settings.

Manic Reactions. Mania and depression appear to be opposite sides of the same coin. Both are reactions to anxiety in situations where reality is untenable to the individual. Both occur in individuals with low self-esteem and a sense of being unwanted, unloved, and unimportant. The depressed person attempts to cope with these feelings by saying, in effect: "I am weak, helpless, unprotected, and unloved; protect me and love me." The manic individual sets up a reaction formation against the feelings by denying their existence. In mania, self-esteem is artificially high. The individual is overconfident; to him all things are possible. He may make grandiose plans, invest money unwisely, and get involved in all sorts of unsound activities. His elated mood is a denial of hopelessness, grief, or rejection.

Like depression, mania may occur at various levels. *Hypomania*, at a nonpsychotic level, may involve a mild state of euphoria, increased activity, restlessness, and a mild impairment of judgment and planning. The person appears to be gay, speech and conduct may be somewhat uninhibited, and he or she is not too concerned with risks or practicality. To a casual observer, the individual may appear to be quite normal and constructive. Indeed, some hypomanic individuals may accomplish a great deal at times, although usually they do not do things well.

Mania, at a psychotic level, is characterized by elation and expansiveness, excitement, distractibility, irritability, increased motor activity associated with flight of ideas, and uninhibited speech and behavior. Delusions, with a content of grandiose achievement, power, or possessions, may be present. The individual may go for long periods of time without rest or food, ultimately running himself down physically. Unrealistic optimism and self-assertiveness are commonly found. Yet, the manic is sensitive and intolerant of criticism. At times, he may be destructive, particularly when an attempt is made to restrain or curb his ideas and behavior. Transitory depressive reactions may intervene, or a full-blown depression may succeed the mania.

NEUROTIC DISORDERS

While there is much disagreement and confusion in the classification of the neuroses (psychoneuroses), the term is generally used to refer to a variety of symptomatic emotional disorders, less severe than the psychoses, characterized by overt anxiety, or a broad spectrum of *manifestations* of anxiety. In contrast to the psychoses, there is generally no gross disorganization of the personality, and while the neurotic may perceive external reality in a somewhat warped or distorted way, there is no gross break with the outside world. Despite the fact that the neurosis represents a more moderate reaction than the psychosis, it can be equally incapacitating at times.

The neurotic probably has had a greater degree of security in his formative years than the psychotic. As a result, he has greater ego strength; he is better able to cope with people and situations. The internal conflict or external stress must be greater than for the psychotic before he develops symptoms; when they do develop they tend to be more limited and easier to reverse.

Neurotic reactions are precipitated by an intensification of anxiety or by weakening of the defenses against anxiety. As indicated, anxiety may be intensified by growing *internal conflict* (for example, sexual drive versus "morality") or by *external factors*—experiences and relationships that are symbolically threatening. Defenses may be weakened by illness, fatigue, brain injury, and other realistic (nonsymbolic) pressure (for example, loss of income), particularly when these are cumulative. Except for the symptoms of unstructured anxiety, the symptomatology of the neurosis will largely reflect the personality structure or patterns of the individual. Unstructured anxiety indicates the presence of more anxiety than the individual can handle—a form of disequilibrium between anxiety and defense. Unless it is reduced in some way, a retrograde reaction can be anticipated. Examples of this would be personality disorders developing into symptomatic neuroses, psychosomatic disorders, or psychoses; neuroses developing into acute psychoses (probably not too common a phenomenon); or acute psychoses becoming chronic psychoses. The converse is equally true; supportive situations and relationships tend to reduce anxiety, to decrease symptomatology and regressive trends.

One more phenomenon is worthy of note. Certain defenses against, or symptoms of, anxiety "bind up" or channel the anxiety. Obsessive compulsive reactions, conversion reactions, but not psychosomatic reactions (see below) sometimes will reach a state of "balance," at least for brief periods. When this occurs, the individual shows little apprehension or concern and has no great motivation to change things since he is aware of no acute discomfort.

Emotionally determined behavior is frequently manipulative in nature—that is, it represents, among other things, an attempt to influence or control others. This process is sometimes referred to as a "power operation." An example would be the "martyrlike" mother who constantly points out to her children the sacrifices she has made for them, and the obligations they therefore have to her. In many ways, neurotic reactions may bring neurotic satisfactions or gains. In addition to the primary gain of reducing the sense of anxiety, secondary gains such as a dependent status or the opportunity to express hostility safely may accrue to the individual. Illness and disability lend themselves very well to neurotic gains in our culture, since they can be used as socially acceptable alibis for many things. The individual who resorts to this, however, usually finds it necessary to narrow down his world and to sacrifice a considerable amount of his individuality, freedom, and self-respect.

ANXIETY REACTION. This term, sometimes referred to as "anxiety state," is used to designate reactions where diffuse or free-floating anxiety is the outstanding symptom (see above) because the defenses are not adequate to handle anxiety. It is not usually a static thing; the individual is likely to improve or grow worse in a relatively brief period of time, depending on circumstances, availability of help, and so on.

DISSOCIATIVE REACTION. Dissociated activities are those that are carried on outside of awareness; they are motivated by repressed material— by the subconscious or unconscious. In a sense, "the left hand doesn't know what the right hand is doing." Segments of the personality seem to operate independent of each other. *Amnesia* (loss of memory for certain events), *fugue* (an amnesic state often characterized by flight, running away from reality), *somnambulism* (sleep-walking), *depersonalization,* and *multiple personality* are examples of dissociative reactions. While classified as neurotic disorders, dissociative reactions may occur in psychotic processes.

CONVERSION REACTION. In conversion reaction, also referred to as *conversion hysteria,* an emotional reaction is converted into a physical symptom. As in the case of dissociation, repression (dynamic forgetting) is a major defense. However, the anxiety is bound up in functional symptoms that are usually sensory or motor in nature, occurring largely in parts of the body that are under voluntary control. Sensory symptoms may include blindness, deafness, or loss of sensation (anesthesia) in various parts of the body; motor phenomena may be manifested by a variety of paralyses, loss of voice (aphonia), and tics.

Conversion symptoms may sometimes occur in a limb or organ that has previously sustained an injury; this may occasionally present a problem of differential diagnosis. Theoretically, conversion reactions should be completely reversible; in fact, prolonged disuse of a limb may bring about permanent atrophy or contracture and a degree of permanent physical disability.

These symptoms, since they involve a "physical disability," generally offer considerable secondary gain to the individual. For a period of time they may bind up anxiety so efficiently that the individual may appear to be quite indifferent to his impairment.

Conversion reactions should not be confused with psychosomatic disorders (see below). The former have a symbolic origin (for example, the hand that would strike the parent becomes paralyzed), there is considerable reduction of anxiety, they tend to occur in parts of the body subject to voluntary control, and there is relatively little true organic impairment or threat to life. Psychosomatic disorders are caused by prolonged visceral and somatic tensions that accompany anxiety, there is little diminution of anxiety, they occur in organs innervated by the autonomic (involuntary) nervous system, and if untreated, they may produce irreversible lesions in the involved organs which may pose a threat to life.

The incidence of conversion reactions appears to be less now than during the time of Freud. Perhaps this is due to the fact that the so-called hysterical personality develops in an individual who was limited or overprotected in earlier years, and thus has grown up rather naïve and unworldly. Immature emotional patterns are characterized by credulity and suggestibility. Thus, conversion sysmptoms represent the individual's uninformed concepts of the functioning of the body, rather than a true neurological picture (for example, "glove" or "stocking" anesthesias that do not correspond to neural pathways). Emotional reactions tend to be histrionic—artificial and overdramatized—calculated to influence the observer. As indicated, true physical disability lends itself rather well to this pattern of coping with life and relating to people. However, the greater sophistication of our generation and the increased sociocultural freedom we enjoy do not appear to be as conducive to the development of the hysterical personality as in the past.

PHOBIC REACTIONS. A phobic reaction appears to represent an attempt to localize or encapsulate anxiety by fixating it on an object, place, or situation. This is in contrast to an "anxiety reaction" where the anxiety is diffuse and not attributed to anything specific. The phobia may be fixated on something that symbolizes an unconscious unacceptable wish, such as a sexual symbol, or on substitute objects related to anxiety, such as knives or bridges. By displacing anxiety on to a phobic object which in itself is quite harmless, the individual delimits the sense of threat; instead of everything being dangerous, only the phobic object is sensed as dangerous. If this is avoided (for example, high places, closed places, certain animals), the individual is able to carry on most activities without a pervasive sense of dread. In other words, by narrowing down his world a little, the individual is able to cope with other aspects of reality a little better, at least temporarily. Since this defensive reaction actually is not really a rational effective way of dealing with the anxiety-provoking situation, the individual becomes less able to handle other pressures, internal or external, so that further withdrawal of one sort or another may be necessitated with time. Eventually, phobias may be complicated by obsessive, constantly recurring thoughts of the phobic object, which may incapacitate the individual almost as much as if he were faced with the actual object. Since symbolic meanings of a subjective nature play an important role in the selection of phobic objects, a great variety of phobias have been described.

OBSESSIVE COMPULSIVE REACTION. Ideas of an irrational nature that keep recurring (obsessions) and repetitive acts of an irrational nature that the individual feels compelled to do (compulsions) are the chief symptoms of the *obsessive compulsive neurosis*. The acts stem directly from the ideas, although not all the ideas are transformed into action. Symptoms often appear to combine aggressive, sexual, or other anti-social ideas and opposing moralistic or corrective behavior reflecting guilt, which reacts against or attempts to atone for the thought. Cleanliness, rituals of undoing, and orderliness are examples of the reaction formations that are quite common. In some individuals, obsessional material such as preoccupation with numbers predominates; in others, compulsions such as hand-washing rituals are seen most frequently. Either situation can be incapacitating to the extent that little or no constructive work can be carried on. Ideas and acts are used in a magical way to ward off threat; if they stop, the individual is overwhelmed by anxiety. Rituals may represent the defense of undoing— a symbolic attempt to annul or cancel the effect of one's behavior or thought, comparable to the common superstition of throwing a pinch of spilled salt over one's shoulder to prevent bad luck. Through the defense of *isolation,* ideas are divorced from their emotional content, thus permitting the individual to repress the anxiety that accompanies his thoughts.

Obsessive compulsive symptoms appear in many other forms of disorders. Similarly, elements of obsessive compulsive personality structure (described below) appear in some schizophrenic, depressive, and psychosomatic reactions, apparently reflecting the reaction of the individual to certain forms of authoritarian, overmoralistic parental figures.

DEPRESSIVE REACTIONS. As indicated under "Affective Disorders," depressions may occur at any level, with dynamics that are similar but varying in intensity. At the neurotic level, anxiety is handled by self-criticism and depreciation, inactivity, and a lack of drive. Discouragement and dependency go hand in hand. A sense of guilt frequently reflects ambivalent attitudes toward a significant individual (for example, hostility and love toward a parent or spouse who has died). Delusions, hallucinations, and other severe symptoms are absent. There is usually a precipitating factor in the environment that initiates the reaction. However, it should be noted that reactions of grief and mourning to loss, deprivation, and disability are quite normal; they can only be considered neurotic when they are unduly prolonged.

PERSONALITY DISORDERS

Personality disorders, as the term indicates, are manifestations of the basic personality structure of the individual. They represent lifelong patterns of adaptation and behavior; they are therefore highly resistant to change. Unlike the symptomatic disorders, they are not experienced as alien or anxiety provoking, so that there is little motivation for improvement or change. Moreover, they are so deeply ingrained that they are virtually a part of the person, so that while they may be modified to some extent, there is little likelihood of fundamental change.

To some extent all individuals have personality disorders built into their personality structure. Usually they represent minor maldevelopments, misinterpretations of reality, deficiencies or distortions of thought and behavior manifested by such things as inefficiency, self-defeating activities, inadequacies, and negative or antisocial attitudes. They form part of the individual's patterns for relating to others and coming to grips with his environment. To him they are "right" or sound, although others may see them as odd, queer, mean, weak, belligerent, suspicious, withdrawn, improper, and so on. The term "character disorder," which may be considered synonomous with personality disorder, does not reflect a moral judgment, but rather refers to the characteristics of the individual. In this sense, we speak of some people as "characters." However, it should be noted that personality or character disorders may manifest themselves through antisocial behavior. For example, individuals whose sense of inadequacy combines with distorted values and resentment of society to produce chronic lying, cheating, stealing, sexual deviation, addiction, are classified as having sociopathic forms of personality (character) disorders.

As with other diagnostic classifications, personality disorders are not clear-cut, mutually exclusive entities. Generally, they take their name from personality structures or types, which in turn reflect some of the major characteristics of the group, such as *schizoid personality, inadequate personality, compulsive personality.* While each of these labels subsumes a fairly consistent constellation of characteristics and dynamics, the label gives a stereotyped inadequate picture of an individual. Moreover, the various theoretical schools use different terminology reflecting their varying theoretical orientations. Thus, a compulsive personality in one system might be labeled an "anal character" in another system.

Personality structure forms the foundation for emotional development, healthy or unhealthy. Thus, when symptomatic disorders occur, their nature and manifestations are influenced to a large extent by the underlying personality structure. The symptomatic disorder will show many dynamics that are similar to the basic personality structure of the individual. For example, the fussiness and cleanliness of the compulsive personality may appear as a hand-washing ritual in the obsessive compulsive neurosis. But note also that the overconscientiousness of the compulsive personality, the self-criticism, and intrapunitive attitude of the symptomatic depression, and the projection of unacceptable feelings in the paranoid schizophrenic, all represent expressions of guilt induced originally by authoritarian figures, as well as ways of handling the concomitant hostility. Thus, there may not necessarily be a one-to-one relationship between a personality structure (or disorder) and a symptomatic disorder, although a relationship exists invariably.

Is an individual with a personality disorder "sick" or disabled? The question is of more than academic interest. For example, in order to be eligible for services from the federal-state programs of vocational rehabilitation, an individual must be disabled. If the person with a personality disorder is not considered disabled, he is not legally eligible for such services. The answer is not an easy one. Some personality disorders, for example, the compulsive personality, are not usually obstacles to gainful employment. Others, such as the schizoid personality or the inadequate personality, may have severe vocational (and other) handicaps. Many welfare recipients, criminals, delinquents, and addicts, to name just a few, suffer from personality disorders. While these are often difficult groups to work with and rather unresponsive to psychotherapy, they do often respond to environmental manipulation—placing the person in a supportive setting—particularly when this is in the context of a comprehensive rehabilitation program.

Where the question of the existence of a disability is of importance, it would seem desirable to evaluate each case on its own merits, rather than establishing an overall generalization.

Since personality disorders are discussed in other sections of this chapter they will be treated only briefly here.

COMPULSIVE PERSONALITY. The compulsive individual is a rigid, highly inhibited type of person with an excessive concern for morality and authoritarian standards. Driven by a sense of guilt and a need for conformance, he is preoccupied with such things as orderliness, detail, perfection, punctuality, cleanliness, and economy. Overtly conscientious, idealistic, and considerate, he is likely to be basically critical and intolerant in his relationships with others. Spontaneous feelings are highly repressed; intellectualization and pedantry are substituted for emotional reactions. Inclined to drive himself hard, the compulsive individual finds it hard to relax. Work may be one of the few activities that offers him a release from guilt feelings and self-criticism. He is often a good worker, particularly when careful attention to detail, accuracy, and good workmanship are important.

HYSTERICAL PERSONALITY. Repression of anxiety-producing material is the primary defense of the hysterical personality. Thus, dynamic forces, pushed out of awareness (and therefore out of conscious control), are responsible for certain important aspects of behavior. Through overprotection, dominance, geographic or cultural isolation, the hysterical individual has been kept emotionally immature, unsophisticated, and with limited ability to accept responsibility. Naïveté and credulity produce a high degree of suggestibility. Dramatized histrionic behavior is common. Emotional reactions may be highly exaggerated. Similarly, symptoms of bona fide illnesses and disabilities may be built up and perpetuated to provide secondary gains for the hysteric, since illness and disability lend themselves quite readily to hysterical manifestations.

PARANOID PERSONALITY. The dynamics of the paranoid personality are similar to, but less extreme than, the paranoid schizophrenic. The former has established a more stable *modus vivendi,* free from overt psychotic symptomatology, although this may develop under great stress. Highly sensitized to others, he tends to react to people with suspiciousness, envy, and hostility. Attitudes and motives of those with whom he comes in contact are often distorted and misinterpreted as he projects his own resentment and hostility on to them. Litigious or belligerent behavior is frequently the result. Since he trusts no one, rationalizes his own behavior, and is relatively unaware of a sense of anxiety, this person is not easy to work with in a counseling role. Extreme frankness and clarity are necessary on the part of the counselor. Since the paranoid personality is usually a master at rationalization and intellectualization, he can turn any counseling situation into a verbal duel with the odds all in his favor. Logic, debate, and persuasion are likely to have little effect if the counselee does not accept his need for help.

There are a number of occupations requiring a suspicious nature into which the paranoid personality can fit quite well. Similarly, this type of personality is often able to operate businesses that are financially successful.

SCHIZOID PERSONALITY. Developing in childhood, the schizoid personality may represent a lifelong pattern of adjustment, or it may be the prelude to a schizophrenic break, occurring often in late adolescence or early adulthood. An early sense of rejection has taught the schizoid to detach himself emotionally from others in order to avoid further hurt and loss of self-esteem and to reduce anxiety. He becomes a highly repressed individual, inwardly quite sensitive, but to the observer emotionally aloof or flat, impersonal and withdrawn. His relationships are highly superficial; there is little overt hostility or even self-assertion. An active inner life, autistic in nature, is substituted for the healthier, externalized world of striving and coping. If there is no psychotic break—the schizoid personality is sometimes mistake for an inactive chronic schizophrenic—the schizoid personality may go through life as a rather detached, introverted, or eccentric individual. A satisfactory vocational adjustment is quite possible in a setting that does not require close interpersonal relationships.

PASSIVE-AGGRESSIVE PERSONALITY. This pattern represents one type of reaction to an overly protective or restrictive upbringing. The individual, who has never learned to stand on his own feet, grows up to be highly dependent. Along with this goes a considerable degree of resentment, which the individual, because of his dependent needs, fears to express overtly. Instead, it is expressed by passivity, helplessness, and a lack of accomplishment, resulting in clinging, manipulative relationships where others are used to pull one's chestnuts out of the fire. Thus, overt passivity and dependence combine with disguised hostility, uncooperativeness, and obstructionism. Aggressive reactions may become overt where there is prolonged frustration of passive-dependent needs.

INADEQUATE PERSONALITY. A long history of marginal adjustment to society which is not due to mental retardation, cultural deprivation, physical limitations or symptomatic emotional disorders characterizes the inadequate personality. Lack of adaptability, accomplishment, and the capacity for sustained effort combined with poor judgment, ineptitude, and social inadequacy result in a "Sad Sack" or "Nebbish" type of adjustment. Relatively little self-direction or self-sufficiency can be expected, but in a structured, supportive setting this type of individual could be productive at simple routine activities.

SOCIOPATHIC PERSONALITY. Behavior patterns that are against society or unacceptable to society (in the absence of symptomatic disorders) are the common element in this broad category that would include many delinquents, criminals, alcoholics, addicts, and sex deviants. In this category would be cases sometimes given the more controversial label of "psychopathic personality." The psychopath is an individual who lacks moral standards, is indifferent to the rights and feelings of others, and runs afoul of the laws and mores of society. Lacking acceptable social standards and values, his antisocial behavior produces little sense of anxiety and guilt or desire to change.

Sociopathic personalities generally lack any real identification with parental figures (the representatives of society), or else they are in rebellion against them. However, certain forms of sociopathic behavior represent primarily the value systems of subcultures, out of harmony with or opposed to the values of the predominant culture, rather than emotional disorders. An example might be the confidence games of the gypsies, often described in the newspapers, practiced on *other* ethnic groups. As workers, parents, and functioning members of the community, sociopaths leave something to be desired. Other than this, the subgroups should not be considered as necessarily having similar personality dynamics.

While it is true that as a group sociopathic personalities are reported to show relatively little response to psychotherapy, case work, and rehabilitation procedures, this is an overgeneralized stereotype of limited validity. Decisions with respect to providing treatment and services should be made on an individual basis, without prejudgments and bias. There are many instances, in all diagnostic subcategories, of individuals who have eventually made constructive adjustments to society.

PSYCHOSOMATIC DISORDERS

Both the term "psychosomatic" and its implications are highly controversial. The term is unacceptable to some because it implies to them an untenable dichotomy between mind (psyche) and body (soma). To others, particularly with a strict biological-organic orientation to disease, the idea that emotional reactions can produce organic dysfunction is both unscientific and unproved. Even among those who accept this premise, there is a considerable lack of agreement as to the nature of the process and the preferred treatment (as shown in other chapters of this book). In medicine, the term "psychophysiological autonomic and visceral disorders" is considered more suitable than "psychosomatic disorders" because the former refers to specific medical entities while the latter refers more to an approach or a point of view. Neither term, *per se*, gives adequate recognition to the impact of social, cultural, and economic factors on emotions and human well-being.

Most disease processes can be exacerbated or intensified by emotional factors. In turn, disease processes and disabling conditions are likely to provoke emotional reactions in individuals (somatopsychic reactions). "Psychosomatic" usually refers to physical disorders (excluding conversion reactions) that are *caused or precipitated*, in whole or in part, by emotional factors. It is important to recognize that other etiological factors, in addition to emotional, may be involved in psychosomatic disorders. For example, emotional stress and strain may precipitate epileptic seizures or asthmatic attacks, in individuals prone to these disorders, by lowering the body threshold or tolerance to these reactions. Environmental factors, allergic sensitivities, the presence of infections, lesions, and structural weaknesses may all play a causative role. Conversely, a specific disorder may be largely of psychological origin in one individual and of infectious, allergic, or traumatic origin in other individuals.

Psychosomatic disorders occur in organs or body systems that are under the control of the autonomic (involuntary) nervous system. This would include the cardiovascular, gastrointestinal, genitourinary, musculoskeletal, and respiratory systems, the skin, the endocrine glands, and the eyes. Rheumatoid arthritis, asthma, colitis, peptic ulcers, hypertension, menstrual irregularities, headaches, backaches, neurodermatoses, and urticaria are some of the more common disorders considered to have an important emotional component.

Many other disorders have been described at one time or another as psychosomatic, not always with adequate evidence. Prolonged reactions such as a nervous stomach or spastic colon may be prodromal to full-blown syndromes and warrant early psychological and medical evaluation on a preventive basis. Some symptoms such as vomiting, constipation, frigidity, palpitations of the heart, and vertigo which are often emotionally determined do not lend themselves easily to classification. Frequently they are symbolic in nature—for example, vomiting as an attempt to get rid of something unwanted—so they are classified as conversion or hysterical reactions. However, they are not usually under voluntary control, and they do not usually reduce anxiety. Sometimes these are referred to as "anxiety equivalents" in psychoanalytic terminology. In the same terminology, organic changes occurring without psychic meaning—that is, not on a symbolic basis—are referred to as organ neuroses.

Wartime experiences suggest that even individuals with strong egos may develop physical symptoms under severe emotional stress. However, usually only certain personality types somatize their emotions. Generally, some combinations of the following factors are present: personality is rather immature, dependent needs are fairly strong, anxiety is mobilized rather easily, emotional patterns are moralistic, self-restrictive and limiting, reflecting parental authoritarian standards taken over by the individual, emotions are deeply repressed so that the individual is unaware of their existence, and there is a high level of hostility which rarely is expressed overtly except to subordinates or children.

Psychosomatic symptoms are the somatic expression of repressed emotions. Instead of the more normal expression and discharge of feelings and the physiological tension that goes with them, there is a constant source of internal stress unrelieved by expression or action. In this connection, it should be remembered that the individual carries the source of most of his anxiety and hostilities within him always. Prolonged innervation of the body systems for "fight or flight" that never takes place may lead eventually to organic changes, possibly on the basis of excessive, unremitting "wear and tear." The question of why one organ or another is selected has never been satisfactorily answered.

There is a rather wide range in the severity of emotional reactions represented by somatic symptoms. Such symptoms may occur from a neurotic level to an acute psychotic level. While some schizophrenic individuals may have psychosomatic symptoms, the psychotic withdrawal usually reduces overt anxiety and its somatic expression. Since anxiety is not alleviated by psychosomatic symptoms, the disorder may grow progressively worse with time unless it is treated effectively.

Probably an appreciable number of psychosomatic disorders could be prevented if psychotherapy could be brought to bear upon the individual or if his environment could be suitably modified before lesions develop in the various end organs. Once organic pathology has developed, competent medical care is needed, possibly including surgery in more advanced cases of some disorders. Psychotherapy alone is not likely to reverse the organic process. Conversely, medical care and surgery may alleviate the physical symptoms, but they do not usually affect or correct the emotional factors. In my opinion a combination of medical treatment and psychotherapy is the approach of choice whenever possible. This is true even when the diseased condition is corrected by surgery. Unless the emotional factors are modified, new symptoms may, and often do, develop in other parts of the body.

The very fact that certain individuals develop physical symptoms in response to emotional stress suggests that they are not willing or able to face their emotional problems directly. As a result, they do not usually seek psychotherapy, and even when it is made available to them, they tend to be resistant. This attitude is often abetted by some physicians who do not see any value in, or need for, psychotherapeutic procedures. Regardless of the rationale, it is rather amazing to see the number of individuals who prefer the relatively radical approach of surgery (where they are passive recipients of treatment), to the much more conservative approach of psychotherapy (where they must assume some responsibility for their improvement). It should also be noted that for some individuals it is more appealing to be able to attribute all of one's difficulties to an organic impairment than to face the implications (however the individual sees them) of a psychogenic disorder.

Despite the factor of resistance, psychotherapy, counseling, case work, and environmental changes can influence the course of psychosomatic disorders. Major modifications of personality structure are not needed to improve the symptomatic picture; if the individual can be helped to externalize his feelings, his susceptibility to somatic symptomatology will decrease accordingly. A more ambitious objective, and therefore more difficult, would be to decrease the amount of anxiety and hostility in the individual, while building up self-confidence and self-acceptance. Just removing him from a stressful situation at home or on the job—for example, through hospitalization—may result in a dramatic, though frequently temporary, decrease in symptoms. Group psychotherapy is sometimes effective when individual therapy fails. This may be due to the fact that it is easier to see immature behavior in others than in oneself. At a later stage, it may be easier to see similar reactions in oneself, supported by the group.

Since the individual's employment, or lack of employment, may contribute to the overall emotional stress, vocational counseling with the aim of harmonizing vocational activities and personality factors may be quite helpful. Similarly, the skills of the case worker can be of considerable benefit in improving family relationships and reducing friction and conflict within the family unit. The multidisciplinary approach of a rehabilitation center could lend itself very well to the multiple problems invariably found in psychosomatic disorders.

EMOTIONAL REACTIONS TO DISEASE AND DISABILITY

Physical disease and disability are problems of life to which man reacts emotionally. In many instances, the emotional reaction may be more disabling than the primary disorder. Indeed, from the rehabilitation point of view, a disability *is* emotional as well as physical. It follows then that a program of services for the chronically disabled is incomplete unless it provides for the psychological needs of patients.

A physical disability is usually seen as a loss by the disabled person. The normal reaction to loss is grief or depression (reactive depression), which may last for a few weeks or for a few months. Depressions tend to lift when the patient has had a chance to take stock of his situation and regain a ray of hope for the future. A persistent depression indicates that the patient is not able to accept what he sees as the catastrophic aspects of the disability. Oddly enough, the complete absence of a depressive reaction following the onset of disability indicates the same thing—the reality of the situation is ignored through the defense of denial. A possible exception might occur in the case of the guilt-ridden individual who sustains a disability. Here the disability may be seen as a form of punishment representing atonement for past sins; since this wipes the slate clean, depression does not occur.

Once past the depressive phase, a heightened level of anxiety is apt to set in. In part this reflects the individual's recognition of his new limitations, limitations which will make it more difficult for him to adapt to the outside world and compete with others. In addition, the anxiety will be a manifestation of the symbolic meaning that disability has for the individual. Loss of body integrity, loss of manhood or womanhood, and punishment for sins are examples that are frequently encountered. It is important to realize that the reaction may have little relation to reality; a minor disability may be seen as a major calamity. The skilled worker learns the meaning of the disability to the patient and, where it is distorted, helps him to develop a more valid reality-based conceptualization of himself.

Some individuals may use illness and disability to defend against anxiety. For those who do not want to face responsibility, compete and cope, or seek positive satisfaction and reward, illness and disability offer a socially acceptable rationale or alibi for passivity, inactivity, and lack of accomplishment. Moreover, in our society the sick person gets added attention, protection, and frequently income in the form of compensation or pension. In some subcultural groups, where unremitting hard work is the individual's lot, illness provides the only respite from a life of toil. In short, weakness and incapacity lend themselves to a variety of gains, not all of which need be neurotic.

A similar pattern is seen in the hypochondriac who retreats into illness that exists largely in his own mind. The hypochondriac is usually guilt-ridden and self-restricting. Feeling unworthy and not entitled to love or satisfaction, he seeks attention and protection through "illness." At the same time, a withdrawal from the "threat" of social, sexual, or vocational activities is possible.

Ignorance, misconceptions, and misinterpretations of medical data and their implications may produce adverse emotional reactions in patients. This may be due to superstition, cultural beliefs, or simply limited comprehension on the part of the patient. On the other hand, disorders may be induced in a patient (iatrogenic disorders) by a too studious preoccupation with a point of view, by a lack of empathy with the patient, or by a careless word or action on the part of a physician or other professional worker.

Despite all generalizations, the meanings of disease and disability are highly subjective for each individual. Programs of treatment and rehabilitation should be based on this premise rather than preconceived ideas. Meanings can be changed with new insights and new perspectives. The onset of a disabling condition is often a turning point in a person's life, not always in a negative direction. Many individuals, who led "lives of quiet desperation" before becoming disabled, have gone on to lead satisfying lives despite their disabilities.

EMOTIONAL REACTIONS TO BRAIN INJURY

Two related reactions are involved in the emotional symptomatology of brain injury. One is the response of the individual to the motor, sensory, communicative, and intellectual impairment that may result from brain injury; the other is the emotional disinhibition caused by impairment of the control mechanisms of the brain, acquired through learning and experience, that have structured emotional patterns and regulated emotionally dictated behavior in the past. The emotional symptoms, like the physical and intellectual symptoms, may range from minimal to severe.

Free-floating anxiety seems to be fairly common following many brain injuries. Part of this is undoubtedly due to the fact that the individual realizes that he is not able to cope with his environment as well as he did in the past. There is awareness at some level of increased impotence, helplessness, and incapacity. There is also the psychological reaction to loss of integrity and loss of function that may accompany any physical disability. Finally, there is the likelihood that typical defense mechanisms (which have a cognitive element) are impaired when the brain is injured. Thus, anxiety that was formerly repressed or channeled is now present on a conscious level, often quite visible to the naked eye. With the anxiety goes restlessness, impatience, and low frustration tolerance, all of which have to be taken into account when planning programs of retraining and rehabilitation. Faced with a situation he cannot handle—that is, when his low level of frustration tolerance has been exceeded—the brain-injured patient's behavior is apt to become highly chaotic and disorganized; Kurt Goldstein has called this a "catastrophic reaction."

There is a strong need for closure—for things to be finite, tangible, concrete, present here and now. In an effort to make objects more available to his senses, the brain-injured person may resort to a compulsive orderliness. The easily distracted hemiplegic, learning to walk, stays close to a wall or a person; he tends to freeze up if he has to cross an open place. Unable to act on an "as if" basis, to project himself to another place or ahead in time, anything that he might need (but does not need here and now) is a cause for anxiety unless he can see it or feel it.

Depression, with its usual implications, is a frequent finding. This may be overt, or it may lie just below the surface, appearing at times of stress. Euphoria is a much less frequent finding in my experience, although it does occur.

Reduced ability to think abstractly is common following brain injury; the loss may be minimal or it may be severe. Impairment of judgment, memory, comprehension, and perceptual ability may occur singly and in combination. The patient may be disoriented for time, place, and person; that is, he may have no knowledge of the time and date, of his physical location, or of the people with whom he comes in contact daily. Perseveration—persistent repetition—of words, ideas, and behavior is frequent. This is a manifestation of the rigidity of the brain-injured person, his difficulty in making mental shifts or trying new approaches. Virtually any function of intelligence may be impaired to some extent, depending upon the nature, location, and size of the lesion as well as the age of the individual at the time of injury. The intellectual impairment cannot help but influence the emotional reaction.

The impairment of emotional control and inhibition produces some distinctive behavior. In some instances, there is an "impulse disturbance"; as soon as a thought enter consciousness it is acted upon. There is no pause for consideration of the consequences of the action. At times, this type of behavior can be destructive. Generally, there is a lowered emotional threshold. Slight stimuli that in the past would never have produced a visible reaction in the individual, now produce crying or laughing—somewhat of a "sham reaction." Emotionality, which is easily aroused, tends to persist abnormally long. Covert or repressed elements of personality may become overt; the brain-injured person may behave in some ways that were quite foreign to him in the past.

There is a tendency for the brain-damaged person to become quite self-centered. He may demand considerable attention from staff or members of the family. Realistically, his dependent needs are greater as a result of his limitations, but the demands may reach an irrational level.

Psychotic reactions, characterized by hallucinations or delusions, may occur in conjunction with brain injury. It is difficult to say if they are caused by brain damage or released by brain damage. Periods of agitation, confusion, or disorientation are not necessarily indicative of a psychosis. Similarly, the jargon and other communicative difficulties that occur with aphasic disorders are not indicative, *per se*, of emotional symptomatology. At times, with combinations of motor, sensory, intellectual, communicative, and emotional symptoms present, the question of whether or not a psychosis is present may be purely academic.

Symptomatology in brain injuries varies considerably, depending upon the extent of the damage, on the one hand, and the previous personality of the individual, on the other. Even when the primary condition is chronic and irreversible, it is quite possible to restore a considerable degree of function and adaptability through rehabilitative services of a coordinated nature.

TREATMENT

Treatment of emotional disorders, as one might expect, is influenced to a large degree by the theoretical background, training, and professional affiliations of the practitioner. Too often, emphasis on one theoretical orientation or one form of treatment results in professional myopia, with other valid approaches to patient care being neglected or excluded. The existence of considerable dogmatism, rigidity, and professional rivalry is unfortunate from at least two points of view: new approaches are now being developed that offer considerable hope for the future, and if they are to be successful there is a great need for cooperation among workers and for integration of services.

If emotional disorders are not to be understood as typical disease processes, then the concept of cure is inappropriate. Rather, changes of various sorts are brought about by a diminution of stress, by improvement in the individual's capacity for tolerating stress, by reducing the number of irrational factors that cause anxiety, by dulling the individual's perception of the outside world and of himself, or by some similar approach. Obviously, some methods are effective through relief of symptoms only; others operate in a much more ambitious way by attempting to increase the competence or emotional strength of the individual. Some are aimed at the soma, some at the psyche, and still others focus on the environment. The applicability and effectiveness of a given form of treatment will vary, depending on a variety of factors such as age, education, and socioeconomic background of the patient; the severity and duration of the disorder; the skill and personal attributes of the practitioner. Even simple forms of treatment may have excellent results if they reverse a chain of unfortunate events for an individual and permit him to move in a constructive direction again.

SOMATIC TREATMENT

Drug therapy and shock (convulsive) therapy are the two major forms of somatic treatment in current use, with the success of the former being responsible for decreased reliance on the latter. Tranquilizing drugs, applicable to the treatment of anxiety, turmoil, confusion, and tension, are used to calm patients without putting them to sleep. One important result of the use of tranquilizing drugs is that staff members are better able to work with patients who in the past were decidedly unappealing. Since the advent of tranquilizers, there has been a steady decrease in the use of restraints—strait jackets, isolation cells, locked wards—with hospitalized patients. Hospital wards changed dramatically for the better as patients' behavior became less extreme. As is the case with medications in general, proper dosage of the tranquilizers is important; an inadequate dosage may be ineffective, while an overdosage may produce undesirable side effects.

Antidepressant drugs appear to have some value in treating milder cases of depression. Their efficacy has not been demonstrated as clearly as that of the tranquilizers.

Electroshock treatment which induces seizures has been used extensively for the treatment of depressions where it has been moderately effective. For some physicians, it has been the treatment of last resort; for others it has been the first choice, particularly with older patients. While its use is diminishing, it still is of value in treating depressed patients who cannot be reached by other methods. Both drug therapy and shock therapy have the value of making certain patients amenable to other forms of therapy. Relaxant medications are used in the various forms of shock therapy to lessen the danger of fractures from the seizure.

Insulin shock treatment, although still used widely in some countries, is generally declining as a form of treatment, particularly in the United States. It is more complicated and difficult to administer than electroshock treatment, producing a hypoglycemic state and coma. Moreover, the attendant dangers are greater, with the possibility of prolonged coma or circulatory collapse. Used in the treatment of schizophrenia, there is some indication that it produces more lasting benefit than electroshock, although neither has clearly been demonstrated to be of value in this disorder. However, the ease, simplicity, and relative safety of drug therapy, as well as its success, appear responsible for the decreased use of insulin treatment in schizophrenia.

PSYCHOTHERAPY

The term psychotherapy is generally applied to a verbal form of interaction between therapist and patient. Based essentially on psychoanalytic theory, there are many variations, many schools of thought, and a variety of practitioners. The objectives generally are to have the patient understand himself and gain insight into the irrational aspects of his personality, see himself in a more positive way, and deal more effectively with people and problems.

It is a conservative form of treatment, and when it is successful, its benefits are probably more sustained than any other form of psychological treatment. However, there are many obstacles and difficulties in its use. To name a few: a high level of skill is needed by the therapist; only a handful of people can afford or obtain this type of treatment; it requires a lot of motivation and drive, which is very often missing in the people who need help the most; it moves slowly; it is not too effective with the lower socioeconomic groups and with the mentally retarded; and to many people, particularly those with limited intellectual and verbal ability, it is a meaningless activity. When effective, psychotherapy increases the individual's ego strength and efficiency, reduces anxiety (and accompanying symptomatology), and increases tolerance for frustration and pressure.

ENVIRONMENTAL MODIFICATION

The two traditional forms of treatment described above are focused on the individual—somatic treatment on the body and psychotherapy on the psyche or mind. Environmental modification attempts to change the emotional reaction of the individual by influencing or changing the environment in which he operates so that his problems will be decreased and he will be subject to less stress and strain. There is no expectation that it will increase his ego strength or his problem-solving ability for the future. Neither is there any particular attempt to explore the subconscious mind or bring about the development of insight. The method is simple, the goals are modest. With a decrease in external pressure, brought about by the active intervention of a case worker, a counselor, or an agency, some temporary decrease in anxiety accompanied by a corresponding improvement in adjustment is anticipated. Along these lines, it should be remembered that there are many complex situations in life that make demands which even the emotionally mature person has difficulty in meeting. Helping a person to overcome a realistic obstacle may be all that is needed to keep him on an even keel indefinitely. Providing living accomodations, arranging for financial aid, or finding a disabled person a job would all be examples of environmental modification.

WORKING WITH THE FAMILY

Treatment of the family unit, if successful, can be of considerable value, particularly in the functional disorders. Families tend to set up patterns of interaction among the various members which are consistent and enduring. Disturbed parents tend to bring up disturbed children. When disturbed adults marry, they usually select disturbed spouses. Therapeutic measures aimed at only one member of the family unit tend to be ineffective if he or she is continuously exposed to the usual pressures and power operations of the family. Therefore, treatment is frequently aimed at the most important members of the family unit in an effort to improve the interrelationships and lessen pressures. In some disturbed families, one member, made a scapegoat by the rest of the family, ends up in a mental hospital. If the patterns in this family cannot be modified, the patient may have a greater chance to get along in the community if he does not return to the family. The family, which is the unit of living, should also be considered the unit of treatment.

MILIEU THERAPY

Milieu or environmental therapy combines elements of psychotherapy and environmental modification. Based on the theory that all aspects of one's environment can be helpful or harmful, all relationships and activities of the daily cycle are structured, as far as possible, for maximum therapeutic benefit. Medical routines and the traditional hospital hierarchy of professional staff and maintenance personnel are deemphasized. Instead, the objective is to set up a "therapeutic community," patterned after the one described by Maxwell Jones in England, where meals, living arrangements, work and social activities all contribute to emotional growth. This informal approach, based upon a 24-hour-a-day program, is somewhat in contrast to the more formal programs of treatment where the various therapeutic modalities are scheduled on a regular basis for a given period of time, following which treatment ceases until the next day's schedule resumes. It is also different from therapy based on the traditional doctor-patient relationship, since it is based on a variety of concurrent relationships involving professional workers, maintenance workers, volunteers, and patients, with none being the primary treatment agent.

Milieu therapy has never really been dignified by having a well-developed body of theory to explain its operations or provide a basis for research and teaching. Recently, however, Elaine and John Cumming, in their book *Ego and Milieu,* have provided such a rationale. They state that ego growth takes place when an individual successfully resolves a crisis or problem in his life situation. This would suggest that controlled situations in the person's environment can be structured to provide considerable emotional growth. While this type of therapy requires highly competent direction, it has the advantage of being able to make excellent use of relatively untrained, relatively inexpensive personnel who are more readily available than trained professional workers.

REHABILITATION

Rehabilitation, in its brief history, has had the objective of minimizing residual disability while increasing function and adaptive skills. If, as stated earlier, emotional disorders are expressions of man's inability to cope effectively with the demands, responsibilities, and problems of life, it follows that rehabilitative procedures are at the same time therapeutic procedures. As a person functions better and develops skills—be they vocational, social, educational, recreational, self-care, communicative, use of the community—he is better able to cope with life.

This has been demonstrated in recent research projects with chronic hospitalized schizophrenics who until recently were considered hopeless. Using comprehensive activity programs focused on meaningful work, these projects have been able to bring an appreciable number of bottom-of-the-barrel schizophrenics to the stage where they were able to be discharged and accept full-time gainful employment in the community with a remarkable degree of stability.

Rehabilitation in the institutional setting focuses on the reality orientation of work activities graded in terms of difficulty and responsibility. These activities, which could include training in work skills or work habits, institutional maintenance work, subcontract work, day work outside the hospital, and so on, should provide reimbursement to the patient when his work warrants it. They, in turn, are integrated with all other activities in which the patient participates. In effect, rehabilitation concepts and milieu therapy are combined; Hyde and associates have called this *milieu rehabilitation.* All facets of institutional life are structured so that the patient moves forward through his activities gaining skills and self-confidence as he does. Increased rewards are earned with acceptance of increased responsibility. The various interpersonal relationships of the patient are used to help him learn how to get along with a variety of people in a variety of settings. Going into the community and learning how to use it effectively—that is, to travel, shop, bank, socialize, work—is an important part of the program. Living arrangements are also graded so that the patient can gradually move from ward life to independent living. The patient is helped to develop a bank account and to learn to use money so that he can care for himself financially when he is discharged. Throughout there is respect for the individual, and the expectation that he can assume responsibility for himself.

This type of program brings about comprehensive growth in the individual—emotionally, socially, vocationally, and financially. It appears to have widespread application to disorders, both acute and chronic, that are psychosocial in nature. It may be anticipated that considerable research will be devoted to this approach in the years to come.

BIBLIOGRAPHY

American Psychiatric Association. *Diagnostic and Statistical Manual of Mental Disorders.* Washington, D.C.: American Psychiatric Association, 1952.

Cumming, Elaine, and John Cumming. *Ego and Milieu.* New York: Atherton Press, 1962.

Ewalt, J. R., E. A. Strecker, and F. G. Ebaugh. *Practical Clinical Psychiatry,* 8th ed. New York: McGraw-Hill Book Co., 1957.

Fenichel, Otto. *The Psychoanalytic Theory of Neurosis.* New York: W. W. Norton and Co., 1945.

Hollingshead, A. B. and F. C. Redlich. *Social Class and Mental Illness.* New York: John Wiley and Sons, 1958.

Hyde, R. W., J. S. Bockoven, H. W. Pfautz, and R. H. York. *Milieu Rehabilitation.* Providence 6, R. I., Butler Health Center, 1962.

Joint Commission on Mental Illness and Health. *Action for Mental Health.* New York: Basic Books, 1961.

Jones, Maxwell. *The Therapeutic Community.* New York: Basic Books, 1953.

Sullivan, Harry Stack. *Conceptions of Modern Psychiatry.* Washington, D.C.: The William Alanson White Psychiatric Foundation, 1947.

Szasz, T. S. "The Myth of Mental Illness," *The American Psychologist,* 15:2, 1960.

White, Robert W. *The Abnormal Personality.* New York: Ronald Press, 1948.

XV

MENTAL RETARDATION

The term "mental retardation" conjures up many and varied reactions, not only among lay people who are not supposed to be sophisticated, but even among the many professionals who should know. Lack of understanding, distortions, misconceptions, stigmas, have clouded this disorder from early times. Confusion about definition, terminology, and classification aggravate this distortion.

No discussion of mental retardation should start without reference to the excellent "Report of the President's Panel on Mental Retardation."

Mental retardation ranks as a major national health, social, and economic problem:

. . . It afflicts twice as many individuals as blindness, polio, cerebral palsy, and rheumatic heart disease, combined. Only four significant disabling conditions—mental illness, cardiac disease, arthritis, and cancer—have a higher prevalence, but they tend to come late in life while mental retardation comes early.

. . . About 400,000 of the persons affected are so retarded that they require constant care or supervision, or are severely limited in their ability to care for themselves and to engage in productive work; *the remaining five million are individuals with mild disabilities.* [Italics added.]

. . . Over 200,000 adults and children, largely from the severe and profound mentally retarded groups, are cared for in residential institutions, mostly at public expense. States and localities spend $300 million a year in capital

By Patrick J. Doyle, M.D., and Morton A. Seidenfeld, ph.d., Vocational Rehabilitation Administration, Department of Health, Education, and Welfare, Washington, D.C. This chapter was written by Dr. Doyle and Dr. Seidenfeld in their private capacity, and no official support or endorsement by the Vocational Rehabilitation Administration of the Department of Health, Education, and Welfare is intended or should be inferred.

and operating expenses for their care. In addition, they spend perhaps $250 million for special education, welfare, rehabilitation, and other benefits and services for retarded individuals outside of public institutions. In the current fiscal year, the Federal Government will obligate an estimated $164 million for the mentally retarded, about three-fourths for income maintenance payments and the rest for research, training, and special services. Federal funds for this group have nearly doubled in five years.[1]

DEFINITION AND DISTRIBUTION

There are many definitions of mental retardation. The President's Panel defined it as follows:

The mentally retarded are children and adults who, as a result of inadequately developed intelligence, are significantly impaired in their ability to learn and to adapt to the demands of society.[2]

Of the estimated 5,400,000 individuals who are mentally retarded, only 4 to 5 per cent are institutionalized; the remainder are in the community. The retarded represent slightly more than 3 per cent of the total population. While the assumption is frequently made that intelligence has a normal or "bell-shaped" curve of distribution, there is a greater frequency of severe retardation than would be expected in terms of normal probability. Roughly 400,000 individuals are estimated to be moderately or severely retarded, with the former outnumbering the latter by about 2 to 1.

Mental retardation is somewhat more prevalent among males than among females; there is no clear-cut explanation for this. Organic forms of retardation are of approximately the same order of magnitude in upper and lower socioeconomic groups. However, nonorganic or nonbrain injured forms, sometimes referred to as "subcultural," are much more frequent in the lower socioeconomic groups. Among the lower socioeconomic groups, mental retardation (and other disorders) tend to "nest" in certain families. This is sometimes attributed to a hereditary factor, but in this connection it should be remembered that mental deficiency, when it is genetically influenced, frequently results from characteristics transmitted as recessive traits, with normal parents producing some abnormal offspring. A wide variety of environmental factors would appear to be implicated in the familial distribution of nonorganic forms of retardation.

Several surveys have shown that the highest distribution of retardation is in the age range 10–14, followed by ages 15–19. Younger and older groups show a sharp drop in prevalence. These findings seem to represent an artifact of the school setting related to academic ad-

[1] President's Panel on Mental Retardation, A Proposed Program for National Action to Combat Mental Retardation, October 1962, pp. 1–2.
[2] Ibid., p. 1.

justment. Many individuals classified as retarded during school years appear to be able to make an adequate adjustment to the community in adulthood.[3] It is obvious that highly accurate epidemiological data are lacking. The *Perinatal Collaborative Study* under way at the National Institutes of Health may help clarify some of the problems related to incidence, prevalence, and distribution.

MENTAL RETARDATION AS A PSYCHOLOGICAL PROBLEM

THE NATURE OF MENTAL RETARDATION

It has been pointed out frequently that "mental retardation" is not a disease, not a single categorical entity. It is a symptom much the same as a headache or a pain located anywhere in or on the body. It is a symptom derived from many etiological sources, some of which have become pretty well identified, a few of which are already known to be preventable, most of which we know relatively little about.

Mental retardation may have a primary biological cause—particularly the severe and moderate cases—or the primary cause may be non-biological in nature. Let us consider the latter group. For the most part, these are of social origin and very little factual information exists regarding them. We can at least review the progress that has been made so far in exploring these areas. Perhaps the leading social factor is poverty and its handmaiden cultural lag, or what is today often erroneously called cultural deprivation. As a matter of fact, no human being who lives among other people can truly be called culturally deprived; rather he lives in a subculture that has not yet evolved to a sufficient degree ways and means of being accepted by or accepting standards established in a surrounding superculture. Thus, among the impoverished in Appalachia, in many rural and geographically isolated areas, and in certain ethnically established subcultures within the United States, the cultural level of the country as a whole prevents or inhibits certain isolated subgroups from taking on the cultural characteristics of the broadly predominant cultural pattern. These isolated subcultures take on the characteristics of groups denied the opportunity for meeting the demands that their economy, education, and ethnic origin forces upon them. They in turn suffer the insecurity and uncertainty associated with the process of acculturation until ways can be found for them to make the transition. Unfortunately, this may require a generation or more to pass before it can be accomplished even under the most favorable circumstances.

[3] For a more complete discussion of distribution see Paul V. Lemkau, "Epidemiological Aspects of Mental Retardation" in *The Evaluation and Treatment of the Mentally Retarded Child in Clinics*. New York: National Association for Retarded Children, 1956.

For a variety of reasons, but most especially because of social and economic factors, these areas of cultural lag contain within them many etiological sources associated with the occurrence of mental retardation. Among these are faulty nutrition, inadequate diet, lack of prenatal preparation and obstetrical care, prematurity, lack of postnatal care, and the gamut of medical problems discussed elsewhere. On the psychosocial side may be found such factors as lack of funds for clothing, lack of transportation to school, lack of in-home stimulation to intellectual development, excessively large family size, inadequacies of schools and lack of school personnel, lack of contact between home and school, and many others, including the all-important lack of sensitivity on the part of family to signs of intellectual retardation.

We know that it takes much more than provision of money to relieve poverty; besides changes in living conditions and improved economic conditions, it takes provision of jobs so that people may feel independent, may attain a sense of self-worth, and may create for their children a sense of something more than waiting for the relief check or gift baskets of food. People must feel that they have earned what they get, that increased effort on their part brings greater and better opportunity for themselves and their children. These changes do not come packaged in a form that we can give to people; they must create them out of their own conviction that they are worthy and have earned what they have.

From the standpoint of mental retardation this is a most important factor. Somewhere between 50 and 75 per cent of the mentally retarded as of the moment appear to have mental deficits that are associated with no known pathology of the brain. Perhaps as our scientific knowledge increases, some of these disabled people will be found to have organic causes. However, the indications are that the majority of them are the victims of an environment that fails to provide sufficient opportunity, adequate motivation, or enough stimulation to make them want to learn how to effectively participate in active living. Like a green plant denied access to sunlight, a vital catalyst remains dormant, and the plant soon becomes withered and lifeless.

Difficult and slow moving as modern scientific research has been in providing an answer to inborn errors of metabolism and other psychophysiological problems, the need for a solution to the psychosocial errors that are responsible for the failure of retardates of today to attain full use of their mental capacity is even greater. It is difficult to overcome the effects of actual brain damage or faulty brain development, because there is no known means of replacing or adding brain tissue. Therefore, we must do the best that modern skill will permit in the utilization of the undamaged portion of the brain. Early detection of certain biochemical factors or physical factors in some instances may prevent the damage from taking place. When actual cellular damage does not occur, so that the brain is intact and quite capable of functioning if we but knew how to get it started, we have the possibility of reversing the process and developing an individual who is able to make his own way. Since such appears to be the case among those in the most common category of retarded, we stand in an excellent position to correct a major disability, as soon as we can establish methods by which this form of disability can be overcome.

To accomplish this we need to institute some rather startling changes in our concepts of the care and treatment of mental retardation. Considering here only the most significant of these needed changes we note, for example:

1. We need to correct our thinking of the mentally retarded as hopeless, uneducable, and socially unacceptable. So much success has been attained by patient, understanding human beings working with the retarded that often even the more severely damaged can be improved. Clinically, one sees such severely damaged rather infrequently because they do require much more prolonged and continuous help than can ordinarily be given in a noninstitutional environment. Fortunately, this group is but a very small minority. The majority are children and adults who when promptly and properly identified can be made totally or very nearly totally useful and adequate members of society. When recognition and treatment are delayed, the results may be less satisfactory but can be, and usually are, sufficient to improve the individual's outlook significantly.

The nature of the services rendered are described by Gunzburg, who states: "Only by tackling directly and realistically those life situations which the defective has either not been taught or which he has not understood when at school, can we hope to remove confusion, irritation and panic born from ignorance. In this form Education will have become perhaps the most valuable single therapeutic factor in the work of rehabilitation."[4] When the approach described by Gunzburg has been used, very remarkable inroads have been made in bringing retardates to effective levels of independence, social and vocational competency with consequent employment and responsible placement in community life.

2. In a somewhat similar vein, our thinking has been distorted by the belief that the retardate is likely to be a bad child, a delinquent who gets into all sorts of trouble. Of course, there have been retarded children and adults who have been in trouble with the law, with

[4] N. C. Gunzburg, "The Place of Future Education in the Rehabilitation of the Adult Subnormal," in *Proceedings of the London Conference on the Scientific Study of Mental Deficiency, 1960,* Dagenham, England: May and Baker, Ltd., 1962, pp. 251–257.

their schools and their communities, but for the most part when this has occurred it has not been because of any desire to do evil or flaunt society, but rather because of their poor judgment and high degree of suggestibility. Unfortunately, when their training has not prevailed long enough to help them learn how to select their friends and associates, or when social factors already discussed have thrown them into environments where they come into frequent company with gangs who offer them at times the only opportunity for social recognition they get, then they do become victims of a leadership that uses them as tools to do their more distasteful chores. The retarded seldom embark on a criminal career on their own. As Margaret Mead has observed: "The individual is born with greater or lesser capacities for certain types of behavior, but whether these behavior patterns will appear will depend on the culture, and on his exact place within the society." [5] Retardates who grow up in homes where the behavior of the family invites conformity, regard for law, and respect for each other are not likely to allow themselves to indulge in antisocial behavior unless they fall into hands determined to teach them otherwise.

Stern has recently pointed out that in the past it was thought that a high correlation existed between delinquency and low intelligence.[6] However, a 1951 report of the World Health Organization entitled "Psychiatric Aspects of Juvenile Delinquency" indicates little or no relationship.

As a matter of fact, we agree with Stern's comment: "The severely retarded are too greatly handicapped even to be able to attempt delinquency; likewise, by and large, so are the moderately retarded. Even the mildly retarded are not ring leaders. They lack initiative and tend to be dupes, falling in with 'the gang' because in the face of social and academic failure they so pathetically need to 'be somebody.'"

3. Another misconception that creates problems in attaining opportunities for the mentally retarded to gain their rightful place in society, to find employment and acceptance by their peers, is the belief that as a group they not only are lacking in intellectual skills, but also are mentally ill.

Actually, there is every reason why certain mentally retarded should be expected to suffer from mental illness, much the same as the non-retarded public may become the victims of mental illness. When this occurs we can relate the illness to the excess pressure of life on the retardate. These pressures that create frustration for all people are many times magnified for the retarded where the threshold of frus-

[5] Margaret Mead, "Culture and Personality" in *The Encyclopedia of Mental Health,* New York: Franklin Watts, Inc., 1963, p. 419.
[6] Edith Stern, "Mental Retardation," *ibid.,* p. 1200.

tration tolerance is at times depressed when the individual has fewer ways of coping with demands of his environment.

In discussing the dimensions of mental illness among the mentally retarded, O'Connor reported that 6 to 12 per cent of feebleminded patients (mean IQ = 70) at Darenth Park suffered from "severe neurotic handicap" and no less than 40 per cent suffered from "mild neurotic tendency" or "instability." [7] The same source reports that Penfield diagnosed "neurotic" in 17 per cent and "psychotic" in 6 per cent of 627 patients classified as feebleminded or dull.

There is no doubt that the mentally retarded often have emotional problems related to poor emotional control and excessive frustration, and as one approaches the lower intellectual levels, these do appear to be more severe in nature. In the higher level of retardates, the frequency of emotional problems increases, oftentimes may even reach double the number,[8] but in the majority of such cases the involvement is neither very serious nor permanent.

In the area of vocational activity of the retarded, good supervisory relations following adequate work preparation appears to be quite enough to maintain the retardate "on the job."

The more severe mental disorders associated with mental retardation are, of course, more complicated. The psychoses of childhood, especially childhood schizophrenia, often provide symptoms that cause the individual to act in such a fashion as to prevent normal contact with his environment. This is a built-in mechanism that leads to reduced learning and altered behavior closely approximating that of simple mental retardation. As a result, those involved are often mistaken by the less experienced professional for retarded rather than psychotic children. Others regress as a result of their psychosis. It is virtually impossible to obtain reliable figures on the frequency of the association between the mentally ill and retarded in the population of children. The best that can be said is that it is not a rare occurrence.

4. A final source of environmental approach to meeting the problems of the retardate that deserves attention and some repetition is the necessity to see the situation as less of a genetic dilemma and more of a problem in correction of faulty environment. It is difficult to say how much of the mentally retarded population derives from genetic causes. Surely those with inborn errors of metabolism, with familial diseases that include mental retardation as a symptom, with certain genetic disease capable of producing physiological effects that damage or prevent normal brain development, do represent a portion of the retarded

[7] N. O'Connor, quoted by J. Tizard, "Individual Differences in the Mentally Deficient" in A. M. Clarke and A. D. B. Clarke, *Mental Deficiency: The Changing Outlook*, New York: The Free Press of Glencoe, 1958, p. 167.

[8] Clarke and Clarke, *loc. cit.*

population. It has been variously estimated, but 25 per cent seems close to a consensus figure. Those who are in this category, again, seem to represent the more severe forms of mental retardation. The process in some instances is preventable and to some extent, if caught early enough, reversible. For the most part, they still represent the more or less permanently damaged retardates.

By far the majority classed as mentally retarded do not appear (as yet) to be damaged genetically but rather appear to be the result of poor environment. Admittedly, there may at times be other genetic factors such as speed of performance, rigidity and instability as personality factors, and even such factors as limitations in the rate and amount of learning of the individual may have certain genetic components; but environment, especially if it is favorable environment, may be able to overcome or minimize the genetic aspect of this form of retardation.

Once we appreciate the great importance of environmental factors, we can develop much more optimism, better programs for training and preparation of most retarded individuals. This is our goal.

INTELLIGENCE AS A FACTOR IN MENTAL RETARDATION

There is little doubt that some characteristics commonly associated with intelligence are significantly involved in our conception of mental retardation. But what these specific characteristics are appears to be far from clear once we remove the veneer that superficially hides the facts.

Historically, mental retardation first became a subject of serious consideration when it was found necessary to fit a given child into a group of seemingly similar-aged children, all of whom were expected to conform to certain externally imposed rules and regulations. It was his experience with formal education that most often brought the child with faulty learning characteristics to the attention of others, as well as difficulty in conforming to demands of the formalized milieu.

Let there be no mistake—the dullard, the slow-witted, the clod, and the foolish were known long before the period of mass education began, but they were seen only as people to be pushed about, to be used, or to be misled by connivers and the dishonest, quick to seize upon the dim-witted as their toadies because they could and would follow directions without asking "Why?"

But it was the formal processes of education that lead Binet and Simon to develop their early instruments for scaling the competency of individuals in the pursuit of academic knowledge, and thus it has been ever since. It is hardly necessary to point out how very important a place the IQ occupies in modern appraisal techniques. This index is applied to school, to vocational preparation, to the work situation, to legal rights, and to life as a member of the local, state, and federal community.

Before we go further it would seem wise indeed to take a searching look at just what intelligence and mental retardation have to do with each other. Perhaps we may find that too much of what is assumed about the mentally retarded is either incorrect or somewhat distorted from the facts by modern usage. As the Englishes so aptly state regarding intelligence:

> There is more agreement on the behaviors referred to by the term than there is on how to interpret or categorize them. Three concepts recur frequently in attempts to state its connotations:
> 1. Ability to deal effectively with tasks involving abstractions;
> 2. Ability to learn;
> 3. Ability to deal with new situations.[9]

You as an individual may have selected some other definition which you prefer and for which you are obligated to provide supporting evidence. In our opinion the above definition most nearly supports existing evidence of what intelligent behavior actually requires.

The more commonly used intelligence tests are exceedingly weighted with learned information and with approaches to the solution of problems in a manner that has been taught in the more formal educational situations. Language usage, arithmetical skills, spelling, factual information, and social conformity are the products of learning. If all of us were given equal training by equally good teachers in equally stimulating environments, our differences in performance might truly provide at least inferential evidence of differences in our intelligence. Unfortunately, the if factor seldom applies in the wide variety of opportunities afforded our children. Thus, what we are measuring is most often an index of what the individual has acquired in his milieu and not what he could do were he given optimal opportunities with those against whom he is competing.

Now what has all this to do with mental retardation? In part, it is related to what we are talking about when we speak of mental retardation. If we use the American Association for Mental Deficiency definition of mental retardation we are referring first of all to "subaverage general intellectual functioning"; secondly, to the fact that this "originates during the developmental period" (from birth to 16 years of age), and thirdly, to the fact that these behavioral impairments occur in three primary areas—namely, (1) maturation, (2) learning, and (3) social adjustment.

It is apparent that our society, and, for that matter, most of the

[9] H. B. English and A. C. English, *A Comprehensive Dictionary of Psychological and Psychoanalytical Terms*, New York: Longmans, Green and Company, 1958.

modern cultures of the world, apply the categorical stereotype "mental retardation" to all members of the society who for one reason or another are unable to compete intellectually, without extra help, with those who do not require such assistance. We often act as though "mental retardation" should be defined as "the lack of ability to do well on an intelligence test." Some of our school systems, as well as public and private agencies who serve the retarded, appear to base their selection for categorical placement simply upon the IQ or on the mental age without corroboratory evidence.

In our opinion, the error of this approach to categorical "mental retardation" does not rest in the testing instruments nearly so much as it does in the failure of testers to pay heed to the fact that the test of intelligence does not, and never will, measure more than the instrument is capable of measuring. Such tests measure what they have validly been intended to measure—namely, those facets of intelligence which their subtests have been shown to measure—no more and no less. Furthermore, tests can truly measure these only when adequate information exists about the individuals' background. If the retardate has been denied similar opportunity to attain intellectual levels accorded to those whose norms are being applied to him, he can hardly be expected to perform in a comparable fashion. As Anastasi points out: "The same score obtained by persons varying widely in education, socio-economic level or cultural milieu may have different connotations in the prediction of subsequent performance in training, on a job, or in other criterion situations." [10] This may very well be the reason that IQ's are such poor predictors of rehabilitation outcomes. The fault lies not so much in the test as in the test interpreter's conceptual reaction when he fails to recognize that the individual being measured has not had the benefit of experience comparable to that accorded the normative group. How seldom indeed does the psychologist or others using test results include in their report even mention of this fact.

If "test intelligence" is not the *sine qua non* of the categorical status "mental retardation," what should be the determinants? Probably they should consist of a number of component factors: the evaluation of the individual's background including his birth history, his behavioral evaluation during infancy, his preschool development history, his school behavior, his home adaptation, his social development in relation to his family, his peers, and his milieu in general. There is no substitute for a well-developed history procured from the patient, his family, and any other reliable source. There is no available test that one can apply that will not need to be interpreted in the light of all we

[10] Anne Anastasi, *Fields of Applied Psychology*, New York: McGraw-Hill, 1964, p. 45.

can learn about what the presumed retardate has experienced. The individual's background serves as the matrix against which we must decide whether the statistical assumptions we shall make truly apply to him.

This approach to the diagnostic appraisal of the retardate is admittedly much more difficult than merely putting him through an intelligence test, but it has the advantage of dealing with his problem in a clinically trustworthy fashion instead of using a psychologically approved crystal ball, which at best is always a bit cloudy. The application of a measure of intelligence or intellect is essential, but it must be combined with an adequate developmental, social, familial-cultural appraisal so we can see what the individual has done in utilizing the capacities he possesses as related to the opportunities he has encountered.

This approach provides us with a measure, subjective at worst, but more often at least partially objective, to appraise the differences between what the individual's potential level of intellectual functioning may be and what realistically his environment has allowed him to attain. If we find he has a modest or limited ability and he has attained maximal goals in keeping with his capacity, then we know that he is making the best use of his potential, and we can plan a program paralleling the growth of potential we have reason (both observed and statistically supported) to believe may be expected. We may utilize his present environment with confidence that it can support his future endeavors. If, on the other hand, we find that his abilities far exceed his level of attainment, we know with equal certainty that the environmental deterrents must be sought out and removed or corrected before efforts are made to help him attain his potential goals. We know that our efforts cannot be fixed upon training in education alone, but must concomitantly be directed to parental counseling and improvement of cultural factors as they impinge on the retarded individual. This method of approach has the advantage of assuring us that we are focused upon the factors that need to be specifically corrected.

DIAGNOSIS

It is imperative that a complete medical evaluation, neurological history and physical examination be done on all patients suspected of having mental retardation.

MEDICAL DIAGNOSIS

THE HISTORY. In order to bring out the pertinent data for a complete understanding of the problem, many areas must be probed in the taking of the history. For example, one must ask for as complete a medical genealogy as possible. Did parents, grandparents, aunts, uncles, and other relatives have any birth defects, retardation, problems in school related to learning or behavior, or any type of mental or neurological disorder? The history taker must go very deeply into the prenatal history of the mother, looking for information related to infections, trauma, bleeding, or any disorder during the gestational period. Did the mother take any form of medication? What about the birth itself? Was labor or delivery delayed? Did the baby have to be resuscitated or placed in an incubator? Was the baby premature?

For the postnatal period the physician will want to know how well the baby fed and developed the first year of life. Were there any convulsions, unusual lethargy or hyperactivity? What about motor or speech delay? Were there any unusual illnesses? Did the baby have to be hospitalized for any reason?

These, of course, are only a few of the questions one would ask in taking a history.

THE PHYSICAL AND NEUROLOGICAL EXAMINATION. The following brief outline will demonstrate some of the important items to be considered in the examination.

General Appearance. There is, of course, a fairly typical appearance to some specific types of retardation, for example the child with Down's syndrome (mongolism). The latter name was applied earlier in a descriptive sense because of the slanted appearance of the eyes. In addition, most of these children have round faces, poor muscular tone, and short thick necks, to mention but a few characteristics that may be overt.

The child with *microcephaly* (congenitally small head) presents a rather striking appearance. Those with *hydrocephalus* (excess fluid on the brain) will present an opposite appearance—a large head out of all proportion to the rest of the body.

It must be fairly stated, however, that *most cases of retardation will show no exterior stigmas nor will they present any gross changes in appearance distinguishable from normal children.*

Activity. Many retarded children are very quiet and withdrawn. Others are hyperactive. In infancy many are "good" babies with little or minimal crying. Many of the older retarded, especially those with associated demonstrable brain damage, often will be overactive at times with little ability to handle their impulses (impulse disturbance).

Voice, Speech, Language Development. The retarded have more than their share of articulation and language difficulties. Many show delay in speech and language development. A careful evaluation must be made of the hearing of these children. If possible, any child showing difficulties in articulation and language development should have a specialized speech and hearing evaluation.

Height and Weight. Many retarded children are smaller in size than nonretarded of the same age. Many show a history of premature birth.

Nervous and Locomotion Systems. The examiner looks for evidence of paralysis, weakness, abnormal gait or reflexes, poor balance, poor use of hands and fingers. The neurological examination is more difficult to evaluate during infancy. The physician checks the grasping reflex, the righting reflex, and other signs for abnormal neuromuscular function.

Associated Defects. A large percentage of the retarded have additional handicaps such as perceptual difficulties, impaired vision (including blindness), orthopedic difficulties, epilepsy, cerebral palsy, and the speech and hearing difficulties cited above. Many will have associated congenital anomalies, especially heart lesions. Such lesions are associated, at times, with Down's syndrome.

Approximately 40 to 50 per cent of patients seen in a cerebral palsy clinic will manifest some degree of retardation. The cerebral palsy is more often of the spastic type. Similarly 30 to 45 per cent of patients seen in a children's seizure or epilepsy clinic will be considered to have secondary or organic epilepsy and will manifest various degrees of retardation. The prognosis for the seizures is not so good as with the child who shows no evidence of retardation. In large urban clinics the retarded show up in cerebral palsy and seizure clinics because the cerebral palsy and seizures are more of a problem than the retardation. In the better hospitals, however, these children may be seen in several clinics including the mental retardation clinic. It is a tragic combination but many children will manifest all three major handicaps: epilepsy, retardation, and cerebral palsy.

THE LABORATORY EXAMINATION. The following laboratory procedures are used fairly commonly as aids in diagnosing the syndromes causing mental retardation:

- Blood test for hemoglobin, syphilis, inborn errors of metabolism (the Guthrie test for PKU).
- X-rays of skull and spine, long bones and wrists.
- Radioiodine uptake studies to rule out cretinism (thyroid deficiency).
- Urine tests to rule out inborn errors of metabolism (PKU, galactosemia), lead poisoning; tests for coproporphyrins, amino aciduria.
- Chromosomal studies.
- Spinal fluid examination is helpful if the patient has convulsions, bulging fontanels, suspected syphilis, or hydrocephalus.

CHROMOSOMAL STUDIES. Because of the current interest in the genetics of mental retardation, it might be of interest to discuss this subject briefly. The recent discovery of chromosomal aberrations in Down's syndrome (mongolism) has highlighted this interest.

Varying degrees of emphasis are placed on heredity as a cause of retardation. In the not too distant past, virtually all forms of retardation were attributed to genetic factors. Currently there exists a growing tendency to attribute a much smaller percentage of cases to them. Three forms of genetic influence have been described as follows:

1. *Multiple Inferior Genes.* This is the most highly controversial category, purporting to cover 60 to 80 per cent or more of the retarded population—the lower segment of the "normal" distribution curve for intelligence. This form of retardation is variously referred to as physiological, subcultural, or familial. One school of thought says that this form of retardation is caused by environmental and not genetic factors. An opposed school of thought claims that this group, although not suffering from a single genetic defect, seems to have inherited multiple genes which determine their inferior intelligence (multiple because what we label "intelligence" appears to be made up of many factors rather than being a single inheritable entity). Neither point of view can be completely supported with clear-cut evidence.

2. *Conditions due to Mutant Genes.* This is a smaller group under which can be placed several dozen conditions, some well-defined, others suspected. Each of these is caused by a single mutant gene or pair of mutant genes at a single locus. Tuberous sclerosis is transmitted as an autosomal dominant trait with marked variation in expressivity. Other conditions, including PKU, Tay-Sachs disease, and infantile Gaucher's disease follow the laws of autosomal recessive inheritance.

3. *Conditions Associated with Chromosomal Aberrations.* The works of Tjio and LeJeune between 1956 and 1959 demonstrated that in certain cases Down's syndrome (mongolism) was associated with changes in the number of chromosomes. One of these changes increases with the age of the mother. These chromosome changes can be distinguished by a relatively simple laboratory test. It is important in terms of family counseling for the physician to know whether these specific aberrations exist. In 1960, another discovery relative to chromosomal aberration and Down's syndrome was reported. It was disclosed that some mongoloids, particularly among the children of younger mothers, have only 46 chromosomes due to a process called translocation. This is a joining of a portion of an extra chromosome-21 into another. Further genetic aberrations discovered include mosaicism and others.

It is therefore necessary in certain cases to do chromosome studies in order to bring intelligent genetic counseling services to prospective parents.

DIFFERENTIAL DIAGNOSIS (Medical). There are conditions that can give professional workers the impression that a child is retarded when, in fact, there is another condition. Also, some of the following conditions can aggravate retardation.

1. Infantile autism. This is a psychosis manifested by bizarre behavior, withdrawal, loss of emotional affect, and even mutism. Competent psychiatric diagnosis is necessary.

2. Deafness.
3. Visual difficulties.
4. Extreme emotional disorder.
5. Severe cerebral palsy with speech defects.
6. Aphasia.
7. Miscellaneous speech or reading disorders.
8. Certain neurological conditions such as amyotonia congenita.
9. Uncontrolled seizures.

These are only a few of the conditions the professional worker must be aware of before making a final diagnosis of mental retardation. The differential diagnosis from a psychological standpoint must also be considered.

PSYCHOLOGICAL DIAGNOSIS

Mental retardation being a symptom or complex of symptoms rather than a disease, diagnosis is dependent upon the ability of the clinician or the observer to provide means by which the individual can reveal characteristics that are specifically identifiable, either directly or indirectly, with mental deficit. Since early diagnosis is of the utmost importance, ideally we would look largely to the pediatrician, the pediatric neurologist, the pediatric psychiatrist, and the pediatric psychologist to provide us with information leading to prompt recognition of this disability. As a rule, the psychologist is called upon to determine the presence and degree of mental retardation. However, as Michal-Smith and Kastein point out: "The final diagnosis of mental retardation cannot be made by any one discipline, but rather should be the result of a formulation by a multi-discipline approach." [11] The presence of organic damage to the brain, psychic disturbances, and related behavioral abnormalities may serve to complicate the picture. No attempt is made here to delineate the test procedures in the psychologist's armamentarium. These are manifold and are well described in the literature.

Mental retardation in the older individual—the adolescent and the young adult—represents, in a sense, a different diagnostic problem, because the hope for prevention or minimization of the effects of this disabling symptom complex has been largely lost. By the time the child has become deeply involved in the process of socialization and has already begun to experience stigmatization at the hands of peers, parents, and the population in general, much damage will have taken place. Furthermore, deprivation of stimulation from his environment due to his inability to properly communicate will have cost him a

[11] Harold Michal-Smith and Shulamith Kastein, *The Special Child: Diagnosis, Treatment and Habilitation,* Seattle, Washington: New School for the Special Child, Inc. 1962, pp. 7–9.

great deal in motivation, in self-regard, and in his drive to attain status in an environment that can only be regarded as hostile.

Diagnostic evaluation in this group must include not only assessment of intellect, but appraisal of social adaptation in home, school, and broad social contacts, including work experiences. As Heber so well indicates there has been a failure "to consider the effects of the sociocultural milieu of low income families in reporting and interpreting findings" [12] in current status studies based on income, type of job, length of time on the job, marital and court records, and so forth.

CLASSIFICATION. A careful review of all factors should allow at least a tentative classification of the individual in terms of probable cause of his disability. This could be conceptualized as follows:

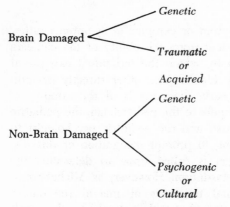

Brain Damaged	*Genetic*	Factors that prevent normal brain development
	Traumatic or Acquired	Factors that destroy or impair essential parts of the brain
Non-Brain Damaged	*Genetic*	Factors that influence the central nervous system such as sensory, neuromuscular, physiological, and prevent or disturb normal learning
	Psychogenic or Cultural	Environmental factors that reduce normal acquisition of learning as educational, emotional, economic, social

EDUCATIONAL EVALUATION. The educational evaluation is a major screening element. This should include due consideration of the history, medical and psychosocial assessments, as well as the past and present performance of the individual in a variety of learning situations.

It is not always easy for the teacher or the school as a whole to provide the kind of educational background that will be most valuable to the individual. Too frequently, the practice has been to provide a fore-shortened, watered-down version of the curricular offering characteristic of the chronological age and grade of the children. Standards are dropped, but the pupil goes through the same program as he might be expected to do if he were just another mediocre child among other mediocre children. At other times, a false assumption is made that since the retarded child lacks intellectual skills, he is ideally suited to work with his hands, and he is shunted into a mechanical training program. Unfortunately, the facts do not bear out this assumption.

[12] Rick F. Heber, "The Educable Mentally Retarded" in Samuel Kirk and Bluma B. Weiner, *Behavior Research on Exceptional Children*, 1963 Council for Exceptional Children, NEA, p. 89.

This is a shortsighted policy which sells both the learner and the school short. The school is supposed to prepare the child for life. Many of the skills taught and intellectual offerings do just that for the normal child, but there are many things that are far from essential for those who cannot profit from them. Too many empirical concepts that are not supported by research remain in the programs of schools and institutions dealing with retarded learners. A careful reappraisal of the educational programs that apply to modern concepts developed out of modern study and investigation is badly needed.

One of the areas of preparation for life that most assuredly should begin in the formative years of schooling is that of vocational preparation. Ordinarily, it is not until quite late in the academic program that the child is given any orientation to his vocational life. This is probably quite satisfactory under ordinary circumstances, but for the child whose learning is considerably slower than average, it falls far short of his needs.

We agree with Elise Martens when she states:

Because a deficient child can by the time he is 16 years old learn a little of a given school subject, it by no means follows that such learning should become the goal of his education. It would be a far wiser investment of time to center his education on the activities which will be of greatest use to him . . . under the system of school progress by grade, retarded children are frequently subjected to tasks which they cannot possibly understand or perform; and frequently they are permitted to go from grade to grade without achieving anything of satisfaction to themselves or to their teachers.[13]

While we echo Martens' plea for providing the child who is retarded with the kind of education that will lead him to a useful and satisfying socioeconomic life, we join her especially in reiterating the concept that: "It is just as important to educate the mentally retarded child to be happy and efficient in his social relationships as it is to make him able to earn a livelihood." In fact, we would go one step further, for on the basis of experience we believe he is unlikely to be able to earn a sustained livelihood unless he can maintain his social relationships effectively.

From the vocational standpoint, one might well seek a good deal more emphasis than is supplied by Martens' approach. While there is certainly a great deal more realism in her approach than is ordinarily seen in the regular school curriculum, there is somewhat less than one might hope for if we wish to place these young people in competitive labor after leaving school. As a matter of fact, if similar emphasis could be given industrial preparation or preparation for service jobs

[13] Elise H. Martens, *Curriculum Adjustments for the Mentally Retarded*, Washington, D.C.: Government Printing Office, U.S. Office of Education, Bulletin #2, 1950, p. 100.

as that which is given to preparation in food and household sciences, Martens' curriculum would more nearly approach a level that would permit state vocational rehabilitation services to serve these young people more effectively.

A few steps along this educational route have been made and already provide considerable promise for the future. In the state of Texas an agreement between the state vocational rehabilitation agency and the special education department of the state has led to the establishment of coordinators in approximately 40 schools who tie in an educational work program with vocational rehabilitation, and end in vocational placement of well over 50 per cent of the students involved. In Milwaukee, Wisconsin, Detroit, Michigan, and Dayton, Ohio, similar working relationships between the school system and the vocational rehabilitation programs have already resulted in producing better training, better social adaptation, and community acceptance of retarded young people who are getting the most from their education because it ties in with the social and vocational program. Much more remains to be done in this area. This is merely pointing the way for a collaborative program between education and vocational rehabilitation to render maximum services to the retarded individual at a time when he can profit most from it. Education and preparation for life are virtually synonymous. This indicates that a modern educational program for the mentally retarded cannot long be maintained unless it is serving its clientele properly by closely coordinating its plans with vocational rehabilitation services and with community agencies so as to provide for recreational, religious, and social needs.

VOCATIONAL EVALUATION, JOB PLACEMENT, AND HABILITATION

Habilitation, as well as rehabilitation, is a process rather than treatment, philosophy rather than technique. When properly developed it is hard to conceive of these processes as being phasic or chronologically regulated on a step-by-step basis. Of course, diagnosis will precede other elements in the process, but only because there has to be a commitment in someone's mind that a given individual is not functioning in a normal fashion. On the other hand, even diagnosis is subject to revision, as indeed are other aspects of the habilitation-rehabilitation program during the process. Actually, the treatment of a disability, physical or mental, involves so many different kinds of preparatory or corrective activities that one cannot really say that there is an established order. The only exception is the necessity of carrying out lifesaving efforts ahead of all others. Realistically, many of the component elements of rehabilitation can and do go on simultaneously.

Although vocational habilitation and/or rehabilitation is often described as though it is the final step in the total treatment process, it should occur throughout. Maximum emphasis, of course, is delayed to the time when the retarded individual is ready for it. It has already been indicated that a great deal of prevocational orientation and preparation can begin during the formative years when the retarded child is acquiring his basic education. Similarly, with proper counseling and guidance, the parents and the community can work together to not only provide the child with an appreciation of the values and satisfaction in vocational performance, but also help develop patterns of behavior that will provide a basis for acceptable work behavior.

As a matter of fact, in a manner that emulates the concepts of "Activities of Daily Living" (ADL), one could posit a list of "Activities of Daily Working" (ADW). While not all mentally retarded individuals may attain them, a very sizable proportion can and should be encouraged to reach them. Among the items in such a list we might include the following:

1. Can adapt to and accept the impact of interpersonal relationships with people on the job.

2. Can successfully get to and from work on some regularly available form of transportation.

3. Can understand and perform all the regular activities of the job on which he is placed and has sufficient flexibility to perform and emotionally tolerate at least two other related jobs to which he may be displaced.

4. Understands the importance and carries out time and attendance obligations of the job.

5. Possesses sufficient initiative to maintain his job performance at acceptable levels with no more supervision than the employer or supervisor deems feasible.

6. Possesses sufficient emotional stability to remain on the job until work merits advancement or until supervisor can correct annoyances.

7. Possesses sufficient basic educational skills to manage himself without undue dependence on others to interpret or explain what is expected of him.

8. Possesses sufficient self-control and social judgment to prevent others from taking advantage of his mental limitations.

9. Can manage all his ordinary financial activities without help from others.

While this is by no means intended to be an exhaustive list, it is intended to reflect some of the areas that are most troublesome in the vocational adaptation of mentally retarded people. Peckham has pointed out that school and vocational rehabilitation counselors could, by close cooperation, do much to insure the attainment of these functions by the mentally retarded.[14] A failure to develop most of these to an acceptable level would be a reasonably good criterion to prognosticate failure in work ability in competitive vocational fields, though not necessarily denying the potentiality of working in a sheltered environment.

Like the ADL, the ADW list is not intended as an absolute or restricting guide to vocational potential, but merely as a basis for appraising and developing potential for independent work performance.

Similarly, and of even greater importance to ultimate vocational adaptation, is the importance of developing acceptable interpersonal relationships. In childhood this is relatively easy; postponed to adolescence or adult life it is difficult and sometimes impossible to attain.

It has been observed, for example, that the mentally retarded child who has suffered from a lack of psychological stimulation associated with tender loving care (TLC), lack of expressed warmth and love from parental or other sources, and the failure to establish a continuing relationship with any one adult, has an increased concept deficiency, impaired development of normal inhibitory patterns (self-control), affect hunger (excessive need for attention and affection), emotional imperviousness (superficial interpersonal relationships), lack of normal tension and anxiety following hostile, aggressive behavior, and significant social regression.[15]

It is altogether obvious that not only is supplying TLC, warmth, and love to a mentally retarded child the decent, humane, and sensible behavior toward the child, but it can have a very decided effect on his vocational, social, and educational behavior. That is why it is of such vital importance to deal with the problems of the parent even before we start to cope with the retarded child's problems.

Management

MEDICAL AND SURGICAL

One of the current problems related to management of medical aspects of retardation is the widespread feeling among physicians that medically nothing can be done. In the strictest sense this has some validity. However, the physician has the following aids:

[14] Ralf A. Peckham, "Problems in the Job Adjustment of the Mentally Retarded," *American Journal of Mental Deficiency*, 56:448–452, 1951.

[15] W. Goldfarb, cited by L. Kanner, "Emotional Disturbances Simulating Mental Retardation" in J. Magary and J. Eichorn, *The Exceptional Child: A Book of Readings*, New York: Holt, Rinehart and Winston, 1960.

1. Use of psychotrophic medication. This would include the use of psychic energizers such as Dexedrine and deanol and tranquilizers such as reserpine. The phenothiazines and meprobamate are also useful. Psychotrophic medications are helpful in calming the agitated and toning down the hyperactive child. These medications must be used with caution.

2. Other medications. Many children with retardation have either cerebral palsy, epilepsy, or both. In these cases the use of appropriate anticonvulsants and/or muscle relaxants is indicated. The diet for phenylketonuria is now well known. In general, it seems to be a good method for preventing brain damage. Within a few years we shall have more valid statistical proof of this.

3. Surgical treatment. Early neurosurgical management of hydrocephalus, craniostenosis, and subdural hematoma in selected cases helps prevent some of the secondary brain damage associated with these conditions.

4. Psychiatric treatment. The retarded and their families perhaps have more attendant emotional problems than any other group of disabled. Prompt and prolonged psychiatric attention is required. This may be especially true in the older, milder retarded child.

RESIDENTIAL CARE

From 4 to 5 per cent of the 5.4 million mentally retarded are in institutions. Many of these institutions are antiquated and overcrowded. Future trends show more emphasis toward smaller community-based residential facilities with comprehensive medical and psychological services to insure that the retarded are given all advantages in terms of general health, vision, speech, hearing, and so on.

However, there will always be a need for good custodial care, and future institutions must be specially designed for the retarded.

COUNSELING WITH PARENTS

One of the most difficult tasks with which professional workers will be faced is that of providing the family of the retarded with interpretive counseling and guidance when the diagnosis is firmly established. The emotional impact on parents of this knowledge about their child can be most devastating. Professional workers must use great tact, warmth, and sympathy, yet at the same time be objective. Suggestions regarding the child's care or placement obviously depend on many factors: attitude and intelligence of parents, degree of retardation, associated handicaps, siblings, economic factors, and the availability of community or residential facilities.

Many conferences will be necessary. Feelings of guilt, inadequacy, anxiety, hostility, suspicion, and fear of the future must be faced openly. Too often hasty recommendations are given to "Put the child away." This can be a serious mistake in many cases. The use of a visiting nurse can help parents greatly with systematic habit training and the teaching of self-help techniques. Consultations should be arranged between the parents of the educable and trainable and the appropriate school authorities. Supplemental therapy, such as psychiatric, speech, and hearing, should be arranged. A great aid to most parents is the realization that they are not alone with this problem. Local affiliates of the National Association for Retarded Children can be most helpful in mobilizing community resources. The clergy should be brought into the picture at the earliest possible time. It should be emphasized that during their first six or seven years most mentally retarded children do better with the love and security afforded only by their parents and family. Institutionalization directly from the nursery or in early infancy should be discouraged in most instances. It is obvious then, since only 4 to 5 per cent of the retarded can ever be placed outside the home, mental retardation is primarily a problem of the home and the community.

Regardless of degree of economic status, regardless of their ability to "hire" or "purchase" services for their retarded child, parents have an essential role to play in giving their retarded youngster the love, warmth, understanding, and support any child has a right to expect. The value of parental understanding of the retarded child cannot be overestimated. As a matter of fact, in many ways this is the single most important determinant in the attainment of maximal habilitation of the mentally retarded. Parents or parent substitutes who understand, accept, and work with their child can be of great help in encouraging, stimulating, and strengthening his efforts to make full use of his abilities, whatever they may be. Furthermore, they bring to the child needed environmental experiences which are immensely valuable in helping him gain control of his life milieu. Social, educational, and psychological preparations for life can be successfully utilized only when the child is able to feel confidence and trust in his environment. This comes largely as a result of the confidence he has developed in his most important contact with the environment, namely, his parents!

The old concept that those who conceive and bear children necessarily are well adapted to caring for them, as a matter of fact, seems unwarranted. The biological process that results in the conception of a child is hardly a selective device, and one cannot assume maturity, understanding, or love of the product of the womb. Too often the events that lead up to conception are based upon motives that are completely the reverse of these desirable characteristics. Children are produced for many reasons—for the satisfaction of emotional demands, for the resolution of personal problems, to promote security, and many others, including thoughtlessness. We hope, of course, that these less acceptable factors are distinctly limited to the few, but we cannot ever be sure of the motivations that lead to childbirth.

Strangely enough, in spite of all our modern scientific advances, we have done relatively little to elevate the standards of preparental and parental education, especially with reference to that which is provided for the parents of the mentally retarded. The tendency still continues to be that of assuming that a few soothing words, a compassionate pat on the shoulder, a brief, sometimes even brutally terse summing up by the physician or some other professional worker regarding the state of their child's mental development and his prognosis are all that these parents require. Sometimes they get even less and are not given even a brief explanation.

This is a tragic oversight, since it may destroy or at least seriously aggravate the emotional burden of parents and siblings, as well as the retarded individual. The effect of such errors in the orientation of parents is likely to last the duration of their lives and that of their children.

There is probably no "royal road" to parental understanding, nor is there a clear-cut formula that can be used to stimulate its development. Of one thing we may be sure: it takes a great deal more time and effort than are now generally being expended by most workers in the field to achieve it. We may also be quite sure that the beginning or parental orientation to their specific problems relative to their mentally retarded child should begin soon after the condition has been recognized, or better yet, even before this occurs, in a prenatal guidance clinic. Parents should be aware that sometimes children are born with defects and that when this occurs, neither parent nor child is to blame. Parents should be trained to avoid self-blame and to overcome this by attaining self-fulfillment in helping their child to attain the measure of his potential ability.

Some parents, perhaps the majority, will need considerable strengthening of their own ego-structure before they are prepared to face the fact that they have produced a less than perfect child. They will need to be relieved of guilt feelings before they can even begin to understand what may be said to them about their child. Obviously, this cannot be accomplished in one brief session.

Thus, for some parents it may take weeks, even months, of consistent, effective counseling to get them to a point where they can do what is expected of them. Others may attain understanding at a much more rapid rate and achieve at least a basic level of insight accompanied by self-control, to such an extent that they can successfully assume the proper parental responsibilities for their child.

Whatever the requirements may be to bring parents to a readiness point to effectively care for their retarded child, they must be achieved by appropriate preparation and not by guess or faulty assumptions. Our present-day approach of discussing the problems of the retarded child with the parent appears to be far too abbreviated and to lack sufficient appraisal of the parents' ability to tolerate the child's limitations and use their knowledge in his interest. Before discussion proceeds very far, we should know a great deal about the parents' personality, their own mental competency, and their ability to use and understand the information that is being provided them.

Wille has stressed the importance of the preliminary preparation of the parent. She states:

> Regardless of where the social worker finds the parents of the retarded child, the emphasis should be focused on release of guilt and tension, a healthier psychological separation of the parent from the retardate and strengthening of self-confidence through a series of successful experiences in handling the child. . . . The majority of parents need help in extracting themselves from their emotional involvement with the retardate. . . . The parents must psychologically separate themselves from the child, and with better perspective be able to think in terms of the child's future, as well as their own satisfaction in life.[16]

Michaels and Schueman illuminate another aspect of the parental behavior that emphasizes the need for sound therapeutic assistance to the parent even preceding our attack on the problems of the retardate. They say:

> In general, the initial impact of awareness of having a retarded child brings with it a period of shock, bewilderment, and disbelief . . . frequently followed by a time during which the parents vacillate between unrealistic despair and equally unrealistic hope. They run from one "expert" to another, in search of someone who can give authoritative denial to the bitter facts. At the very least, feelings of realistic sorrow and disappointment are inevitable.[17]

In the face of this picture of what takes place in parental reaction, obviously the parent is hardly prepared to accept much counseling until he has overcome his initial period of grief. Then we may anticipate the need for considerable guidance and counseling before the emotional conflicts can yield to a sound, more objective appraisal in which the parental role assumes its proper perspective.

We have deliberately expanded on the concept of counseling of the parents under the heading of "Management" because we feel that this is one of the most important aspects in the overall care of the retarded.

---

[16] Blanch M. Wille, "The Role of the Social Worker," *American Journal of Mental Deficiency*, **66**:3:464–471, 1961.

[17] Joseph Michaels and Helen Schueman, "Observations of the Psychodynamics of Parents of Retarded Children," *American Journal of Mental Deficiency*, **66**:4:568–573, 1962.

PREVENTION OF MENTAL RETARDATION

There are many forces working diligently to foster more and better research, basic and applied. Among these are the United States Department of Health, Education, and Welfare, private foundations such as the Joseph P. Kennedy, Jr., Foundation, the National Foundation, the National Society for Crippled Children and Adults, the Association for Aid to Crippled Children, The American Association on Mental Deficiency. Strong leadership has been given by the National Association for Retarded Children, Inc.

The concept of research should be broadened to include more applied research and research within community settings. However, the greatest potential contribution of research is prevention. In this vein, the President's Panel Report has suggested specific biological and medical preventive measures such as the following:

- Improved obstetrical practice to avoid damage of anoxia, mechanical and other brain injuries during delivery.
- Elimination of congenital syphilis by blood tests and effective therapy during pregnancy.
- Prevention of viruses and infections of pregnancy, such as rubella, toxoplasmosis.
- Careful screening to identify infants with inborn errors of metabolism—phenylketonuria and galactosemia; use of special dietary treatment for both disorders; identification of the carrier state in both mother and father in case of galactosemia.
- Strict enforcement of standards in the use of medical and nonmedical equipment such as x-ray which produces ionizing radiation.
- Laboratory detection of particular types of chromosomal aberration.[18]

In general, as our knowledge increases we are able to provide more effective preventive measures through parental counseling on genetic factors, maternal and child care, and early screening and treatment of disease. Based on current knowledge, certain observations are pertinent:

1. Programs of prevention should be aimed at the high risk groups—namely, those where maternal care is frequently inadequate, as in colored, rural, or low income groups.

2. Hospitals should adopt and use every measure for the prevention of perinatal brain damage.

3. There should be wider surveillance on the use of drugs by pregnant women.

[18] President's Panel on Mental Retardation, *A Proposed Program for National Action to Combat Mental Retardation*, October 1962, pp. 48–49.

4. More funds should be available to study means of preventing or reducing accidents resulting in head injuries.

Preventive measures must also be aimed at the correction or amelioration of adverse environmental conditions. The slum areas breed thousands of children who show lack of stimulation or motivation toward achievement and toward standards of high performance. Many come from a family organization or structure that is emotionally crippling to the child.

A sociological note in prevention was expressed by Dr. Lloyd M. Dunn at the recent White House Conference on Mental Retardation. He points out one of the trying problems that constantly bother serious workers in this field—namely, environmental deprivation. Dr. Dunn says:

> As to the 96 per cent of the retarded who live in the community and are largely culturally disadvantaged, education has a special challenge and responsibility to provide outstanding educational opportunities.
>   . . . Existing behavioral science research indicates that an inadequate environment has a debilitating effect on intellectual development. Furthermore, it suggests that the intellectual development of a child is significantly influenced by the motivational and value structures to which he has been exposed, and by the sensory, educational, psychological, and cultural conditions which he experiences. Thus, it is my belief that improvements in intellectual functioning of underprivileged children through environmental enrichment will be appreciable. . . .

THE FUTURE OF THE MENTALLY RETARDED

What the future is likely to hold for the mentally retarded is to a very large extent going to depend upon what can be done to alter preconceived ideas, rigid practice, policies, and concepts embraced by responsible leaders in the field at the present time. If we sincerely want to advance toward optimal gains for the retarded, we must stop temporizing and develop realistic approaches to their problems. Furthermore, we shall have to stop departmentalizing our services. We cannot give education the sole right to persons age 4 to 16, implying that these children constitute a vocational rehabilitation problem only after that age, and expect to achieve very effective results.

Realistically, we should begin to think of team work in rehabilitation extending into the formative years as well as adult life. The training in good work habits begins in childhood, not in adult life. A retardate who fails to develop habits of promptness, dependability, and attention before he is 16 may not acquire them in the years that follow. Yet proper early preparation during his school period will make it relatively easy for him to carry over this habit into the working world. To say that this is not vocational rehabilitation is to ignore the fact that the very lack of these essential work habits is one of the single most predominant factors in his failure to hold a job after he has been trained. In fact, he is fired much more frequently for deficits in work habits than for failure to be able to do the work expected of him.

Inability to read, inability to adapt socially, faulty behavior on the job, are all deficits that are contributing to work failure. Yet the school, far more than any adult training program, has the time, the resources, and the responsibility for such training. If this training can be related to life activities, including work, the child may emerge better equipped to cope with reality.

Thus, the early introduction of a counseling and guidance program—say at least the eighth or ninth grade—is bound to be much more effective than later when the child's behavioral pattern has been allowed to gel.

Thus, it is clear that early training must be vocationally oriented, and while it may deal less with specific job peparation, it is fundamentally concerned with shaping generally correct work attitudes and abilities. Vocational rehabilitation, in the eyes of state directors of vocational rehabilitation agencies, may at times seem far separated from the public and private elementary and secondary school. Perhaps many state educational directors feel the same way. Yet, if these responsible leaders can be brought to see him, much more can be done for the future life development of the mentally retarded child. These contributions in both areas of education and vocational rehabilitation could be increased many fold.[19]

There is indeed a hopeful note as recently expressed by the late President Kennedy:

We as a Nation have long neglected the mentally ill and the mentally retarded. This neglect must end, if our Nation is to live up to its own standards of compassion and dignity and achieve the maximum use of its manpower.

This tradition of neglect must be replaced by forceful and far-reaching programs carried out at all levels of government, by private individuals and by state and local agencies in every part of the Union.[20]

[19] Morton, A. Seidenfeld, "Mental Retardation, A Further Assessment of the Problem," Rehabilitation Service Series No. 63–62, June, 1962, U.S. Department of Health, Education, and Welfare, Vocational Rehabilitation Administration, Washington, D. C.

[20] "Special Message to the Congress on Mental Illness and Mental Retardation," by President John F. Kennedy, February 5, 1963.

XVI

MENTAL RETARDATION SUPPLEMENT

CATEGORY DEFINITIONS [1]

I. MENTAL RETARDATION ASSOCIATED WITH DISEASES AND CONDITIONS DUE TO INFECTION

This grouping is to be used for the classification of those cases in which mental retardation is the result of residual damage from an intracranial inflammation due to an infection. Within this division diseases are subgrouped in terms of whether the infection occurred prenatally or postnatally as follows:

ENCEPHALOPATHY ASSOCIATED WITH PRENATAL INFECTIONS. All of the prenatal maternal infections are classified under the major division of *due to infection*. Though there is some controversy as to whether maternal infections may result in congenital cerebral defect in the absence of direct infection of the fetus, there is sufficient evidence to indicate that in many of these conditions a direct fetal infection involving the brain does occur. It should be noted that, in rare instances, prenatal infection of the fetus may occur in absence of recognized clinical disease in the mother.

Cytomegalic Inclusion Body Disease, Congenital. This is a maternal virus disease which is usually mild or subclinical in the mother. Infection of the fetus, however, results in hepatosplenomegaly, erythroblastosis, jaundice, and disorders of the brain and other organs. It may be recognized by the presence of inclusion bodies in cellular elements in the urine, cerebrospinal fluid, and tissues.

[1] Code numbers have been omitted.

Excerpted, with permission, from *A Manual on Terminology and Classification in Mental Retardation*, Monograph Supplement to *American Journal of Mental Deficiency*, 2nd ed., 1961, prepared by Rick Heber, pages 20–43. The American Association on Mental Deficiency, P.O. Box 96, Willimantic, Connecticut.

Rubella, Congenital. Some of the offspring of mothers contracting rubella in the first trimester of pregnancy exhibit a variety of congenital anomalies including deafness, cataract, cardiac malformations, and mental defect.

Syphilis, Congenital. The fetus of a mother with syphilis may suffer transplacental infection by the disease. The child may show a meningovascular type disease or a diffuse encephalitis leading to juvenile paresis. Diagnosis is based on the history of maternal infection, positive serology in the mother, and signs of congenital syphilis such as Hutchinson teeth, interstitial keratitis, chorioretinitis, pupil anomalies, rhagades, bossing of frontal bones, and persisting positive serology. Clinical signs and serological reactions are not consistent but either finding in conjunction with evidence of maternal infection is presumptive evidence of congenital infection.

Juvenile paresis shows an onset at any age before adolescence. The child may or may not be mentally retarded before the onset of symptoms which include progressive impairment of gross and fine motor skills, personality disintegration, delusions, and deterioration. The cerebrospinal fluid shows a positive specific reaction for syphilis, a paretic gold curve, and increased protein.

Toxoplasmosis, Congenital. This condition is due to infection by *Toxoplasma*, a protozoan-like organism. It is contracted *in utero* from the mother where the infection is ordinarily subclinical. Wasting, convulsions, spasticity, chorioretinitis, and hydrocephalus or microcephaly may be evident at or shortly after birth. There are several serological tests for both mother and infant which are helpful in establishing a diagnosis.

Other, Congenital. Occasionally, fetal damage from maternal epidemic cerebrospinal meningitis, equine encephalomyelitis, etc., has been reported. The mere history of a maternal infection is frequently coincidental, however, and should never rule out consideration of other possible etiologies.

ENCEPHALOPATHY DUE TO POSTNATAL CEREBRAL INFECTION. All postnatal cerebral infections are to be classified in this category regardless of the nature of the infecting agent. Both focal and generalized types of cerebral infection are included. In these . . . postnatal infections . . . the type of infecting agent . . . may be virus, bacteria, or other micro-organism.

II. MENTAL RETARDATION ASSOCIATED WITH DISEASES AND CONDITIONS DUE TO INTOXICATION

All cases of mental retardation associated with cerebral damage due to serums, drugs, or other toxic agents are classified in this division as follows:

ENCEPHALOPATHY, CONGENITAL, ASSOCIATED WITH MATERNAL TOXEMIA OF PREGNANCY. Though somewhat controversial, it is believed that mental retardation may be attributable, in rare instances, to maternal toxemia of pregnancy. Diagnosis in this category must not be made without reliable evidence of a severe and prolonged toxemia of pregnancy.

ENCEPHALOPATHY, CONGENITAL, ASSOCIATED WITH OTHER MATERNAL INTOXICATIONS. Cerebral pathology resulting in mental retardation, on occasion, may be due to maternal intoxications such as carbon monoxide, lead, arsenic, quinine, ergot, etc.

BILIRUBIN ENCEPHALOPATHY (Kernicterus). Kernicterus may follow severe jaundice in the newborn and is characterized by a yellow bilirubin staining of brain areas, especially the basal ganglia, cerebellar nuclei, hippocampus, and medulla. Advanced stages of the condition are marked by demyelination, gliosis, loss of cells in the cortex, globus pallidus, and corpus luysi. Choreoathetosis and mental retardation are common sequelae.

This condition is frequently due to Rh incompatibility between fetus and mother but also may be caused by A, B, O, or some of the more rare blood type incompatibilities. Kernicterus, in the absence of blood incompatibility, may result from prematurity and severe neonatal sepsis or any condition producing a sufficiently high level of serum bilirubin.

POST-IMMUNIZATION ENCEPHALOPATHY. The post-serum and postvaccinal encephalitides are tentatively classified under *due to intoxication* though there is no general agreement as to whether the neuropathology in these cases is due to an allergic reaction, the vaccine virus, or another virus activated by the vaccine.

Inoculation with serum, especially anti-tetanus serum, or vaccines such as smallpox, rabies and typhoid may result, occasionally, in nervous system reactions. Such a reaction usually involves the peripheral nerves but, in rare instances, takes the form of encephalitis. When this is the case, signs of meningeal, focal cerebral, cerebellar, and cord involvement may be present. Convulsions, stupor, coma, and motor dysfunction are common during the acute phase. Permanent neurological impairment may be represented in behavior disorders, dyskinesias, convulsions, and mental retardation.

ENCEPHALOPATHY, OTHER, DUE TO INTOXICATION. Permanent damage to nervous tissue may result from a wide variety of intoxicants including lead, carbon monoxide, tetanus exotoxin, botulism exotoxin, etc. Lead has been the most significant of these for mental retardation. Lead may be absorbed from paint, lead toys, lead acetate ointment, and cosmetics.

Symptoms include irritability, loss of appetite, abdominal colic, constipation, headache, vomiting, convulsions, delirium, neck rigidity, papilledema, and coma. Blue lines on the gums, a punctate basophilia, and a lead line on bone x-ray confirm the diagnosis.

III. MENTAL RETARDATION ASSOCIATED WITH DISEASES AND CONDITIONS DUE TO TRAUMA OR PHYSICAL AGENT

Cases of mental retardation associated with injury of the brain due to trauma or mechanical or physical agent are classified in this division. Further specification within this category is made as follows:

ENCEPHALOPATHY DUE TO PRENATAL INJURY. On very rare occasions encephalopathy may occur as a result of prenatal injury. Prenatal irradiation leading to encephalopathy is an example. Pregnant women exposed to large amounts of irradiation of the uterus produce a highly increased incidence of offspring showing a wide variety of congenital abnormalities including cerebral defects associated with severe mental retardation. The types of malformation are related to the developmental stage of the fetus at the time of irradiation and to the amount of irradiation given. Irradiation of the uterus during the first trimester of pregnancy may result in microcephaly, malformations of the eyes and extremities, and mental retardation of varying degrees of severity.

Prenatal asphyxia is also included in this category. Maternal anoxia, anemia, and hypotension are believed to cause prenatal anoxia and result in congenital encephalopathy.

ENCEPHALOPATHY DUE TO MECHANICAL INJURY AT BIRTH. Difficulties of labor due to malposition, malpresentation, disproportion, or other complications increase the probability of damage to the infant's brain at birth.

The immediate signs of severe injury include nystagmus, retinal hemorrhage, pallor, inability to make sucking movements, high-pitched feeble cry, respiratory disturbance, and a tense or depressed fontanel. Lesions that are commonly produced by birth injury include tears of the meninges, blood vessels, and brain substance. Bleeding within the brain tissue is common following birth trauma. While small amounts of blood may be absorbed, any considerable hemorrhage is likely to be followed by softening and cyst formation.

Tears of the falx cerebri or the tentorium may result in hemorrhage into the subarachnoid or subdural space. The brain itself may also be lacerated. This type of injury may follow difficult forceps deliveries. Other types of lesions in birth injury include venous-sinus thrombosis and arterial embolism and thrombosis.

The structural evidence of birth injury tends to diminish with time and in the brain of the older retardate may be evident only in non-specific changes of gliosis, cavitation, and abnormal myelination. The more gross effects of birth injury of the brain, obvious neurological disabilities and mental defect, are easily recognized through psychological examination of behavior and neurological examination of motor and sensory function. Sensory examination may demonstrate abnormalities of touch, pressure, pain, temperature, vision, and hearing.

It is now believed that brain injury may result not only in neurological disability of the classical variety but also in more subtle disorganizations and defects of motor, sensory, perceptual, emotional, and integrative behavior. A brain-injured child may be either hyperkinetic or hypokinetic. There may be fluctuations in muscle tone, synkinesias, impairment of associated movements, bursts of primitive reflex activity, defects in ocular convergence, mixed cerebral dominance, and a general clumsiness in motor activity.

Impairment of postural behavior may be evident in the child's tendency toward exaggerated use of supports, in his difficulties in learning complex motor skills such as climbing, cycling, and skating, in the frequency with which he loses his balance and falls, especially during the first years after learning to walk, and in the tense, anxious way in which he responds to anti-gravity play. This postural impairment may also manifest itself in a general clumsiness and immaturity of coordination and balance such as when the child is asked to stand on one foot or hold his arms forward in extension while his attention is distracted. In the latter instance choreiform movement, synkinesia, convergence, or wide drift of the arms reveals impairment. Rotation of the head of the brain-injured child may produce wide arm drift, convergence, or persistence of the tonic neck posture. The child may show exaggerated resistance to any externally induced change in posture or equilibrium. Disturbance in the coordination of respiratory and speech movements also may be present.

Perceptual processes of the brain-injured child may be impaired so that he is unable to respond normally to stimuli. Visually, the child may have difficulty in isolating foreground from background. Problems of auditory perception may be manifest in an inability to remember sounds, to discriminate their pitch, or to localize their source. The brain-injured patient may also show specific or generalized difficulties in perceiving and understanding spoken language. Kinesthetically, there may be an impairment in the ability to discriminate tactual stimuli.

The social-emotional behavior of these patients may be deviant, presumably as a result of confusion and frustration. While the more frequent tendency is toward aggressive, hyperkinetic behavior, some of these children become passive and withdrawn. A tendency toward ritualistic, compulsive behavior on the part of some brain-injured patients has been noted also.

Not all of the organic and behavioral symptoms and sequelae of brain injury described above will be found in any one patient. Nor is there one feature of brain injury which will be present universally. Some brain-injured patients demonstrate general retardation in intellectual behavior while others evidence segmental disabilities in specific aspects of behavior as described. The range in severity of impairment varies from minimal to gross and is based on such factors as the locus and extent of the cerebral damage. The clinical picture of brain injury given here also applies in instances of neonatal asphyxia or cerebral injury due to post-natal factors occurring during infancy. The presence of these manifestations of brain injury do not, therefore, necessarily imply a birth injury. Confirmatory historical evidence in the nature of the delivery and neonatal period should be present.

ENCEPHALOPATHY DUE TO ANOXEMIA AT BIRTH. Anoxemia as a basic cause of cerebral damage can be presumed in instances where there has been asphyxia due to difficulties in respiration during the neonatal period. This may be due to interference with placental circulation as is the case, for example, with premature separation from the placenta, with massive bleeding with placenta previa, or with prolapse or compression of the cord. Excessive use of depressive drugs or anesthetic agents may delay onset of respiration and produce asphyxia.

ENCEPHALOPATHY DUE TO POSTNATAL INJURY. In a small proportion of the mentally retarded, the behavioral defect may be attributed to postnatal cerebral injuries of various kinds. The type of head injury sustained in falls from high chairs, cribs, tables, etc., cannot be accepted, however, as the cause of mental defect unless accompanied by evidence of severe trauma (fractured skull, prolonged unconsciousness, etc.) followed by a regression in rate of development. Postnatal asphyxia, infarction, thrombosis, laceration, and contusion of the brain resulting in mental defect are to be classified in this category.

IV. MENTAL RETARDATION ASSOCIATED WITH DISEASES AND CONDITIONS DUE TO DISORDER OF METABOLISM, GROWTH, OR NUTRITION

All conditions, associated with mental retardation, directly due to metabolic, nutritional, or growth dysfunction are to be classified in this category. This includes the cerebral lipoidoses, disorders of carbohydrate and protein metabolism, and nutritional deficiencies. Conditions classified in this division are to be specified as follows:

CEREBRAL LIPOIDOSIS, INFANTILE (TAY-SACHS DISEASE). This is a progressive lipid dystrophy predominantly affecting the nervous system and characterized by an accumulation of lipid substance in the nerve cells.

The disease is transmitted as a single recessive gene. The parents are normal but both are carriers with a probability of having one child out of four affected. Marriages producing affected children show an increased incidence of consanguinity. The majority of cases are from Jewish families though non-Jewish families occasionally are affected also.

The infantile is the most common form of cerebral lipoidosis. The infant usually appears normal at birth but clinical signs of the disease become readily apparent between one and twelve months. In the usual clinical course, the child who has been developing normally for perhaps three to six months becomes apathetic, shows muscular weakness, is unable to maintain his posture, to hold his head steady, and regresses in his ability to grasp objects. This motor loss is accompanied by progressive visual deterioration. Examination of the retina shows degeneration in the macular area through which the choroid vessels reveal the pathognomonic "cherry-red spot." Occasionally one observes squint and nystagmus. Though retinal involvement varies, blindness is usually present giving rise to the name infantile amaurotic family idiocy. Death usually ensues within one to three years of onset but may be much later.

In extremely rare instances a congenital form of the disease has been noted.

ENCEPHALOPATHY ASSOCIATED WITH OTHER DISORDERS OF LIPOID METABOLISM. All disorders of lipoid metabolism except for the infantile form of cerebral lipoidosis are to be classified in this category. . . . These conditions are specified further as follows:

Cerebral Lipoidosis, Late Infantile (Bielschowsky's Disease). The late infantile form of cerbral lipoidosis has its onset from the second or third year and is more common in non-Jewish families than the infantile form. Paralysis, mental deterioration, and amaurosis [blindness] progress with death ensuing in a few years. Retinal examination may reveal optic atrophy rather than the "cherry-red spot" characteristic of the infantile form.

Cerebral Lipoidosis, Juvenile (Spielmeyer-Vogt Disease). In the juvenile form of cerebral lipoidosis signs of the disease become evident between the ages of five and ten. Loss of mobility of facial expression, difficulties with vision, or impairment of balance and coordination may be the first indications of the disease. The patient may develop a peculiar gait, leaning forward with bent knees. The involvement of pyramidal, extrapyramidal, and cerebellar systems is more obvious in the juvenile than in either of the infantile forms. The paralysis is partly flaccid and partly spastic in nature and progresses to complete disability. Epileptic seizures are common in this form of the disease.

Pigmentary ("pepper and salt" appearance) degeneration of the retina leading to blindness is usually present. The mental deterioration may be complicated by psychotic reactions, delusions, and hallucinations. The course of the disease is from five to ten years with death generally occurring by intercurrent infection or status epilepticus.

Cerebral Lipoidosis, Late Juvenile (Kufs' Disease). The late juvenile form develops between the fifteenth and twenty-fifth years and shows progressive mental deterioration and motor disability characterized by rigidity, tremors, and ataxia of the cerebellar type. Convulsions are usually present. Only when the onset of the late juvenile form is at an earlier age level would a case generally be classified as mentally retarded.

Lipid Histiocytosis of Kerasin Type (Gaucher's Disease). This condition is characterized by deposition of kerasin in the reticuloendothelial cells of the spleen, liver, and other organs of the body, and occasionally in the ganglion cells of the cerebral cortex, cerebellum, and basal ganglia. Diagnosis is by splenic puncture, aspiration of marrow, or biopsy of a lymph node showing Gaucher's cells.

The nervous system in this disease is generally not involved except in infants. In the infant, onset of the disease is usually about the fourth or fifth month. There is much enlargement of spleen and liver, a regression in developmental level, and a general physical deterioration. The child becomes apathetic, unresponsive, and spastic. There is a hypochromic anemia, leukopenia, and thrombocytopenia. The disease is fatal within a few years of onset. When onset is delayed until later childhood, the nervous system and intellectual functioning are rarely affected.

Lipid Histiocytosis of Phosphatide Type (Niemann-Pick Disease). This condition is characterized by deposition of lipophosphatides in the reticuloendothelial system, particularly involving the liver and spleen. The condition generally develops at three to six months with the infant showing abdominal distention and general physical deterioration. Liver, spleen, and lymph glands become enlarged and the mouth may show a blue-black pigmentation. The child may become deaf. Frequently, cerebromacular degeneration and a "cherry-red" spot similar to Tay-Sachs disease are found.

Special investigations of the blood show hypochromic anemia, leukocytosis, and thrombocytopenia. Splenic puncture, lymph node biopsy, or marrow examination show characteristic foam cells containing lipid droplets. The foam cells in the pulmonary alveoli result in "snow storm shadows" on x-ray. In the majority of these cases death ensues within a few years. A distinction between Neimann-Pick and Tay-Sachs disease is made on the basis of the enlargement of liver and spleen in the former condition.

PHENYLKETONURIA. Phenylketonuria is a disorder of metabolism, genetically transmitted as a simple recessive, which prevents the patient from converting phenylalanine into tyrosine. This results in an accumulation of phenylalanine and other intermediary metabolities. The excessive phenylalanine is deaminated to phenylpyruvic acid and is excreted in the urine.

Clinically, these children tend to be less pigmented. There may be a history of eczema and dermatitis. There is usually some degree of microcephaly present, the incisors are broad and spaced widely, and there is often an odd posture in which the head and trunk are bent and the arms and legs held somewhat flexed. The patient walks on a broad base and in an awkward manner with somewhat short steps.

Apart from brisk tendon reflexes, neurological findings are absent except in severe cases which may show cogwheel rigidity and hypertonicity. Some phenylketonurics are hyperactive and many show digital mannerisms. Though they range from mildly to severely retarded, the greatest percentage of cases demonstrates severe retardation. There is now evidence to indicate that mental retardation in phenylketonuria may be greatly lessened in its degree of severity or prevented altogether through early diagnosis and treatment. The diagnosis of phenylketonuria is easily confirmed by testing the urine for phenylpyruvic acid or for elevation of serum phenylalanine.

ENCEPHALOPATHY ASSOCIATED WITH OTHER DISORDERS OF PROTEIN METABOLISM. All disorders of protein metabolism, except for phenylketonuria, are to be included in this category. In the expanded classification they are to be specified as follows:

Hepatolenticular Degeneration (Wilson's Disease). This condition, genetically transmitted as a simple recessive, is characterized by a decrease of copper in the blood stream due to inability of cerulo plasmin to bind the copper. The increased copper concentration damages the tissues of the liver, brain, and other organs. In the central nervous system the basal ganglia are principally affected but, to a lesser extent, the cortex, cerebellum, and other levels are also involved. There is a nodular cirrhosis of the liver. Most cases are not manifest until the second and third decades but onset in early childhood is reported on occasion.

Evidence of neurological involvement includes gross tremor, muscle spasms, Parkinsonism, rigidity, torticollis, dysarthria, dysphasia, convulsions, and mental impairment. Most cases eventually show the Kayser-Fleischer ring, a brown or greenish-brown deposit of pigment in the cornea adjoining the sclera. It is most easily found on slit lamp examination.

The course of the disease is generally slow with the patient succumbing within ten years. Rarely, cases may terminate in a few weeks or last as long as three or four decades.

Porphyria. Porphyria, genetically transmitted as a dominant, is a metabolic disorder characterized by the excretion of porphyrins in the urine. The intermittent excretion of burgundy-colored urine or urine which darkens on exposure to light is diagnostic of the condition.

Symptoms of acute porphyria, which include paroxysmal colic, convulsions, polyneuritis, and a variety of delirious or psychotic mental reactions, generally affect middle aged persons but, rarely, may occur in children causing irreversible mental deterioration.

GALACTOSEMIA. Galactosemia is characterized by a congenital disorder of carbohydrate metabolism which results in an accumulation of galactose in the blood stream. The infant is in good condition at birth but on a milk diet soon begins to show symptoms. Jaundice and vomiting are common and in spite of an insatiable appetite the child shows evidence of malnutrition. Histological changes are found in the liver and lens of the eye. This is reflected, clinically, in enlarged liver, cataract, and mental deterioration which is usually severe in degree. The death rate is high and persons who survive generally show some cirrhosis of the liver. The high galactose blood level produces an increased output of insulin from the pancreas and a reduced discharge of dextrose from the liver which results in hypoglycemia. In infants on a mild diet, reducing substances are found in the urine with Benedict's reagent. This may be identified as galactose by chromatography or fermentation tests.

ENCEPHALOPATHY ASSOCIATED WITH OTHER DISORDERS OF CARBOHYDRATE METABOLISM. All disorders of carbohydrate metabolism, except for galactosemia, are to be included in this category. In the expanded classification these conditions are specified as follows:

Glycogenosis (Von Gierke's Disease). Glycogenosis is a disease which appears to be due to a deficiency in glycogen-metabolizing enzymes. It is characterized by a deposition of glycogen in the liver, heart, kidneys, muscles, and occasionally in the central nervous system in which case mental retardation and convulsions are commonly associated.

Hypoglycemosis. Hypoglycemosis may result from a variety of conditions including adenoma of the pancreas, administration of insulin, liver disease, adrenocortical insufficiency, starvation, islet cell overactivity, and galactosemia. Hypoglycemia occurring secondary to galactosemia would be classified, however, according to the latter condition rather than the former. A familial variety has been described in which hyperinsulism did not seem to be present but in which the administration of protein or of leucine or isovaleric acid produced a hypoglycemic reaction.

The hypoglycemic attack is characterized by sweating, shaking, tachycardia, pallor, weakness, headache, vomiting, and visual disturbances including diplopia. Hemiplegia or convulsions may occur. Psychic reactions include fear, depression, irritation, agitation, difficulty in concentrating and, occasionally, hallucinations. There may be confusion terminating in unconsciousness. In the infant the condition may manifest itself in a combination of epilepsy and mental defect. Confirmation of the diagnosis may be obtained by glucose tolerance tests. The protein-sensitive familial variety may be detected by a blood sugar curve following a casein test.

Hypoglycemia may occur without any mental impairment. Severe, repeated attacks, however, produce cerebral damage which, though reversible for some months, eventually tends to become permanent.

ARACHNODACTYLY (MARFAN'S SYNDROME). The principle feature of this condition is a tendency toward a long, narrow body configuration. Fingers and toes are thin, elongated, and spidery. The thorax is narrow and generally kyphotic. The head is also long and narrow. Frequently associated with the skeletal abnormalities are coloboma, dislocation of the lens of the eye, and congenital heart defect.

Mental retardation is not always an associated feature. The characteristic manifestations show considerable variation in individual cases with elongation of the digits being a major essential in making a differential diagnosis. The basic etiology of the condition, which represents a defect in connective tissue metabolism, is unknown though some cases are on record which indicate a genetic transmission.

HYPOTHYROIDISM. Hypothyroidism as a cause of retardation may be subdivided into the congenital and acquired types. In goiter areas, congenital hypothyroidism may be due to iodine deficiency in the mother during pregnancy. The congenital type of hypothyroidism also includes cases where there is an absence or hypoplasia of the thyroid gland. The condition may also be associated with a genetically determined enzyme defect which results in a defective synthesis of thyroxine. In such cases the thyroid is morphologically normal though a goiter may develop later. This form is sometimes called biochemical hypothyroidism.

Clinically, hypothyroidism may be recognizable at birth although it does not become particularly manifest until the later months. The hypothyroid infant is dwarfed with his length particularly diminished. There is a thickening of subcutaneous tissue and the features look coarse and heavy. The child's appearance is puffy and dull, the lips tend to be thick and the tongue protrudes. The hair is thin and lusterless, the anterior fontanel is gapped broadly, and the forehead may be wrinkled. The head tends to be of fair size with a well developed occiput as contrasted with the Mongoloid child. Distention of the abdomen with umbilical hernia is usually present. The skin is dry, rather cold, and may be desquamated. The infant may be constipated, sluggish, and apathetic. The pulse of the hypothyroid infant is slow and abnormal neurological signs such as ataxia, rigidity, tremors, and hyporeflexia may be present.

The basic metabolic rate may vary between -20 and -50 per cent, and the uptake of radioactive iodine is considerably reduced except in the biochemical form of the condition. The protein-bound iodine is far below the normal range of 4 to 8 micrograms per cent. The blood cholesterol is usually raised to more than 300 mg/100 cc. Roentgenographic study of the long bones reveals recurrent development of ossification centers and epiphyseal union.

With acquired or juvenile hypothyroidism there is an early period of normal thyroid function and development followed by the onset of symptoms and signs of hypothyroidism at a variable age. These children are stunted, with heavy, puffy features, thin hair, dry skin, a waddling gait, protruding abdomen, and prominent buttocks. The cerebral changes are less pronounced with later onset but the child will still demonstrate sluggish physical and mental reactions. Acquired hypothyroidism is apt to develop during periods of stress, infection, or rapid growth. In such cases the thyroid is presumably congenitally hypoplastic and, as a result, unable to meet the increased demand in the stress situation.

There is great variation in the clinical picture presented in hypothyroidism with delayed growth and skeletal development associated with a low level of protein-bound iodine being the only cardinal feature present in all instances.

GARGOYLISM (LIPOCHONDRODYSTROPHY, HURLER'S DISEASE). This disease is manifested by the deposition of an intermediary metabolite, probably a mucopolysaccharide, in almost all tissues of the body but especially those of the brain, liver, heart, lungs, and spleen. A variety of cells are involved: neurones at all levels; cells in the liver, pituitary, and skin; and reticuloepithelial cells in lymph nodes and spleen. The widespread connective tissue involvement is responsible for the skeletal deformities which characterize this condition. The urine is characterized by increased amounts of polysaccharides. Two forms of gargoylism are usually recognized, one form due to autosomal recessive gene transmission and the other to sex-linked recessive gene transmission.

Clinically, some signs may be evident at birth. These include head enlargement, limitation of joint movement, and later, cloudy corneas. At three months, x-rays may show beginning deformity of the upper lumbar vertebrae and some loss of tubulation of the long bones. Kyphosis of the lumbar spine may become evident about the same time. The characteristic features may be present as early as six months. The gargoyle has a large head with a protruding forehead which is far out of proportion with the stunted body; the eyebrows are bushy, and the nose is saddle-shaped. The features are coarse and heavy with a deep crease between the lower lip and chin, thick lips, large tongue, short neck, and double chin.

Mental retardation which ranges in degree from minimal to severe is usually evident by the time the child is two years of age. By five years of age, wedge-shaped vertebrae and a variety of other bone abnormalities may be distinguished on x-ray. The trunk is short even in relation to the diminished limbs. The belly is protuberant and there is usually an umbilical hernia. Except during infancy there is a characteristic deformity of the hands in which the fingers are short and partially flexed. There may be limitation of movement in wrists, elbows, shoulders, hips, knees, ankles, and toes. The hips and knees are usually partially flexed when the child stands. Examination of the abdomen may show considerable enlargement of liver and spleen. Clouding of the cornea, especially in the deeper layers, is usually found in the autosomal recessive cases. Examination with the slit lamp reveals multiple punctate dots of varying size.

The prognosis is particularly poor in the autosomal recessive cases, most affected children dying before their teens. A few survive into the third decade before succumbing, usually, to heart failure or respiratory disease.

ENCEPHALOPATHY, OTHER, DUE TO METABOLIC, GROWTH, OR NUTRITIONAL DISORDER. This category is for classification of a large number of rare metabolic and nutritional disorders which, on occasion, produce encephalopathy and result in mental retardation and which are not classifiable in any of the preceding categories of this division.

V. MENTAL RETARDATION ASSOCIATED WITH DISEASES AND CONDITIONS DUE TO NEW GROWTHS

This group includes all diseases and conditions associated with cerebral new growths. This does not include those cases of growth which are secondary to trauma or infection or cases involving overgrowth of fibrous tissue resulting from atrophy or degeneration. Neoplastic diseases are to be classified within this division as follows:

NEUROFIBROMATOSIS (NEUROFIBROBLASTOMATOSIS, VON RECKLINGHAUSEN'S DISEASE). Neurofibromatosis is characterized by cutaneous pigmentation and tumors of the nerve trunk and skin, and anomalies of the central nervous system. There are a number of variations in the disease, the major division being into the central and peripheral types which may occur separately or in combination. The disease is hereditary showing a dominant gene type transmission with reduced penetrance and variable expressivity. Some affected persons, therefore, show incomplete forms of the disease in which the overt clinical manifestations may be absent altogether.

"Café au lait" patches which vary greatly in size and in the area of the trunk covered are present in almost all cases. Frequently, pedunculated cutaneous tumors are present on the trunk and perhaps other areas of the body. Neurofibromas within the skull, undoubtedly, are present in all cases associated with mental symptoms and may produce increased intracranial pressure and focal compression of the brain. Epilepsy is a frequent concomitant.

Differential diagnosis is based on the association of the skin discoloration with neurofibromas. The intelligence level may vary from normal to severe retardation. The disease may or may not be progressive.

TRIGEMINAL CEREBRAL ANGIOMATOSIS (STURGE-WEBER-DIMITRI DISEASE). The cardinal feature of this condition is a "port wine stain" or cutaneous angioma on the face usually in the area of distribution of the trigeminal nerve. This is accompanied by a vascular malformation over the meninges of the parietal and occipital lobes. The vessels in the meningeal angioma are generally venous and capillary and do not give rise to a bruit. The cortex underlying the affected meninges is also maldeveloped showing loss of nerve cells, gliosis, and calcification which can be detected by skull x-ray. In the very young infant, before calcification has occurred, the angioma may be demonstrated by arteriogram. There may be tortuosity of the retinal vessels on the affected side.

Neurological signs may include epilepsy, transient or permanent hemiplegia, and bleeding from the meningeal nevus.

TUBEROUS SCLEROSIS (EPILOIA, BOURNEVILLE'S DISEASE). Tuberous sclerosis, a disease transmitted by a dominant gene with reduced penetrance, is characterized by multiple gliotic nodules irregularly disposed through the cerebrum and central nervous system. These are associated with adenoma sebaceum of the face and with tumors in other organs.

The cardinal clinical features are the butterfly-shaped rash of adenoma sebaceum, epilepsy, and variable mental disorder. The butterfly-shaped rash may develop at any time from birth to adult life but usually begins as a few small whitish or brownish nodules or pink spots. The rash spreads from the cheeks to the forehead, head, and neck over a wide butterfly-shaped area. The nodules vary in size from a pinhead to a pea. When small they may be more easily palpated than seen. Later, especially toward puberty, the rash tends to become more red and to spread more widely.

Small yellowish-white nodules or phacomata may be seen on the retina. These phacomata have a mulberry appearance because of the little nodules on them. Tumors are also found in other parts of the body including rhabdomyomata of the heart, kidney tumors, and periosteal thickening of the bones, especially the phalanges. Nodules under the nails are not uncommon. The pathology may involve the lungs resulting in symptoms of respiratory disease.

Sometimes adenoma sebaceum may be present without cerebral involvement or mental deterioration. In other instances, the external skin manifestations may be absent and the case may not be diagnosed until autopsy. In absence of the characteristic rash, x-ray confirmation of the diagnosis may be available. The calcified cerebral nodules may be visualized, with the cranial vault presenting a "moth-eaten" appearance.

Retarded development and convulsions may appear very early. Though these infants may show fair motor development, retardation in social and adaptive behavior will be apparent. Progressive tumor growth and accompanying severe convulsions generally shorten the lives of these patients. However they may survive to adulthood in which case they commonly become psychotic.

INTRACRANIAL NEOPLASM, OTHER. There are a number of relatively rare neoplastic diseases, in addition to those specified above, which may involve the brain and lead to mental retardation. Such conditions are to be included in this category. . . .

VI. MENTAL RETARDATION ASSOCIATED WITH DISEASES AND CONDITIONS DUE TO (UNKNOWN) PRENATAL INFLUENCE

This division is intended only for the classification of those conditions for which no definite etiology can be established but where it can be established that the condition existed at or prior to birth. These are conditions which, otherwise, would be classified under *due to unknown or uncertain cause with the structural reaction manifest.* It will be evident that this category, primarily, has temporal rather than etiological connotations. Its inclusion in an etiological classification is justified on the basis that the temporal information does serve to restrict the range of probable and possible etiologies. It therefore represents a greater degree of etiological refinement than does categorization under *due to unknown or uncertain cause.*

It should be noted that not all conditions which are a result of factors occurring during the prenatal period are classified under this division. Where more definite etiologies can be established for prenatal conditions they are classified accordingly. Examples are *congenital rubella* which is classified under *due to infection,* and *encephalopathy associated with prenatal irradiation* which is categorized under *due to trauma or physical agent.*

Conditions classified in this category include the clinical syndromes involving mental defect which are present at birth but are of unknown etiology, the primary cranial anomalies, and congenital cerebral defects of undetermined etiology. They are to be specified as follows:

CEREBRAL DEFECT, CONGENITAL. This category is intended for the classification of congenital cerebral defects of *undetermined etiology* such as agyria, microgyria, congenital porencephaly, etc. The congenital cerebral defect must be proven and not merely presumed. Many of the specific diagnoses included in this category cannot be established except at autopsy. In some instances the defect can be demonstrated by pneumoencephalography.

Anencephaly (Including Hemianencephaly). This is a condition characterized by partial or complete absence of the cerebrum, cerebellum, and flat bones of the skull.

Malformations of Gyri. Gyral defects such as agyria, macrogyria, and microgyria are classified in this category. In agyria the brain is perfectly smooth with no evidence of secondary fissuration. In this respect the brain is comparable to that of an embryo of four months or less. Patients who survive with this condition exhibit severe mental retardation.

Macrogyria (pachygyria) is a cerebral malformation in which the gyri are few and relatively broad while the sulci are short, shallow and wide. Commonly, the condition is associated with the presence of ectopic groups of cells in the white matter of the cerebellum and ectopic olivary tissue in the tegmentum of the medulla.

Microgyria is a rather common pathological finding in the severely mentally retarded. Macroscopically, the brain is small in size. In the affected areas, which tend to be bilateral and symmetrical, the normal convolutional pattern is replaced by one in which there is a larger number of close-set small convolutions separated by shallow grooves.

Porencephaly, Congenital. Porencephaly is the term applied to cerebral defect characterized by large funnel-shaped cavities which may communicate on the surface with the subarachnoid space and internally with the ventricles or with each other. They may occur anywhere in the cerebral hemispheres but, commonly, are found in a position corresponding roughly to the central fissure. They may be bilateral and are often symmetrical. The walls are usually smooth and lined by a layer of glial tissue. Porencephaly may be associated with other congenital malformations such as arhinencephaly. Microgyria is sometimes present around the edges of the cavity.

Porencephaly which occurs as the result of asphyxia at birth or postnatal trauma should be classified accordingly and is not to be included in this category.

Multiple Congenital Anomalies of Brain. This category is intended for the classification of those cases in which more than one type of cerebral defect is present.

Other. This category is to be used for classifying those congenital cerebral defects not receiving separate notation. The type of defect should be specified whenever possible.

Cerebral Defect, Congenital, Associated with Primary Cranial Anomaly. This category includes those cases where the cerebral damage is associated with a cranial anomaly of unknown etiology. Where the cranial anomaly is secondary to some other condition, the primary condition should be classified. In such cases, *with secondary cranial anomaly* is to be added to the primary diagnosis as a supplementary term.

In the expanded classification, primary cranial anomalies are specified further as follows:

Craniostenosis. Acrocephaly (oxycephaly) and scaphocephaly will be the most common conditions included in this category.

Acrocephaly is characterized by a tower or steeple-shaped skull consisiting of a high narrow forehead which slopes to a point and forms a dome-shaped vertex. The "tower" skull or high vault is the result of premature closing of the coronal suture.

X-ray examination of the skull may reveal irregularities of texture (a beaten copper appearance) known as digital markings. These markings are due to local rarefaction of the bones and do not correspond with the underlying convolutions. Exophthalmos may develop to such an extent, in some cases, that the child becomes unable to close the lids. Vision, hearing, and olfaction may be impaired. When syndactylism accompanies oxycephaly, the condition is referred to as Apert's syndrome.

Some cases of acrocephaly or oxycephaly are genetically transmitted while others appear to be sporadic. Mental retardation may be present at birth or may develop from cerebral damage in infancy or childhood. The presence of oxycephaly is not associated invariably, however, with deficient intelligence.

Scaphocephaly is characterized by a narrow, elongated, "boat-shaped" head which develops as a result of the head tending to grow vertically owing to premature closure of the sagittal suture. The forehead bulges, the occiput is full and the fontanels tense. The line of the obliterated suture is marked. X-rays reveal the digital markings over the vault. Other symptoms which may be present are exophthalmos, divergent squint, papilledema, and optic atrophy. Mild to severe retardation is frequently but not invariably an associated manifestation.

Hydrocephalus, Congenital. Hydrocephalus refers to increased volume of cerebrospinal fluid within the skull. A distinction is made between increased volume with and without increased pressure. When hydrocephalus occurs without increased pressure it is merely compensatory to atrophy or hypoplasia. This type of case should not be diagnosed as congenital hydrocephalus but, rather, should be classified on the basis of the primary condition and *with secondary hydrocephalus* may be added as a supplementary term. When hydrocephalus is accompanied by an increase in pressure it is indicative of a disturbance in the absorption, formation, or circulation of the cerebrospinal fluid occurring either singly or in combination. All of these difficulties may occur as the result of prenatal factors or congenital cerebral abnormalities. They may also occur postnatally as the result of trauma, intracranial neoplasm, or infection.

A diagnosis of congenital hydrocephalus should be given only when the condition is present at birth, or when the head begins to enlarge soon after birth (and can be presumed to be a result of prenatal factors), and when it is not possible to assign a more primary diagnosis. In cases of hydrocephalus beginning postnatally, a primary diagnosis of meningitis, intracranial neoplasm or other specific etiology should be given, and *with secondary hydrocephalus* added as a supplementary term. In those postnatal cases where a primary diagnosis cannot be made, the patient should be classified as *encephalopathy due to unknown or uncertain cause,* and *with secondary hydrocephalus* added as a supplementary term.

Obstruction in the cerebrospinal pathway is a much more frequent cause of hydrocephalus than is failure in the absorption mechanism. A common case of obstruction is occlusion of the aqueduct of Sylvius by a congenital septum or stenosis or by a post-infective or post-hemorrhagic gliosis. In other instances the foramina of Monro, Magendie or Luschka may be obstructed. An obstruction of the foramina of Magendie and Luschka is generally due to an acute or chronic adhesive meningitis but also may be due to a tumor malformation such as a septum extending over the inferior part of the roof of the fourth ventricle.

Failure of adequate absorption can be due to an impediment to the upward movement of the cerebrospinal fluid, as at the level of the tentorium, from post-meningitic adhesions around the basal cisterns. The cerebral subarachnoid space may be occluded by post-meningitic adhesions, hemorrhage, or accumulation of adventitious material in proliferating phagocytic cells as in some cases of gargoylism or Schüller-Christian disease. Deformity of the bones at the base of the skull in such conditions as platybasia and achondroplasia have also been suggested as a possible cause of hydrocephalus.

Hemorrhage at birth has been known to cause hydrocephalus through blockage of the aqueduct of Sylvius or the subarachnoid space. The occlusion in such cases may be immediate or may follow later with the organization of adhesions in the region of the clot. Such cases would be classified as *birth injury of brain* and *with secondary hydrocephalus* would be added to the diagnosis as a supplementary term.

As fluid accumulates in hydrocephalus the skull enlarges and the brain may become paper thin due to its expansion. The sutures gap widely, the fontanels enlarge and the cranial circumference increases. The skull tends to become globular with alteration in the shape of the face so that the eyes become unusually far apart and the bridge of the nose depressed. Some degree of optic atrophy and visual impairment is present. Deafness is an occasional complication which is most apt to be found when hydrocephalus is a sequel of meningitis.

Hydrocephalics may become epileptic, spastic and paralyzed, with the lower limbs usually affected more than the upper. Severity of physical and mental defect varies to such an extent that, while some cases are bedridden and helpless, others are able to participate in normal school activities.

If the onset of hydrocephalus is delayed until after closure of the sutures, there is not likely to be any great enlargement of the head and diagnosis must be made on the basis of air studies and the patient's history. Clinically, a distinction is drawn between expanding and stationary or arrested hydrocephalus. In expanding hydrocephalus there is a progressive mental and physical deterioration usually ending in the patient's death. In arrested hydrocephalus, once the expansion has stopped, the intracranial pressure returns to normal and some degree of improvement may follow. The sutures fill in and the skull may become rigid and thick. It is not clearly understood what happens at this stage but in some way a state of balance between secretion and absorption of fluid is achieved. Regular measurement of the head circumference may provide an indication of whether the condition is stationary or not. This technique is of value only for patients whose sutures are open.

Internal hydrocephalus refers to the excessive accumulation of fluid in the ventricular system as opposed to external hydrocephalus where there is excess of fluid in the subarachnoid space. The external type is often due to compensatory filling following cerebral atrophy in which case it should not be classified as congenital hydrocephalus.

Hypertelorism (Greig's Disease.) Hypertelorism is characterized by abnormal development of the sphenoid bone with an overgrowth of the lesser wing and an undergrowth of the greater wing of this bone. This thrusts forward the whole frontal bone and separates the nasal bones more widely than normal.

The distance between the eyes is increased so that in extreme cases they tend to appear on the sides of the face rather than in the normal frontal position. Hare lip and cleft palate are frequently associated manifestations. The skull is brachycephalic, the occiput flat, the frontal eminences prominent and the bridge flattened. The palate is high and narrow and the teeth maloccluded. There may be associated congenital abnormalities of fingers, hands, heart, etc. Some cases show an unusually large cleft between the first and second toes, disproportionately small little fingers, and amyotonia.

Macrocephaly (Megalencephaly). Macrocephaly is a rare condition characterized by an actual increase in the size and weight of the brain due in part to a proliferative type of gliosis. Enlargement of the skull may be noted at birth though most of the gross increase in size occurs later. The skull tends to be square rather than globular and, as in the hydrocephalic, the frontal prominences are pronounced. The greater circumference is at the level of the superciliary ridges which are well marked. Pneumoencephalography may show the ventricular system to be enlarged only slightly.

Most cases are severely mentally retarded. Headache, convulsions, and poor vision are common. The life span is generally shortened except in those milder cases without severe epilepsy.

Microcephaly, Primary. According to clinical tradition, the term microcephaly is reserved for cases with an adult head circumference of 42 cm (17 in.) or less. The corresponding criterion for children is 13 in. at 6 months, 14 in. at one year, and 15 in. at two years.

"True" or primary microcephaly presents a characteristic clinical picture and is considered to be transmitted as a single recessive gene. In this type of microcephaly the face is not as reduced in size as the head so that a relatively normal nose and chin, and large ears contrast with the receding forehead and low vertex. The head is greatly diminished in width and vertical measurement, and to a lesser extent, in length. The contrast between the small cranium and the relatively well developed face is diagnostic. The scalp is sometimes loose and wrinkled longitudinally as though too big for the skull. The skull may be ridged with bony crests along the sagittal, coronal and, occasionally, the lambdoid sutures.

The primary microcephalic is invariably moderately to severely retarded. There may be associated defects such as epilepsy, cataracts, microphthalmia, coloboma of the retina, and incomplete formation of the optic nerve.

Microcephaly may also occur secondary to exogenous lesions *due to prenatal infections* such as *rubella* or *toxoplasmosis,* or to trauma such as *fetal irradiation, neonatal asphyxia,* or *birth injury.* Secondary microcephaly should be classified according to the primary condition and *with secondary microcephaly* added to the primary diagnosis as a supplementary term.

LAURENCE-MOON-BIEDL SYNDROME. The four cardinal features of this syndrome are (1) retinitis pigmentosa, (2) adiposo-genital dystrophy, (3) polydactyly, and (4) mental retardation. The progressive retinal degeneration may be manifest in infancy by a loss of central vision. Degeneration starting peripherally first gives rise to diminished night vision. In later stages optic atrophy and total blindness occur. As the superficial structures of the retina degenerate, the dark pigmentation of the deep layers can be seen with the opthalmoscope. There may also be an actual enlargement of the pigment cells and evidence of a melanophorotropic substance in the urine.

The adiposo-genital dystrophy is associated with somewhat variable pathological findings in the anterior pituitary. Basophil cells in the anterior pituitary may increase from the usual 10 per cent to more than

40 per cent. There may be a marked decrease in the number of ganglion cells along with gliosis. The cerebral blood vessels may show fibrosis and defects in the muscular coat. The sella turcica may be enlarged and the pituitary tissue destroyed by cysts. The pituitary gland may be normal but the stalk may contain hyalinized areas. The adiposity has a Froehlich-type distribution with localized deposits of fat about the breasts, lower abdomen, mons pubis, hips and upper thighs. The genitalia are small. Rudimentary or complete extra fingers or toes, which may or may not be joined together, are sometimes present.

The clinical features are present in infancy. In the adult, the classical clinical picture is that of marked obesity, skull deformities such as oxycephly or hydrocephalus, stunted growth, sex infantilism, polydactylism, syndactylism, diabetes insipidus, and neurological defects such as nystagmus, ataxia, staggering gate, facial palsies, and ptosis of the eyelids. Deaf mutism and/or congenital heart disease may also be present. The accompanying mental retardation varies in degree from mild to severe.

Mongolism (Acromicria, Fetalism). This is the commonest of the so-called clinical types of mental retardation. Though there are a number of untested hypotheses, the etiology of this condition remains obscure. It may be regarded as a disturbance of growth which begins at an early embryonic age and affects almost every system and organ in the body.

The head of the Mongoloid is slightly subaverage in size with the length being more sharply diminished than the breadth (brachycephalic). The hair is generally sparse and fine. The nasal bones of the skull tend to be underdeveloped resulting in a flat bridge. The chin is also small and the ears often show an incomplete, simplified, and distorted structure such as an excessive over-folding of the helix. Oblique palpebral fissures and sloping eyebrows may suggest an Oriental appearance. The epicanthus may cover the inner canthus or may be represented by a fold running to the upper lid from the area of the canthus. The prominence of this fold tends to disappear with increasing age. Blepharitis and conjunctivitis are common. Small opacities in the adult lens are common in the older child and adult. These opacities may be arcuate, sutural, and flake, the arcuate type being rather frequent in mongolism though very rare in other diseases. Irregular grouping of the pinned pigment appears as a chain of white specks close to the outer border of the iris. These Brushfield spots are more readily seen in blue-eyed Mongoloids. The commonly found squint and nystagmus are due to myopia rather than to neurological disorders or nerve palsies.

The tongue tends to protrude from the small mouth and may be fissured. Dentition is irregular and the teeth are generally small and misshapened with the third molar usually being absent. Malocclusion is very common. The skin of the Mongoloid lacks normal elasticity and roughens easily. Peripheral circulation is poor. The hands and feet are broad and clumsy and the little finger tends to be very short and to curve inward. Rather than the normal two creases on the little finger there may be only one. The cleft between the first and second toes is unusually large. Usually, there is a furrow running back on the sole from the cleft.

Mongoloids have characteristic palm and finger prints. The two main creases fanning transversely across the palm may be replaced by a single crease (simian line). The fingerprints are characterized by L-shaped loops rather than the usual whirls.

The testes may descend late or not at all. The penis is generally small, in the female the vulva is poorly developed, and in both sexes secondary sex characteristics are delayed in their appearance. The voice of the Mongoloid is generally coarse even in childhood. Mongoloids are generally awkward both in gross and fine motor coordination. Their muscles are hypotonic and the ligaments lax. In approximately 10 per cent of the cases, mongolism is associated with congenital heart defect.

Mental retardation associated with mongolism ranges in degree from moderate to severe with infrequent cases of mildly retarded Mongoloids also having been reported. The severity of the retardation, in general, seems to vary with the severity and number of physical concomitants.

VII. MENTAL RETARDATION ASSOCIATED WITH DISEASES AND CONDITIONS DUE TO UNKNOWN OR UNCERTAIN CAUSE WITH THE STRUCTURAL REACTIONS MANIFEST

This category is intended for the classification of postnatal diseases and conditions where the structural reaction is manifest but where the etiology is unknown or uncertain. Those conditions which are presumed to be of an heredity or familial nature, where no other etiology can be assigned, are included in this category. The structural reactions classified here may be degenerative, infiltrative, inflammatory, proliferative, sclerotic, or reparative. . . . Conditions included in this division are specified as follows:

ENCEPHALOPATHY ASSOCIATED WITH DIFFUSE SCLEROSIS OF THE BRAIN. These conditions are characterized by diffuse demyelination of the white matter of the brain with consequent diffuse glia sclerosis. Intellectual deterioration is an accompanying clinical feature. This group of diseases is often familial in character. If the expanded classification is being used they should be specified as follows:

Acute Infantile Diffuse Sclerosis (Krabbe's Disease). Onset is at age

4–6 months with signs of diffuse cerebral involvement which include convulsions, spastic quadriplegia, amaurosis and deafness. The course is toward death within two years.

Diffuse Chronic Infantile Sclerosis (Merzbacher-Pelizaeus Disease, Aplasia Axialis Extracorticalis Congenita). Clinical signs of pyramidal, extra-pyramidal, and cerebellar disease are found in infancy and progress slowly over a period of years, with occasional remissions, even into adulthood. The onset of the disease is generally at the third or fourth month of life.

Infantile Metachromatic Leukodystrophy (Greenfield's Disease). The products of myelin degeneration in this condition are characterized by their metachromatic staining properties. Of diagnostic significance is the fact that metachromatic material can also be isolated from the urine of the patients. The disease usually begins at about the second year of life and terminates fatally in a few years. Symptoms include motor and intellectual deterioration, convulsive seizures and, generally, optic atrophy.

Juvenile Metachromatic Leukodystrophy (Scholz' Disease). The onset is at 6–10 years of age. The disease is manifested by sensory aphasia and cortical deafness followed by basal ganglia involvement, spastic paralysis, and retardation in intellectual function. Death occurs within a few years.

Progressive Subcortical Encephalopathy (Encephalitis Perixialis Diffusa, Schilder's Disease). The onset of this disease may be at any age. The pathology involves a massive demyelinating degeneration of the cerebral hemispheres extending into the corpus callosum, internal capsule, basal ganglia, and cerebellum with formation of products of myelin degeneration which are sudanophilic in staining reaction.

Symptoms include epileptic seizures, disturbances of vision, deafness, cranial nerve involvement, dysarthria, paralysis, cerebellar and extra-pyramidal motor signs, aphasia, apraxia, agnosia, mental retardation, and psychotic reactions.

Encephalopathy Associated with Cerebellar Degeneration. All encephalopathies associated with cerebellar degeneration are to be coded in this category. Where the expanded classification is being used they are to be specified further as follows:

Spinal Sclerosis (Friedreich's Ataxia). The onset of Friedreich's ataxia is between the ages of 2 and 15. Neurological examination reveals loss of deep reflexes, loss of kinesthetic sensation in the limbs, and a Babinski reflex. Clinical signs include ataxia, nystagmus, loss of deep tendon reflexes, speech impairment, and dementia.

In most cases the course of the disease is toward complete disability by the third decade of life. Mild forms of the condition have a better prognosis.

Encephalopathy, Other, Due to Unknown or Uncertain Cause with the Structural Reactions Manifest. Diseases of unknown or uncertain cause with the structural reactions manifest which do not have a separate notation are to be classified in this category. It includes that considerable percentage of cases of mental retardation associated with progressive neuronal degeneration or other structural defect which cannot be classified in a more specific diagnostic category.

ENCEPHALOPATHY ASSOCIATED WITH PREMATURITY. Instances of mental retardation in association with prematurity are to be classified in this category only where a more primary diagnosis cannot be assigned. Prematurity is to be defined by standard birth weight criteria only and is not to include shortened gestation periods.

VIII. MENTAL RETARDATION DUE TO UNCERTAIN (OR PRESUMED PSYCHOLOGIC) CAUSE WITH THE FUNCTIONAL REACTION ALONE MANIFEST

This category is used for the classification of those numerous instances of mental retardation occurring in absence of any clinical or historical indication of organic disease or pathology which could reasonably account for the retarded intellectual functioning. No case is to be classified in this division except after exhaustive medical evaluation. Cases in the group are specified in terms of psychogenic and psychosocial factors which appear to bear some etiological relationship with the retardation in functioning. This specification is as follows:

CULTURAL-FAMILIAL MENTAL RETARDATION. In addition to absence of reasonable indication of cerebral pathology, classification in this category requires that there be evidence of retardation in intellectual functioning in at least one of the parents and in one or more siblings where there are such.

Because of the parental inadequacy in these cases there is usually some degree of cultural deprivation present. This deprivation is not generally of such a severe nature as to warrant classification under *psychogenic mental retardation associated with deprivation of stimulation.* In those cases where the cultural deprivation is of severe degree, classification under *cultural-familial mental retardation* take precedence where there is a familial history of intellectual subnormality.

There is no intent in this category to specify either independent action of, or the relationship between, genetic and cultural factors in the etiology of cultural-familial mental retardation. The exact role of genetic factors cannot be specified since the nature and mode of transmission of genetic aspects of intelligence are not yet understood. Similarly, there is no clear understanding of the specific manner in which environmental factors operate to modify intellectual functioning.

Cultural-familial mental retardates invariably exhibit a mild degree of retardation in measured intelligence and adaptive behavior.

PSYCHOGENIC MENTAL RETARDATION ASSOCIATED WITH ENVIRONMENTAL

DEPRIVATION. In some instances borderline or mild degrees of mental retardation may be attributable to deprivation at an early age of opportunity ·for learning experiences which are essential for adequate functioning in our culture.

Intellectual and social functioning are intimately related to previous learning experiences. With severe deprivation of stimulation at early age levels an individual may not acquire the knowledge and skills that will enable him to function at the level demanded by the culture. Thus the individual's level of functioning may fall within the range of the mentally retarded.

The deprivation of stimulation in these cases, in general, will be more severe than that commonly encountered in *cultural-familial mental retardation*. This type of deprivation may occur as the result of severe sensory impairments such as blindness and deafness, or rarely, as the result of severe environmental restrictions or highly atypical cultural experience. The retardation in these cases is particularly relative to the demands and norms set by the culture and will almost always be of ̄a marginal or mild degree.

PSYCHOGENIC MENTAL RETARDATION ASSOCIATED WITH EMOTIONAL DISTURBANCE. This category is for the classification of cases of mental retardation associated with a history of a prolonged period of emotional disturbance (neurotic disorder) dating from an early age. It is believed that the emotional disturbance must be extremely severe in order to have any causal relationship to the mental retardation.

MENTAL RETARDATION ASSOCIATED WITH PSYCHOTIC (OR MAJOR PERSONALITY) DISORDER. Cases of mental retardation associated with psychotic or major personality disorders such as autism or childhood schizophrenia, where there is no reasonable evidence of cerebral pathology, are to be classified in this category.

MENTAL RETARDATION, OTHER DUE TO UNCERTAIN CAUSE WITH THE FUNCTIONAL REACTION ALONE MANIFEST. This category is for the classification of those cases of mental retardation where there is (1) no evidence of a physical cause or structural defect, (2) no history of subnormal functioning in parents and siblings, and (3) no evidence of an associated psychogenic or psychosocial factor.

SUPPLEMENTARY TERM CATEGORIES [2]

Definitions of categories included in the supplementary term classification of convulsive disorders and motor dysfunctions are presented below. The reader should refer to the American Psychiatric Association

[2] Definitions of supplementary term categories prepared by Herman Yannet, M.D., Medical Director, Southbury Training School, Southbury, Connecticut.

publication, *Diagnostic and Statistical Manual—Mental Disorders,* for appropriate usage of terms comprising the supplementary classification of psychiatric impairment. Terms included in the classification of genetic components, secondary cranial anomalies, and impairments of special senses have standard meanings and do not, therefore, require further elaboration.

CONVULSIVE DISORDERS

AKINETIC SEIZURES. Akinetic seizures occur primarily in infants or very young children. They are characterized by a sudden loss of postural control without associated muscle contractions or activity. The episode is of very short duration and loss of consciousness is momentary. In infants, while sitting, there is a sudden dropping of the head (salaam seizures). In older children, when standing or walking, there is a sudden loss of voluntary postural control and a dropping to the ground.

AUTONOMIC SEIZURES. Autonomic seizures can occur at all ages. They are characterized by symptoms usually attributed to activity of the vegetative nervous system. These include sudden hypotensive states (syncope), salivation, flushing of face or other parts of body, excessive intestinal activity, etc.

FOCAL SEIZURES. Focal seizures imply the limitation of the cerebral seizure discharge to a particular part of the brain. These usually are either motor or sensory in nature depending on cerebral localization. Most commonly, when motor, a single extremity or part of an extremity may be involved with muscular contractions or spasms. Other parts of the body, like the facial muscles, may also be the focal point of activity. When sensory in nature, a variety of sensations may be felt in a limited part of the body such as, pain, tingling, temperature changes, etc. In focal seizures, consciousness may or may not be lost.

MAJOR MOTOR SEIZURES. Major motor seizures are basically grand mal seizures, always associated with loss of consciousness, generalized tonic and clonic muscle activity, and followed by a period of sleep as a rule. An aura which may be sensory, motor, or autonomic in nature frequently precedes the generalized seizure which may last from 30 seconds to some minutes.

MYOCLONIC SEIZURES. Myoclonic seizures are of two types. The most common, known as "mass myoclonic seizures" or "infantile spasms," occurs almost exclusively, as the latter name implies, during infancy or very early childhood and involves a sudden, short generalized muscle contraction. As a rule, the infant will suddenly and forcibly flex the head on the chest and the thighs on the abdomen. The arms either will be bent at the elbows and held against the chest or they will be extended sideways. Occasionally, the spasm will involve an overextension of the neck and arching of the back. While consciousness is invariably lost, the episode is of such short duration that this may not be appreciated by the parent. These may occur once a day or, less frequently, as often as every few minutes.

Less common myoclonic seizures may be confined to isolated muscle groups and in this form are rarely associated with loss of consciousness.

Petit Mal Seizures. Petit mal seizures are essentially very short (a few seconds in duration) episodes of cessation of activity with a fixed staring appearance. They are not associated with falling, although occasionally a slight swaying is evident. Rarely, there may be a slight tremor of the fingers or eyelids. They are almost always accompanied by a bilaterally synchronous, three-per-second spike and wave paroxysmal discharge in the electroencephalogram. Petit mal seizures are highly specific and practically never associated with mental retardation or other evidence of central nervous system disorders. The term must not be used to describe *any short* convulsion or seizure discharge but must be confined to its specific manifestation as described above.

Psychomotor Seizures. Psychomotor seizures are highly organized activities resulting from cortical discharges, probably arising in the temporal lobes, associated usually with *purposeful* motor manifestations which, however, are inappropriate for the occasion. The patient is never conscious of his activities at the time and subsequently shows amnesia for the event. They may vary from such simple movements as lip smacking or slowly turning the head and body, to such complicated activities as moving around and performing definite intricate acts. The latter manifestations are also called automatisms.

Mixed, Unclassifiable, or Other. Mixed or unclassifiable seizures are seizure manifestations that fit into no definite category as herein described or that represent aspects of two or more categories without any one predominating.

MOTOR DYSFUNCTION

The terms herein to be defined are almost exclusively used in describing the motor disabilities of cerebral palsy patients and have their anatomic basis in disorders of the brain.

Ataxia. Ataxia is a disturbance in postural balance and coordination of muscle activity. Usually it is generalized but the disturbance may be confined to one side of the body or even one extremity.

Hypotonia. Hypotonia implies lack of normal muscle tone or tension and is associated with muscle flaccidity and weakness of varying degrees.

Choreoathetosis. Athetosis implies uncontrollable, involuntary, and poorly coordinated movements of the body, face, and extremities which result in bizarre patterns of muscular activities. They are exaggerated when voluntary activity is attempted but are also present to a lesser extent at all times except during sleep.

Chorea is similar to athetosis in that movements are involuntary and uncontrolled but differs from athetosis in that they are more rapid and more random. The individual muscle jerking also involves a shorter range of movement than is the case in athetosis.

Because of the difficulty in differentiating between chorea and athetosis and because the two are frequently present simultaneously, they are both coded under . . . "Choreoathetosis."

Dystonia. Dystonia is closely related to athetosis also but involves a much wider range of movement which is slower in execution.

Rigidity. Rigidity involves the concurrent activity of both the contracting muscles and their muscle antagonists. There is thus a tendency to markedly diminished motion, general muscle inelasticity, and lack of plasticity.

Tremors. Tremors are involuntary movements that follow a regular rhythmic pattern in which flexors and extensors contract alternately.

Spasticity. Spasticity involves a state of increased muscle tension. Its major manifestation is the increased or exaggerated stretch reflex which exhibits itself by an exaggerated contraction of a muscle when it is suddenly stretched.

Diplegia. Diplegia refers to the involvement of all four extremities to an equal degree on both sides but with greater involvement of the legs than the arms.

Hemiplegia. Hemiplegia is the involvement of both the upper and the lower extremity on one side. The arm is usually more involved than the leg.

Monoplegia. Monoplegia refers to a weakness or paralysis of a single extremity.

Paraplegia. Paraplegia refers to the involvement of both lower extremities, usually symmetrically.

Quadriplegia. Quadriplegia involves all four extremities but with equal or greater disability in the arms than in the legs. The impairment may be symmetrical on both sides or asymmetrical.

Triplegia. Triplegia is the involvement of any three extremities.

INDEX

Page numbers in *italics* refer to major treatment of topics in the text.